Pædiatrics

To my best friend James
To my wife, Kay and my daughter, Ella

Concise
Paediatrics

Edited by

Rachel U Sidwell
MRCP MRCPCH DFFP DA

Clinical Research Fellow and Honorary Registrar in
Paediatric Dermatology
Institute of Child Health and Great Ormond Street Hospital,
London, UK

Mike Thomson
MRCP FRCPCH DCH MD

Consultant in Paediatric Gastroenterology
Royal Free Hospital, London, UK

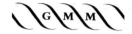

© 2000

Greenwich Medical Media Limited
137 Euston Road
London
NW1 2AA

ISBN 1 84110 027 7

First published 2000

A catalogue record for this book is available from the British Library.

Visit our website at:
www.greenwich-medical.co.uk

Cover artwork by Sam, aged 5½
Typeset by J&L Composition Ltd, Filey, North Yorkshire
Printed by Alden Press Ltd, Oxford

Contents

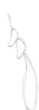

Contributors

James S A Green LLM, FRCS
Specialist Registrar in Urology
Royal Free Hospital, London UK

Paul T Heath FRACP, FRCPCH
Consultant in Paediatric Infectious
diseases
St. Georges Hospital, London, UK

Ahmed F Massoud
MRCP MRCPCH MD
Specialist Registrar in Paediatric
  Endocrinology
Great Ormond Street Hospital
London, UK

Kevin J Murray FRACP
Consultant in Paediatric Rheumatology
Great Ormond Street Hospital
London, UK

Mike Potter MA PhD MRCP MRCPath
Consultant Haematologist
Royal Free Hospital, London, UK

Rachel U Sidwell
MRCP MRCPCH DA DFFP
Clinical Research Fellow and Honorary
Registrar in Paediatric Dermatology

Institute of Child Health and Great
Ormond Street Hospital, London, UK

Mike A Thomson
MRCP FRCPCH DCH MD
Consultant in Paediatric
  Gastroenterology
Royal Free Hospital
London, UK

Michael Waring
BSc FRCS (ORL-HNS)
Consultant Otolaryngologist
St Bartholomews' and
The Royal London Hospitals
London, UK

Callum Wilson FRACP
Metabolic Consultant
Starship Children's Hospital
Aukland, New Zealand

Paul JD Winyard
MA MRCP MRCPCH PhD
Lecturer in Paediatric Clinical Science
Nephro-Urology Unit
Institute of Child Health and
Great Ormond Street Hospital
London, UK

Preface

We wrote this book to fill the gap between enormous post-graduate paediatric tomes and undergraduate paediatric texts with little detail. It is written in a succinct user-friendly style, and has many lists, boxes and annotated diagrams for ease of learning. The aim of the book was to help busy, tired paediatric trainees to learn some of the many paediatric conditions in the least painful and least expensive way possible. It is focused particularly at those contemplating higher examinations, both the MRCPCH and the DCH, but should be useful for quick reference for both those who are further on in training or medical students. We hope that this book will be of help, providing a thorough background knowledge of the subject and aslo give some inspiration for further exploration in the subject of paediatrics.

We would like to thank all who helped with this book. In particular we are indebted to the various specialists who have contributed to the chapters thereby making it as up-to-date as it is. Finally we would like to thank Gavin and Geoff, who have been positive and supportive throughout and fun to work with.

Best of Luck!

R.U.S.
M.T.
June 2000

Acknowledgements

John I. Harper
Consultant in Paediatric Dermatology
Great Ormond Street Hospital
London, UK

Nigel Klein BSc PhD MRCP
Senior Lecturer and Honorary
Consultant in Immunology and
Infectious Diseases Institute of Child
Health and Great Ormond Street
Hospital
London, UK

PG Rees
Consultant Paediatric Cardiologist
Great Ormond Street Hospital
London, UK

Dr. Rod C. Scott MRCP
Specialist Registrar in Paediatric
Neurology
Great Ormond Street Hospital
London, UK

Robin M Winter FRCP
Professor of Clinical Cytogenetics and
Dysmorphology
Institute of Child Health
London, UK

1

Genetics

- Basic cell genetics
- Mutations
- Techniques for DNA analysis and mutation detection
- Chromosomal disorders
- Single gene (Mendelian) defects
- Factors affecting inheritance patterns
- Multifactorial inheritance
- Cancer genetics
- Dysmorphology
- Clinical applications of genetics

Basic cell genetics

THE GENE

The basic unit of inheritance, one gene coding for one feature. Humans are estimated to have between 50 000 and 100 000 structural genes (ie. that code for proteins). Genes are made of deoxyribonucleic acid (DNA), and are organised within chromosomes in the cell.

Somatic cells (*Diploid*)	Contain 22 pairs of *autosomes* (1 pair of *sex chromosomes*)	**46** chromosomes altogether
Gametes (*Haploid*)	Contain 22 *autosomes* (1 *sex chromosome*)	**23** chromosomes altogether

DNA COMPOSITION

DNA is a double helix composed of:

1. *Sugar–phosphate backbone (the pentose sugar* deoxyribose *and a phosphate group)*
2. *Nitrogenous base*
   Pyrimidines: Cytosine (C) and thymidine (T)
   Purines: *Adenine (A) and guanine (G)*

   A always pairs with T } *Complementary* base pairing
   C always pairs with G }

   The sugar–phosphate backbone has a $5'$ and a $3'$ end.
   A **nucleotide** = a unit of one base, one deoxyribose and one phosphate group.
   The DNA is coiled tightly to make up **chromosomes**
   The gene sequence is made of **introns** (code for proteins) interspaced with **exons**

Three bases make up a **codon**, which codes for one amino acid (via the **genetic code**)

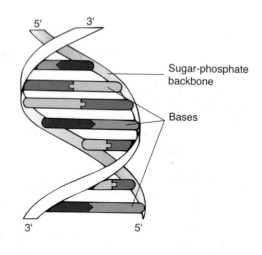

◀ Adenine

▷ Thymine

⊐ Guanine

⊏ Cytosine

Figure 1.1 Structure of DNA

DNA REPLICATION

This occurs in a sequence:

1. *DNA helix splits to form two single strands.*
2. *New complementary base pairs (ie. C with G, and T with A) are added to the single strands at the 3' end (so the new DNA replication grows from 5' to 3').* **DNA polymerase** *enzyme adds the new nucleotides.*

NB. Along a gene, the 5' direction is 'upstream' and the 3' direction is 'downstream'.

Forming proteins from DNA

1. **Transcription.** *The DNA sequence is transcribed into* **messenger RNA** *(mRNA). (mRNA is a single strand like DNA but with a Uracil (U) base replacing all the T bases, and a ribose sugar instead of a deoxyribose sugar.)* **RNA polymerase** *initiates this process. All the exons are removed, so the mRNA is made only of introns. The mRNA then moves from the nucleus to the cytoplasm.*
2. **Translation.** *The mRNA is translated into a protein in the ribosomes (organelles in the cytoplasm).* **Transfer RNA** *(tRNA) attaches to the mRNA. Each tRNA is a clover shape with a three-base pair (anticodon) at one end, which attaches to the mRNA, and a*

three base pair at the other which codes for one amino acid (via the genetic code). Thus a sequence of amino acids is formed which will form a protein.

THE CELL CYCLE

New cells are constantly created. The cell cycle is a continuum of the cell's life, made up of:

1. Interphase. *Most of the cell's life,* **replication of DNA** *and cell contents occur here*
2. Division. *The cell divides into two:*

Diploid cell creation:	**Mitosis** *(nuclear division)*
	Cytokinesis *(cytoplasmic division)*
Haploid cell creation:	**Meiosis**

NB. After the S phase of the cell cycle, the DNA has already replicated, so the cell contains two identical copies of each of the 46 chromosomes. The identical copies are joined together at a centromere and are called **sister chromatids**, making up one chromosome. Because the chromosomes are studied in metaphase of mitosis when they are most condensed, we actually always look at DNA that has replicated, the sister chromatids joined together and appearing as 46 separate chromosome bodies.

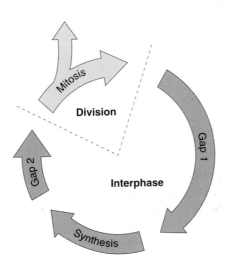

Figure 1.2 The cell cycle

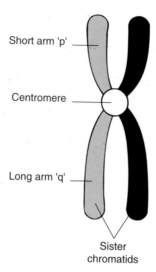

Short arm 'p'

Centromere

Long arm 'q'

Sister
chromatids

Figure 1.3 Chromosome (composed of two identical chromatids). There are two copies of this chromosome in each cell (one from the mother and one from the father).

Mutations

A **mutation** = a change in the DNA sequence. Mutations in germline cells (cells that produce gametes) generally result in genetic diseases. Mutations in somatic cells (normal body cells) may result in cancer (if they occur early on in the zygote, they may result in mosaics).

Genes differ among individuals due to mutations, and differing sequences for the same gene are called **alleles**. If someone has the same allele on both members of a chromosome pair, they are **homozygous**. If the alleles have different gene sequences, the person is **heterozygous**.

A **locus** is the location of a gene on a chromosome.

The **genotype** is the alleles present at a given locus.

A **polymorphism** is a locus with at least two different alleles.

TYPES OF MUTATION

Chromosomal mutations

These are changes that *are large enough to be seen by looking at the chromosomes under the light microscope*. They are studied by **cytogenetic** techniques. (Molecular techniques are now also used to study chromosomal disorders, making the definitions less distinct).

They are due either to changes in the number of chromosomes (eg. trisomy) or large changes in the structure of chromosomes.

Single gene mutations

These are not visible under the microscope and are studied by **molecular genetic** techniques. Examples of single gene mutations:

- **Point mutation**. *One base pair is substituted by another. They may cause one amino acid to change, eg. sickle cell disease*
- **Insertions** *or* **deletions** *of one or more base pairs, eg. cystic fibrosis (a three-base pair deletion)*
- **Whole gene duplications** *eg. Charcot–Marie–Tooth disease (three copies of PMP22 encoding myelin)*
- **Splice site mutations** *Result in abnormal splicing of introns and exons and thus alter the mRNA*
- **Expanded repeats** *An increase in the normal tandem repeats, eg. Duchenne muscular dystrophy*

NB. Polymorphisms may result in *silent mutations* that produce no clinical effect.

CAUSES OF MUTATIONS

- *Spontaneous mutations*
- *Induced mutations (by mutagens):*
  Ionising radiation, eg. X-rays
  Non-ionising radiation, eg. UV light
  Chemicals, eg. nitrogen mustard

Defective DNA repair rate is seen in certain diseases, which consequently have a high rate of tumour formation, eg. Xeroderma pigmentosa, Fanconi anaemia, ataxia telangiectasia, Bloom's syndrome.

Bloom's syndrome
Autosomal recessive, chromosome 15q defect. A syndrome involving increased number of chromosomal breaks, with a sensitivity to UV radiation and increased risk of malignancy.
Features include:

- *Skin* *Butterfly distribution facial rash of telangiectasia and erythema with sun exposure*
  Bullae on lips, hands and forearms
- *Dysmorphism* *Malar hypoplasia*
  Short stature
  Syndactyly, polydactyly, short lower limbs
- *Immunity* *Low antibody levels (IgG, IgM and IgA), recurrent infections*

Techniques for DNA analysis and mutation detection

MOLECULAR GENETIC TECHNIQUES

Polymerase chain reaction (PCR)
This is a technique to make millions of copies of a short DNA sequence very rapidly. It enables rapid DNA analysis for mutation detection from very small amounts of DNA (eg. useful for antenatal chorionic villous sampling).

1. *Double-stranded DNA is denatured to single strands by heating.*
2. *Primers are added and the DNA cooled to enable the primers to anneal to the single DNA strands (The primers are selected because they will attach next to the region of interest on the DNA).*
3. *DNA polymerase is added so the primers are extended along the target DNA, and thus two extra copies are made.*

The cycle is repeated, with doubling of the DNA occurring at each repeat cycle.

Southern blotting

A technique to detect insertions, deletions and rearrangements and also to order DNA fragments into a physical map.

Test DNA is digested by restriction enzymes (eg. EcoR1), the DNA fragments are separated with gel electrophoresis. The DNA is transferred to a nylon membrane and a labelled probe is hybridised to the DNA fragments.

Mutation detection and direct DNA sequencing

Techniques to identify the exact nuclear sequence of a strand of DNA. This is done using chemical cleavage, dideoxychain termination or fluorochrome dye.

CYTOGENETIC TECHNIQUES

Karyotype and chromosome banding

A karyotype is an ordered display of the chromosomes, which are studied during the metaphase part of mitosis. Staining techniques bring out the chromosome bands that may be viewed under the light microscope.

Normal karyotype: 46, XX (female)
46, XY (male)

Fluorescent In Situ Hybridisation (FISH)

This is a technique using labelled DNA probes that are hybridised with the chromosomes being studied. They are then viewed under the microscope. Deletions, excess chromosome material and chromosome rearrangements (eg. translocations) can be detected.

GENE MAPPING TECHNIQUES

Linkage analysis

This is the use of DNA markers to track a gene through a family and to help map a gene. With linkage analysis a specific region of DNA is identified in which the gene is located (the region may contain several million DNA base pairs).

Closely located pieces of DNA (linked DNA) are less likely to be separated by the crossing over process in meiosis and thus are more likely to be inherited together. Linkage analysis is a complex process based on probabilities. The principle is that a region of DNA that can be marked is tracked through generations and if the disease allele is near to this they will generally be inherited together.

A range of known polymorphic DNA markers are used, such as restriction fragment length polymorphisms (RFLPs) and simple tri-, tetra- or pentanucleotide repeats.

Candidate genes

Once a chromosome region has been identified by linkage analysis, this area is cloned and *candidate genes* are analysed to see if they are the gene in question. Candidate genes are those with characteristics that suggest they may be responsible for a disease (eg. code for a particular protein). Candidate genes for a region are then analysed to see if a mutation in them gives rise to the disease.

Chromosomal disorders

ABNORMALITIES OF CHROMOSOME NUMBER

Polyploidy = extra whole sets of chromosomes:

triploidy (69, XXX)
tetraploidy (92, XXXX) } both lethal in humans

Aneuploidy = missing or extra individual chromosomes:

monosomy (only one copy of a particular chromosome)
trisomy (three copies of a particular chromosome)

Non-disjunction

This is the commonest cause of aneuploidy and is the failure of chromosomes to disjoin normally during meiosis.

Down syndrome (trisomy 21)

Karyotype: 47, XY + 21 or 47, XX + 21

Maternal age	Approximate risk of Down syndrome
All ages	1 in 650
30	1 in 1000
35	1 in 365
40	1 in 100
45	1 in 50

Clinical features

General	*Hypotonia* (floppy babies), relatively small stature, hyperflexible joints
CNS	Developmental delay
Craniofacial	Brachycephaly, mild microcephaly
	Upslanting palpebral fissures (Mongolian slant to eyes), *epicanthic folds*, myopia, acquired cataracts
	Brushfield spots (speckled irises)
	Small ears, mixed hearing loss, glue ear, small nose

Protruding tongue, dental hypoplasia
Short neck, (risk of atlantoaxial subluxation with anaesthetics)

Hands and feet	Short fingers, 5th finger clinodactyly, *simian palmar crease* (present in 1% normal population), wide gap between 1st and 2nd toes
Cardiac	CHD (40%): AVSD, VSD, PDA, ASD. Valve prolapse >20 years.
Skin	Loose neck folds (infant), dry skin, folliculitis in adolescents
Hair	Soft, fine: straight pubic hair
Genitalia	Small penis and testicular volume. Infertility common

Genetic causes of trisomy 21

1. *Non-disjunction (95%)*

   The extra chromosome is maternal in 90% of cases and the incidence increases with maternal age.

   After having a child with Down syndrome the risk of recurrence is 1 in 200 under 35 years and twice the age-specific rate if over 35 years.

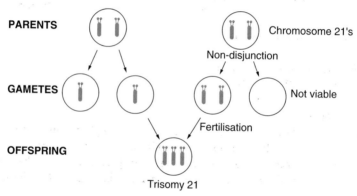

Figure 1.4 Non-disjunction

2. *Robertsonian translocation (4%)*

   Common karyotype: 45, XY, −14, −21, + t (14q21q)

   Here a chromosome 21 is translocated onto another chromosome (14, 15, 21 or 22). This may arise as a new mutation, but in a quarter of these cases one of the parents will have a balanced translocation (see p. 9)

   The risk of recurrence is:

   > 10–15% if the mother is a translocation carrier
   > 2.5% if the father is a translocation carrier
   > 100% if a parent has the translocation 21:21
   > <1% if neither parent has a translocation

3. *Mosaicism (1%)*

   These children have some normal cells and some trisomy 21 cells.

   Karyotype: 47, XY + 21 / 46, XY.

   This results from non-disjunction occurring during mitosis after fertilisation.

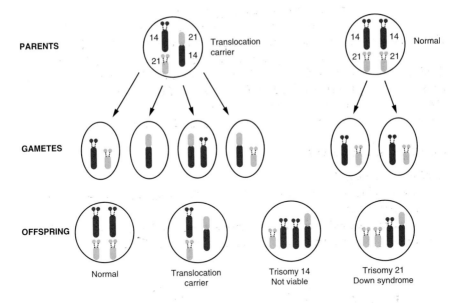

Figure 1.5 Robertsonian translocation

Edwards syndrome (trisomy 18)
Karyotype: 47, XY, +18

Clinical features

General	Low birth weight, fetal inactivity, single umbilical artery, skeletal muscle and adipose hyopoplasia, mental deficiency
Craniofacial	Narrow bifrontal diameter, short palpebral fissures, low-set abnormal ears, small mouth, micrognathia, epicanthic folds, cleft lip and/or palate
Hands and feet	**Overlapping** of index finger over 3rd and 5th finger over 4th. Clenched hand, small nails, **rocker-bottom feet**
Trunk and pelvis	Short sternum, small nipples, inguinal or umbilical hernia, small pelvis
Genitalia	Cryptorchidism (male)
Cardiac	VSD, ASD, PDA, bicuspid aortic and/or pulmonary valves
Other organs	Right lung malsegmentation or absence, renal and gastrointestinal abnormalities

50% die within the first week, and only 5–10% survive the first year. Recurrence risk is low unless parental translocation is present.

Patau syndrome (trisomy 13)
Karyotype: 47, XY, + 13

Clinical features

General	Low birth weight, single umbilical artery
CNS	**Holoprosencephaly** with varying degrees of incomplete fore-brain development. Seizures, severe mental retardation
Craniofacial	Wide fontanelles, microphthalmia, colobomas, retinal dysplasia
	Cleft lip and/or **cleft palate**
	Abnormal low-set ears
Skin	Parietooccipital **scalp defects**
Hands and feet	Simian crease, polydactyly
Cardiac	(80%) VSD, PDA, ASD
Genitalia	Cryptorchidism (male), bicornuate uterus (female)

Most of these children die within the first month (around 80%). Recurrence risk is small unless one of the parents has a balanced translocation.

Turner syndrome (Monosomy of the X chromosome)
Karyotype: 45, X0

Clinical features

General	**Short stature**, loose neck folds in infants
CNS	Mild developmental delay, hearing impairment
Gonads	**Ovarian dysgenesis** with hypoplasia or absence of germinal elements (90%)
Lymph vessels	**Congenital lymphoedema** (puffy fingers and toes)
Craniofacial	Abnormal ears (often prominent), narrow maxilla, small mandible
	Short webbed neck, low posterior hairline
Skeletal	**Broad chest** with **wide-spaced nipples**
	Cubitus valgus
Nails	**Narrow hyperconvex** nails
Skin	Multiple pigmented naevi
Renal	Horseshoe kidney, double renal pelvis
Cardiac	Bicuspid aortic valve (30%), coarctation of the aorta (10%), aortic stenosis, mitral valve prolapse

These children may be given growth hormone, and oestrogen replacement (if necessary) at adolescence.

This is generally a sporadic event and the paternal sex chromosome is the most likely to be missing. NB. Mosaicism is not uncommon and results in milder manifestations.

Klinefelter's syndrome
Karyotype: 47, XXY
Estimated to affect 1:500 males

Clinical features
Features are very variable.

Skeletal   Tall and slim, long limbs, low upper: lower segment ratio

Genitalia Relatively small penis and testes in childhood, most enter puberty normally
Primary infertility, partial virilisation, gynaecomastia (33%)
CNS   Mild mental retardation
Other   Elbow dysplasia

Testosterone therapy may be given from age 11–12 years if deficient.

47, XYY syndrome

Incidence 1: 840 males, though seldom detected as most are phenotypically normal.

Clinical features

CNS   Learning difficulties, poor fine motor coordination, speech delay
common
Behavioural problems (hyperactivity, temper tantrums)
Growth   Accelerated growth in midchildhood
Craniofacial Prominent glabella, large ears
Skin   Nodulocystic teenage acne
Skeletal   Long fingers and toes, mild pectus excavatum

ABNORMALITIES OF CHROMOSOME STRUCTURE

These abnormalities may result from a number of types of chromosome mutation.

1. *Translocations*
   This is the interchange of genetic material between non-homologous chromosomes. There are two types:
   - *Reciprocal translocations. Two breaks on different chromosomes occur and so genetic material is exchanged between the two chromosomes. A carrier of a **balanced translocation** is usually of normal phenotype because they have the normal chromosome complement. However, their offspring may have an **unbalanced translocation**, resulting in a partial trisomy or monosomy, eg. 6p trisomy, 4p monosomy*
   - *Robertsonian translocation (results in altered chromosome numbers – see Down syndrome). The long arms of two acrocentric chromosomes fuse together to make one long chromosome, and their short arms are lost. This only occurs between chromosomes 13, 14, 15, 21 and 22 because these are acrocentric (have very small short arms that contain no essential genetic material.) It can result in Down syndrome for the offspring of a carrier of the Robertsonian translocation.*

2. **Deletions.** *Deletion of a portion of the chromosome occurs, eg. Cri du Chat syndrome (46, XY, del [5p]). Microdeletions (smaller deletions now visible microscopically using new techniques such as high-resolution banding and FISH, or by molecular techniques) include Williams syndrome and DiGeorge syndrome (chromosome 22 microdeletion).*

3. **Duplications.** *Two copies of a portion of the chromosome are present, eg. Charcot-Marie-Tooth disease.*

Cri du Chat syndrome (deletion 5p syndrome)

This is caused by a partial deletion of the short arm of chromosome 5.

Clinical features

General	Low birth weight, slow growth, **cat-like cry**
CNS	Hypotonia, mental retardation
Craniofacial	Microcephaly, hypertelorism, epicanthic folds, down-slanting palebral fissures, abnormal low-set ears
Hands	Simian crease (81%)
Cardiac	Variable CHD (30%)

DiGeorge syndrome

This is due to a microdeletion of 22q. The syndrome overlaps with Shprintzen syndrome, and the two may represent different manifestations of the same genetic defect. It has also been named CATCH-22 (**C**ardiac abnormalities, **A**bnormal facies, **T** cell deficit from thymic hypoplasia, **C**left palate, **H**ypocalcaemia and chromosome **22**.)

The features result from fourth branchial arch development defect (3rd and 4th pharyngeal pouches)

Clinical features

Thymus	Hypoplasia/aplasia, cellular immunity defect
Parathyroids	Hypoplasia/absence, hypocalcaemia and neonatal fits
CVS	Aortic arch anomalies (right-sided aortic arch, interrupted aortic arch, truncus arteriosus, VSD, TOF)
Craniofacial	Short palpebral fissures, short philtrum, micrognathia, ear abnormalities

Shprintzen syndrome

Features include:

CNS	Learning difficulties
Growth	Short stature
Craniofacial	Absent adenoids, cleft palate, prominent nose, long maxilla, small mandible, ear abnormalities
Cardiac (85%)	VSD, right-sided aortic arch, TOF

Williams syndrome

This is due to a deletion of an elastin allele in chromosome 7q11.23.

Clinical features

Craniofacial	Medial eyebrow flare, depressed nasal bridge, epicanthic folds
	Blue eyes, **stellate pattern iris**
	Prominent lips (fish-shaped)
CNS	Mental retardation, friendly manner, **'cocktail party' speech**
	Hypersensitivity to sound
Skeletal	Short stature, hypoplastic nails, scoliosis, kyphosis, joint limitations
Cardiac	Supravalvular aortic stenosis, peripheral pulmonary artery stenosis, VSD, ASD, renal artery stenosis
Renal	Nephrocalcinosis, pelvic kidney, urethral stenosis

Single gene defects (Mendelian inheritance)

Single gene traits are also called Mendelian traits, after Gregor Mendel an Austrian monk who formed some basic genetic principles from experiments with peas. The inheritance of these traits is based on the principles that genes occur in pairs (alleles) in individuals, that only one allele from each parent is passed onto the offspring and that one allele is dominant and the other recessive. There are many factors and exceptions that complicate this pattern.

A *pedigree* is constructed to understand the inheritance of a particular condition.

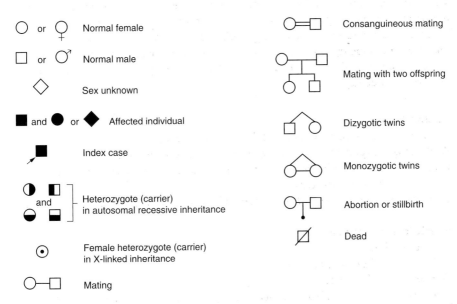

Figure 1.6 Basic pedigree symbols

AUTOSOMAL DOMINANT INHERITANCE (AD)

- *These are often structural defects.*
- *A single allele will exert an effect, thus heterozygotes and homozygotes manifest the disease.*
- *The transmission pattern is* vertical *(disease seen in successive generations).*
- *Offspring of a person with an AD trait have a 50% chance of inheriting the disease. This can be demonstrated diagrammatically (see Fig. 1.7).*

AUTOSOMAL RECESSIVE INHERITANCE (AR)

- *These are often metabolic conditions.*
- *The phenotype only manifests if both alleles are inherited (ie. homozygous individual).*
- *Transmission pattern is* horizontal *(seen in multiple siblings but not parents).*
- *Offspring of parents with an AR trait will have a 25% chance of being affected and a 50% chance of being an asymptomatic carrier (see Fig. 1.8).*
- *Consanguinity increases the chances of a recessive disorder being expressed.*

Examples of Autosomal Dominant and Recessive Conditions

Autosomal dominant	Autosomal recessive
Marfan syndrome	Cystic fibrosis
Achondroplasia	Galactosaemia
Polyposis coli	Homocystinuria
Noonan syndrome	Phenylketonuria
Familial hypercholesterolaemia	Congenital adrenal hyperplasia
Otosclerosis	Friedreich's ataxia

Marfan syndrome

Autosomal dominant, mutations in fibrillin (FBN1) gene on chromosome 15q21.1. There is a very wide variability of expression, and multiple mutations exist so screening cannot be performed. Linkage analysis can be used in families with multiple members affected to identify probable carriers.

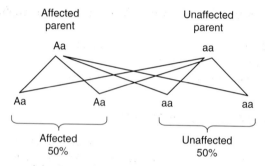

Figure 1.7 Autosomal dominant inheritance

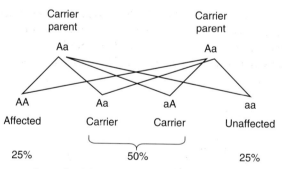

Figure 1.8 Autosomal recessive inheritance

Clinical features

Skeletal   Tall, thin habitus, muscle hypotonia and joint laxity
Decreased upper: lower segment ratio
Arachnodactyly, pes planus, pectus excavatum, **scoliosis**, kyphosis
High arched palate

Eyes   Upward lens subluxation, myopia, retinal detachment

Cardiovascular   Dilatation of ascending aorta, dissecting aortic aneurysm, mitral valve prolapse

The cardiac complications are the commonest cause of death.

Noonan's syndrome

Autosomal dominant condition, usually sporadic.

Clinical features

CNS	Mild mental retardation (25%)
Craniofacial	**Ptosis, epicanthic folds**, hypertelorism, downslanting palpebral fissures, Strabismus, nystagmus, low nasal bridge, low set abnormal ears, prominent upper lip
	Low posterior hairline, **short webbed neck**
Skeletal	Short stature, **shield chest**, pectus excavatum, pectus carinatum, **cubitus valgus**
Cardiac	**Pulmonary valve stenosis**, left ventricular hypertrophy, PDA, VSD, ASD,
	Branch stenosis of pulmonary arteries
Genitalia	Small penis, cryptorchidism
Other	Bleeding diathesis due to a variety of defects

X-LINKED RECESSIVE INHERITANCE

Diseases caused by genes on the X chromosome are X linked, and are usually recessive. The Y chromosome is very small and contains few known genes.

X inactivation

This is a random inactivation of one of the X chromosomes in each cell, which occurs in females. The inactivated chromosome is a dense chromatin mass called a **Barr body**. The theory of X inactivation is the **Lyon hypothesis**.

This explains why X-linked disorders are variably expressed in the female (because females have X-mosaicism).

X-linked recessive disorders

- *Affect males*
- *Carrier females* **may** *be affected (due to Lyonisation)*
- *Sons of female carriers have a 50% chance of being affected*
- *Daughters of female carriers have 50% chance of being carriers*
- *There is no father–son transmission*
- *Daughters of affected males have 100% chance of being carriers*

X-linked dominant disorders

These are uncommon. Females are twice as likely as males to inherit the disorder because they have two X chromosomes. However, the disorder may be lethal in males

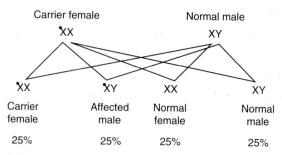

Figure 1.9 X-linked recessive inheritance

and seen only in females (who have one normal X chromosome and thus milder expression of disease), eg. Incontinentia pigmentii.

Examples of X-linked disorders

X-linked recessive	X-linked dominant
Haemophilia A Colour blindness Duchenne muscular dystrophy G6PD deficiency	Familial hypophosphataemic rickets Incontinentia pigmentii

MITOCHONDRIAL DISORDERS

Mitochondria contain their own chromosomes which are maternally derived. A few diseases are the result of mitochondrial mutations. These have characteristic modes of inheritance (not strictly Mendelian) and variable expression. Examples are the mitochondrial myopathies, eg. MELAS and MERRF (see p. 298 metabolic chapter).

Factors affecting inheritance patterns

NEW MUTATION

This is frequent in some conditions (eg. achondroplasia). No previous family history of disease is seen (especially significant in autosomal dominant disorders).

GERMLINE MOSAICISM

A mutation that affects all or some of the germ cells of one parent. Thus a condition that may appear as a one-off mutation recurs in subsequent siblings.

REDUCED PENETRANCE

Some individuals who have inherited the disease do not manifest it phenotypically (eg. retinoblastoma). They can transmit the gene to the next generation.

VARIABLE EXPRESSION

Some individuals manifest the gene mildly and some severely, eg. tuberose sclerosis.

NON-PATERNITY

The genetic picture is confused because the apparent father is not the biological father (relatively common).

ANTICIPATION

This is the development of more severe expression of disease through successive generations. It is seen in diseases that have trinucleotide repeats in their genes. The number of repeats increases through generations and thus the severity of disease.

Examples of diseases associated with trinucleotide repeat expansions

Disease	Repeat sequence	Parent in which expansion occurs
Myotonic dystrophy	CTG	Either parent Congenital form via mother
Friedreich's ataxia	GAA	Either parent
Fragile X syndrome	CGG	Mother
Huntington disease	CAG	Father > mother

PREMUTATION

An example of a premutation is seen in fragile X syndrome.

Fragile X syndrome
An X-linked dominant condition with premutation and expansion occurring via the mother. Seen in approximately 1:1250 males and 1:2500 females.

The term fragile X comes from the fact that the X chromosomes sometimes develop breaks when cultured in a medium deficient in folic acid.

Clinical features
Learning difficulties	(milder in females)
Dysmorphic facies	Large ears, long face
Other	Macroorchidism (large testicular volume), hypermobile joints

Genetics
This condition has unusual genetic features:

- *80% penetrance in males and 30% penetrance in females. (The lower penetrance in females is thought to be due to X inactivation in females.)*
- *Males with the gene who are unnaffected are **'normal transmitting males'**. Daughters of these males are unaffected, but the daughter's sons may be affected*
- *Offspring through successive generations are more likely to be affected*

The gene for fragile X syndrome (FMR1) contains a CGG repeat at one end. Normal individuals have 6–50 copies of this repeat, those with fragile-X syndrome have >230–1000 repeats (a **full mutation**). An intermediate number of repeats (50–230) is seen in normal transmitting males and their female offspring (a **premutation**). Expansions from the premutation to the full mutation do not occur in male transmission. Premutations become larger in successive generations and these are more likely to expand to a full mutation. This explains why males do not give the disease to their sons but the children of the daughters may be affected and this becomes more likely through successive generations.

IMPRINTING AND UNIPARENTAL DISOMY

Genomic imprinting is the differential activation of genes depending on which parent they were inherited from. Examples are Prader-Willi and Angelmann syndrome, and Beckwith-Weidemann syndrome.

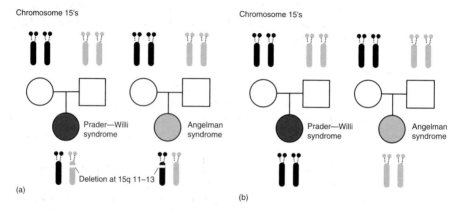

Figure 1.10 Imprinting

Prader-Willi and Angelmann Syndrome

Prader-Willi syndrome	Angelmann syndrome (happy-puppet syndrome)
Neonatal hypotonia	Ataxia
Learning difficulties	Severe learning difficulties
Obsession with food	Happy personality
Obesity	Epilepsy
Micropenis	Characteristic facies (broad smile)

Genetics

The genes for these disorders are found on chromosome 15q11–13.
Failure to inherit the active gene (ie. a deletion) causes the syndrome.
Failure to inherit the paternal copy → Prader-Willi
Failure to inherit the maternal copy → Angelmann syndrome

The deletion may be inherited in two ways:

1. **New mutation.** *Normal parental chromosomes. Gene deletion from one parent.*
2. **Uniparental disomy.** *Normal parental chromosomes. The child inherits both copies from one parent. Thus the normal number of copies are present but there is an effective deletion of the copy from one of the parents. The resulting syndrome depends on which copy is missing.*

Beckwith–Wiedemann Syndrome

Autosomal dominant, variable expression and incomplete penetrance. A minority are caused by paternal uniparental disomy (two copies inherited from the father), with Beckwith-Wiedermann syndrome resulting from *over-expression* of the gene product.

Gene located at 11p15.5, with the maternal copy normally inactivated (imprinted). Imprinting occurs in the insulin-like growth factor 2 (IGF_2) gene on chromosome 11. IGF_2 is active only in the paternal copy (ie. imprinted in the maternal copy). Therefore a double dose of IGF_2 will occur with inheritance of both paternal copies, or loss of maternal imprint (so the maternal gene is activated). The high levels of IGF_2 are thought to result in the following clinical features.

Clinical features

Pregnancy	Polyhydramnions, large for gestational age
Growth	*Macrosomia*, thick subcutaneous tissue, large muscle mass Advanced bone age when infantile.
Craniofacial	*Macroglossia*, prominent eyes, port wine stain central forehead and upper eyelids. *Linear fissures in ear lobule.*
Organ	Large kidneys, fetal adrenocortical cytomegaly, pancreatic hyperplasia, hepatosplenomegaly, large ovaries, cliteromegaly, cardiomegaly
Other	*Infantile hypoglycaemia*, neonatal polycythaemia, *Wilms tumour, hepatoblastoma* (5–10% risk), *hemihypertophy*, umbilical hernia, *omphalocoele*

Multifactorial inheritance

Characteristics that are caused by the combined effects of many genes are **polygenic**. Characteristics affected by genetic and environmental factors are **multifactorial**. Many quantitative traits are multifactorial (eg. BP, height) and are distributed in a symmetrical (Gaussian) fashion.

Many diseases are inherited in a multifactorial fashion and are present only if a liability threshold is reached, eg. pyloric stenosis, cleft lip and palate, neural tube defects.

Recurrence risks for these diseases are based on observation of data gathered on them. For example, the risk of neural tube defect is 1–3:1000 and the recurrence risk is 5% (after one affected child).

Cancer genetics

Cancer occurs when the normal developmental programming of a cell has altered, and the cell is capable of inappropriate proliferation. Cells of a tumour are monoclonal, ie. they all derive from one ancestral cell.

Most cancers are due to genetic changes occurring in somatic cells. Single gene germline mutations are rare and result in inheritable cancers, eg. retinoblastoma. Many cancers are inherited in a multifactorial fashion, eg. breast and colon cancers.

Environmental factors may increase the risk of mutations. **Carcinogens** are environmental cancer causing agents and increase the frequency of genetic cancer-causing events.

Altered genes that predispose to cancer fall into two broad categories: **tumour suppressor genes**, and **oncogenes.**

TUMOUR SUPPRESSOR GENES

These genes are involved in restricting cell proliferation. Their *inactivation* from mutation can result in tumours. The two-hit theory of carcinogenesis is that a tumour occurs only when **both** copies of the tumour suppressor gene are damaged. In inherited cancers the first allele is mutated in the germline, and the second mutation is somatic. Examples are as follows:

Gene	Location	Function	Cancer caused by inherited mutations
RB1 gene	13q14	Cell cycle brake; (binds to E2F transcription complex)	Retinoblastoma, osteosarcoma
APC gene	5q21	Interacts with β-catenin involved in Wnt signalling pathway	Familial adenomatous polyposis
WT1 gene	11p13	Transcription factor	Wilms tumour
BRCA1 gene	17q21	Interacts with RAD51 (DNA repair protein)	Familial breast and ovarian cancers
NF1	17q11	Down regulates pas protein	Neurofibromatosis type 1
NF2	22q12		Neurofibromatosis type 2

ONCOGENES

These are genes whose *product* can lead to unregulated cell growth. Most arise from mutations in *protooncogenes* which are involved in the regulation of cell growth. Mutations occur mostly in somatic cells, though some occur in the germline. Chromosomal translocations may activate an oncogene, eg. the Philadelphia chromosome in CML (a translocation between chromosomes 9 and 22, resulting in the Abl gene joining onto the Bcr gene). Oncogene activation may also be caused by viruses. Examples of oncogenes include the following:

Oncogene	Location	Proposed function	Tumour
N-myc	2p24	DNA-binding protein	Neuroblastoma
Abl	9q34	Protein kinase	ALL, CML
erb-A	17q11	Thyroid hormone receptor	Promyelocytic leukaemia
RET	10q	Tyrosine kinase receptor	MEN, medullary thyroid carcinoma (germline mutation)
SIS	22q12	β subunit of platelet-derived growth factor (PDGF)	Glioma

Dysmorphology

This is the study of abnormal physical development (**morphogenesis**) occurring during embryogenesis, resulting in congenital defects. Congenital defects may be:

1. *major (2–3% newborns): of functional or cosmetic importance*
2. *minor (5–7% newborns): not of functional or cosmetic importance.*

The aetiology of congenital defects is usually unknown or multifactorial. There is an identified genetic component in 30%, and environmental causes are infrequent.

PATHOGENIC PROCESSES

1. Malformation

A primary defect resulting from intrinsic abnormal development during embryogenesis (eg. polydactyly, cleft lip). Causes include:

- *Chromosomal abnormalities*
- *Single gene defects*
- *Multifactorial*

2. Dysplasia

A primary defect involving abnormal organisation of cells into tissues (eg. haemangioma).

3. Deformation

A secondary alteration of a previously normally formed body part by mechanical forces. These can be extrinsic or intrinsic. Causes include:

- *Extrinsic*
  oligohydramnios
  abnormal presentation (eg. CDH)
  multiple pregnancy
  uterine abnormalities
- *Intrinsic*
  congenital myotonic dystrophy
  congenital skeletal defects

Arthrogryphosis is a picture of pre-natal joint contractures resulting from a variety of causes including fetal crowding (oligohydramnios, twins), external constraints (uterine abnormalities) and intrinsic neuromuscular, skeletal or connective tissue defects.

4. Disruption

A secondary defect resulting from extrinsic breakdown of, or an interface with an originally normal developmental process. Causes include:

- *Teratogens*
- *Intrauterine infection*
- *Maternal disease*
- *Limb defect resulting from a vascular event.*

Syndrome. Pattern of multiple primary malformations due to a single aetiology (eg. trisomy 18)

Sequence. A primary defect with secondary structural changes (eg. Potter phenotype, Pierre-Robin sequence)

TERATOGENS

Teratogens are agents external to the fetus's genome that induce structural malformations, growth deficiency and/or functional alterations during pre-natal development.

Human teratogens

Drug	Potential effect	Critical period
Alcohol	**Fetal alcohol syndrome:**	<12 weeks
	Craniofacial: Long philtrum, flat nasal bridge, midfacial hypoplasia, upturned nose micrognathia, ear deformities, eye malformations, cleft lip and palate	
	CNS: Psychomotor delay, microcephaly	
	Other: Cardiac, renal and limb abnormalities	
	Growth retardation and developmental delay	>24 weeks
Isotretinoin	Spontaneous abortion, hydrocephalus, CNS defects, cotruncal heart defects, small or missing thymus, micrognathia	
Warfarin	Nasal hypoplasia, chondrodysplasia punctata	6–9 weeks
	CNS defects secondary to cerebral haemorrhage	>12 weeks
Phenytoin	Craniofacial dysmorphism, hypoplastic nails and phalanges	First trimester
Sodium valproate	Neural tube defects	<30 days
Carbamazepine	Neural tube defects	<30 days
Cocaine	Placental abruption	2nd–3rd trimester
	Premature delivery, intracranial haemorrhage	Third trimester
Lithium	Ebstein's anomaly	<8 weeks
Thalidomide	Limb hypoplasia, ear abnormalities	5–9 weeks
Diethylstilboestrol	Uterine abnormalities, vaginal adenocarcinoma, male infertility	<12 weeks

MATERNAL DISEASES ASSOCIATED WITH NEONATAL DISORDERS

Disease	Malformation/disorder
Diabetes mellitus	Caudal regression syndrome (sacral agenesis) CHD, hypoplastic left colon, renal vein thrombosis, Hypertrophic subaortic stenosis
Hyperthyroidism	Transient neonatal thyrotoxicosis (10–20%) due to placental antibody transfer
Autoimmune thrombo-cytopenia	Transient neonatal thrombocytopenia due to placental antibody transfer
Myaesthenia gravis	Transient neonatal disease, arthrogryphosis (due to placental antibody transfer)
Phenylketonuria	Microcephaly, CHD, mental retardation (if high phenylalanine levels)

Clinical applications of genetics

There are many clinical applications of genetics, including:

- **Antenatal screening.** *This is offered to the general population (eg. antenatal USS), and to selected individuals (eg. amniocentesis if older maternal age). Antenatal screening is useful for selective pregnancy termination, for informing parents of an abnormality in advance of delivery, and to enable any necessary antenatal therapy to be done. (see p. 458.)*
- **Presymptomatic testing.** *Certain diseases that manifest later in life may be screened for (eg. adult polycystic kidney disease)*
- **Genetic counselling.** *Information for couples about hereditary diseases. Antenatal diagnosis. Estimation of risk of transfer of disease to offspring. Information about possible measures to prevent the disease*
- **Gene therapy.** *This is genetic alteration of the cells of individuals with genetic diseases*

GENE THERAPY

Most current techniques involve gene replacement therapy (effective for recessive diseases with missing genes). Gene-blocking techniques are being developed to use in gain-of-function or dominant negative mutations (eg. Marfan syndrome, Huntington disease).

Non-inherited diseases may also be treated with gene therapy, eg. p53 tumour suppressor gene may be inserted into certain tumours.

Most gene therapy techniques are being developed on somatic cells, though work is being done on germline therapy which alters all the cells of the body, and thus the patient *and* their descendants.

Diseases for which somatic cell gene therapy is being tested

Disease	Target cell	Inserted gene
Haemophilia B	Hepatocytes, skin fibroblasts	Factor IX
Cystic fibrosis	Airway epithelial cells	CFTR
ADA deficiency	Circulating lymphocytes, Bone marrow stem cells	Adenosine deaminase
Duchenne muscular dystrophy	Myoblasts	Dystrophin
AIDS	T helper lymphocytes	Dominant negative retrovirus mutations

FURTHER READING

Connor M, Ferguson-Smith M *Essential Medical Genetics*, 5th Ed, Blackwell Science, London, 1997

Larson WJ *Essentials of human embryology*, Churchill Livingstone, New York, 1998

Sadler TW *Langman's Medical Embryology*, 7th Ed, Williams & Wilkins, New York, 1995

Jones KL, *Smiths Recognizable Patterns of Human Malformations*, 5th Ed, WB Saunders, Philadelphia, 1997

2

Immunology

- *Components of the immune system*
- *Clinical features in immunodeficiency*
- *Investigations*
- *Inherited immunodeficiencies*
- *Acquired immunodeficiency*

Components of the immune system

The immune system is subdivided into *innate* and *specific* responses, though there is much interaction between the two.

INNATE IMMUNITY

This involves the elements of the immune system that produce an immediate, non-specific response. The main components involved are

Phagocytes

- *Mononuclear phagocytes* Monocytes (blood), *macrophages* (tissues), *Kupfer cells* (liver). *Antigen presenting cells* (APCs) (see later)
- *Polymorphonuclear granulocytes (PMNs)* Neutrophils (Granulocytes) (95%) Eosinophils (2–5%)

- These cells employ *phagocytosis* (cellular ingestion) of foreign material.
- *Opsonisation* (coating the antigen with antibody and complement) helps ingestion and killing.
- Neutrophils live 2–3 days only. They have granules containing antibiotic proteins, enzymes (eg. lysozyme) and lactoferrin.
  Particularly active against bacteria and fungi.
- Eosinophils produce cytotoxic granules, which are released onto the surface of large organisms (they can employ phagocytosis.) Active against large parasitic infections.

Accessory cells

Basophils and mast cells
Involved in inflammation, parasite immunity and immediate hypersensitivity.

Stimulated by antigens (with IgE) to *degranulate* and release vasoactive substances including histamine. Basophils are in the circulation and mast cells in the tissues.

Antigen presenting cells (APCs)	Present antigens to B and T cells.
Platelets	Involved in inflammation and blood clotting.
Endothelial cells	Involved in the distribution of leucocytes.

Complement

The complement system involves >20 glycoproteins which are activated in a cascade. There are three pathways of activation:

1 & 2.	*Classical (and Lectin) pathway*	Activation via C1q + immune complex (*specific immunity*). (Lectin is antibody-independant).
3.	*Alternative pathway*	Activation via microorganism surface and factors B, D and then properdin (*innate immunity*).

All three result in activation of C3 (to C3a and C3b), and then the final common pathway C5 to C9. Involved in eradication of organisms (via opsonisation, activation of leucocytes and target cell lysis), inflammation and immunoregulation (self from non-self).

Soluble mediators

These soluble messengers mediate inflammation and promote uptake by phagocytosis (opsonisation). They signal their target cells to divide, activate or focus on an area of the body.

Cytokines (those produced by lymphocytes = *lymphokines*):

Interferons (IFNs)	Viral infections. INFα, INFβ, INFγ
Interleukins (Ils)	Il-1 to IL-17. Many functions, direct cells to differentiate and divide.
Colony stimulating factors (CFSs)	eg. G-CSF (granulocyte-colony stimulating factor) GM-CSF-differentiation and division of stem cells.
Others	eg. Tumour necrosis factors (TNFα, TNFβ), transforming growth factor-B (TGFβ),

Antibodies - see later	
Acute phase proteins	eg. C-reactive protein (CRP)

SPECIFIC IMMUNITY

This system involves lymphoid tissue and circulating leucocytes that mount a specific response to an antigen. The main lymphoid organs are:

Primary lymphoid tissue- bone marrow and fetal liver (make B cells), thymus (make T cells)
Secondary lymphoid tissue- lymph nodes, spleen and mucosa-associated lymphoid tissue MALT (eg. tonsils, Peyer's patches).

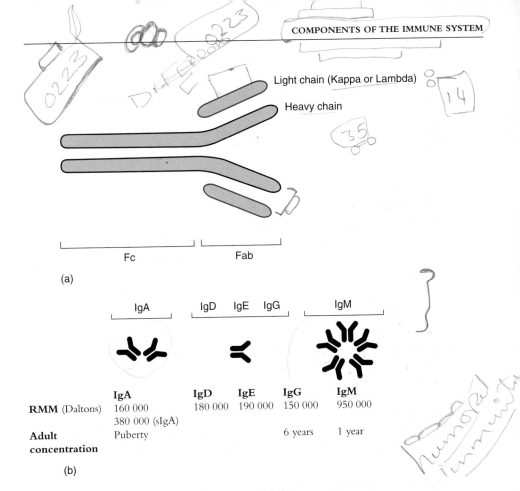

Light chain (Kappa or Lambda)
Heavy chain

Fc   Fab

(a)

	IgA	IgD	IgE	IgG	IgM
RMM (Daltons)	IgA 160 000 380 000 (sIgA)	IgD 180 000	IgE 190 000	IgG 150 000	IgM 950 000
Adult concentration	Puberty			6 years	1 year

(b)

Figure 2.1 (a) Antibody composition. (b) Immunoglobulin structure

Leucocytes have molecules on their surface known as *clusters of differentiation (CD)*, identified using monoclonal antibodies, which are used for identifying subpopulations.

T Lymphocytes

T-Helper cells (TH)   CD4 on their surface. See antigens with MHC class II molecules.
   TH1 subset: Secrete IL-2 and IFN-γ
      Cytotoxicity and inflammation (protect against intracellular organisms eg. viruses, bacteria, parasites).
   TH2 subset: Secrete IL-4, IL-5, IL-6, IL-10
      Stimulate B cells (protect against free-living organisms ie. humoral immunity).
T-Cytotoxic cells (TC)   CD8 on their surface. See antigens with MHC class I molecules. Kill other cells. Down–regulate immune responses.

B Lymphocytes (5–15%)
These produce immunoglobulins (antibodies) and have these on their surface. When activated they become *plasma cells* which make antibody. Carry markers CD 19, CD 20, CD 22 and CD 72–78. Carry MHC Class II antigens for interactions with T cells.

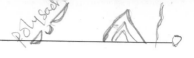

Antibodies

These are serum glycoproteins that are specific to particular antigens. The type of heavy chain determines the class.

IgG	Crosses the placenta (adult levels at birth, transient fall at 3–6 months, adult levels by 6 years)
	Antibody of secondary response
	There are four subclasses:
	IgG1, IgG3 – produced in response to many viruses and tetanus toxin. Complement activation.
	IgG2, IgG4 – produced in response to polysaccharide antigen eg. pneumococcus.
IgM	Major antibody of primary response (elevated in acute infection). Complement activation.
	Seen in the foetus only in intrauterine infection (does not cross the placenta).
IgA	Secretory (sIgA) important in protection of mucosal surfaces eg. respiratory tract, gut
IgE	Involved in type 1 hypersensitivity and against helminthic parasites.
IgD	Present on B cell membranes, precise function unknown.

Natural killer (NK) cells (15%)

CD56 and CD16 surface markings.

Eliminate tumour and virus-infected cells using cytotoxic means.

Lymphokine-activated killer (LAK) cells are cells (NK and certain T cells) that have been activated by IL-2 and particularly target tumour cells.

IMMUNE ACTIVATION AND INTERACTION

The mechanisms of activation and interaction are integral to the immune system and involve:

Antigen presenting cells

- *Langerhans' cells* (skin), *interdigitating cells* (*IDC's*, lymph node) and *germinal centre dendritic cells* (*GCDC*, lymph nodes) – present to TH cells. (These have class II MHCs)
- *Follicular dendritic cells (FDCs)* (lymph nodes, spleen, MALT) – present to B cells
- *Macrophages*
- *B cells* present to T cells

Activation of T and B cells

T and B cells are activated by binding to their specific antigens.

B cells – Bind to native antigens but many need T cells to become activated (many activated B cells then become plasma cells).

T cells – Recognise antigen in association with MHC molecules on antigen-presenting cells.

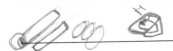

HUMAN LEUCOCYTE ANTIGENS (HLA)

The HLA molecules are encoded for by a set of genes known as the *major histocom-patibility complex (MHC)* on the short arm of chromosome 6.

The MHC genes code for HLA antigens (cell surface glycoproteins) which are present on all tissues and help to identify self from non-self. There are two classes of molecules:

1. **Class I** *HLA-A, B, and C*   – *on all cells except erythrocytes and trophoblast cells*
2. **Class II** *HLA-DP, DQ and DR* – *on T and B cells, monocytes and dendritic cells, inducible on endothelial and epithelial cells*

HLA antigens are important in organ transplantation, where they need to be matched.

Several diseases are associated with specific HLA types (which are being subclassified):

A3	Haemochromatosis	B18	Hodgkin's disease
B5	Behçets syndrome	B27	Ankylosing spondylitis
B8	Tuberculoid leprosy		Juvenile rheumatoid arthritis
B8, DR3	Myaesthenia gravis		Psoriatic arthritis
	Addison's disease		Reiter's syndrome
	Graves' disease		Reactive arthritis
	SLE		Acute anterior uveitis
	Sjögren's syndrome	Bw47	Congenital adrenal hyperplasia
	Membranous GN	DR7, DR2	Goodpasture's syndrome
	Chronic active hepatitis		Multiple sclerosis
	Dermatitis herpetiformis		Narcolepsy
B8, DQ8	IDDM		
DR4	Rheumatoid arthritis	DR7	Minimal change GN
B8, DR3,	Coeliac disease		
DR7, DQw2			

HYPERSENSITIVITY REACTIONS

Reaction	Mediators	Histology	Test	Disease/Condition
Type I Immediate	Free Ag + IgE, mast cells	Vasodilatation Oedema	Skin prick RAST	Anaphylactic shock Atopic diseases
Type II Antibody-dependent Cytotoxic	Cell surface Ag + IgG, ± complement ± K cells	Target cell damage	Coombs' test Indirect immuno-fluorescence Precipitating abs Red cell agglutination	Transfusion reactions Autoimmune haemolytic anaemia Haemolytic disease of the newborn ITP
Type III Immune Complex	Immune complex deposition IgG, IgM, IgA, complement polymorphs	Acute inflammation Vasculitis	Skin test (Arthus reaction) Immune complexes detection (IMF, RIA)	Autoimmune eg. SLE, nephritis Low-grade persistent infections eg. viral hepatitis Environmental antigens eg. farmer's lung

Reaction	Mediators	Histology	Test	Disease/Condition
Type IV delayed	Cell bound Ag + T cells, lymphokines, macrophages	Perivascular inflammation Caseation and necrosis (TB)	Skin test (eg. tuberculin test – induration and erythema) Patch test	Pulmonary TB Contact dermatitis GVHD Insect bites

Skin tests

Type I (prick test) A wheal and flare develop within 20 minutes and resolve in two hours

Type III (intradermal or SC injection) A wheal develops over hours (maximal at 5–7 hours) and resolves over 24 hours (Arthus reaction)

Type IV (intradermal or patch test) An indurated area develops within 2–4 days and resolves over several days

Urticaria and angio-oedema

This is swelling of the skin and mucosa due to capillary leakage. Mechanism may be immunologically-mediated (IgE or complement), or non-immunologically mediated (direct mast cell release, prostaglandin inhibitors). There is release of histamine,± bradykinin causing vasodilatation.

Clinical features

Urticaria Intermittent skin wheals, may itch, last 12–14 hours (dermal swelling from leaking capillaries), recurrent crops may occur. *Chronic urticaria* = lasts >6 weeks

Angio-oedema Swelling mouth, eyes, genitalia, GIT, upper respiratory tract (sub-mucosal and subcutaneous involvement).

Causes

Cause is not often found.

Ingestion	Foods eg. cow's milk, drugs
Contact	Insects, plants
Infections	Viral, bacterial, parasitic
Physical	Cold, sun, heat, mechanical force
Cholinergic urticaria	Sweating (exercise, hot water, anxiety)
Systemic disease	Leukaemia, collagen-vascular disease
Genetic	Hereditary angio-oedema (see p. 40–41), urticaria pigmentosa

Management

Self-limiting disease, usually resolves over weeks or months
Avoid known triggers
Antihistamines (H1 ± H2-receptor blockers)
Adrenaline (severe reaction, anaphylaxis)

Atopy

Atopic individuals have the following:

- *A predisposition to form IgE-mediated (type 1) reactions to common environmental allergens*

- *Susceptibility to asthma, hay fever (allergic conjunctivitis ± rhinitis) and atopic eczema*
- *A family history of atopy*

See p. 135 (asthma) and p. 312 (atopic dermatitis).

INFECTIONS SEEN WITH SPECIFIC IMMUNODEFICIENCY

Deficiency	Organisms	
Humoral (antibody)	Bacteria	Staphylococci, streptococci, haemophilus, *M. catarrhalis*, mycoplasma, campylobacter
	Viruses	Enteroviruses
	Protozoa	Giardia
Cellular (T cell)	Bacteria (intracellular)	Myobacteria, listeria, legionella
	Viruses	CMV, HSV, RSV, measles, EBV, VzV
	Fungi	Candida, aspergillus
	Protozoa	*Pneumocystis carinii*, toxoplasmosis
Combined	Bacteria	Intracellular and extracellular
(cellular and humoral)	Viruses	CMV, HSV, measles
	Fungi	Candida
	Parasites	Cryptococcus, cryptosporidium
	Protozoa	*Pneumocystis carinii*, toxoplasmosis, giardia
Neutrophils	Bacteria	Staphylococcus, gram-negative bacteria
	Fungi	Candida, aspergillus
Complement	Bacteria	Neisseria

Clinical features in immunodeficiency

HISTORY

Infections Frequent, unusual severity, opportunistic, involving multiple sites, poor response to therapy, atypical symptoms and signs
Unusual organisms
Recurrent skin infections, abscesses, sinopulmonary infections, periodontitis

Autoimmune features Arthropathy, rash

Family history Neonatal deaths (particularly male)
Immunodeficiency, parental tonsillectomy
Consanguinity

Other Adverse reaction to vaccines,
Persistent diarrhoea, prolonged wound healing

EXAMINATION

The following may be present on examination.

Failure to thrive
Dysmorphism
Lymphoid tissue May be absent or enlarged (eg. lymph nodes, tonsils, thymus)

Skin	Eczema? Petechiae? Infections? Granulomas? Telangiectasia?
Hepatosplenomegaly	
Eyes	Retinal abnormalities
CNS	Ataxia?

INVESTIGATIONS

INITIAL

FBC with differential count	Neutrophils, lymphocytes, monocytes, eosinophils, basophils
Immunoglobulins	IgG, IgM, IgA
	IgG subclasses
	IgE
Antibody response to vaccines	eg. diphtheria, tetanus, Hib, killed polio
Isohaemagglutinins	(IgM to red cell antigen)
Complement	C3, C4, THC (total haemolytic complement)
Neutrophil function	Nitroblue tetrazolium dye reduction (NBT test) see below.
Lymphocyte subsets	
HIV testing	

SPECIFIC

Cell mediated

Quantitative	T cell subsets (CD3, CD4, CD8, CD4: CD8 ratio, etc)
	NK cells (CD16 and CD56)
	Monocytes (CD14)
Qualitative	Phytohaemagglutinin stimulation (PHA)
	Candida, PPD stimulation
	Mixed lymphocyte reaction
	Response to IL-2 stimulation
	Class II expression (DR expression)
	Activation status (CD25, IL-2 receptor)
Specific	Adenosine deaminase (ADA) purine nucleotide phosphorylase (PNP) enzyme activity.
	Surface expression of CD40 ligand and CD3 intensity

Humoral

Quantitative	B cell markers (CD19, CD20)
	Immunoglobulins (IgA, IgG, IgM, IgE and IgG subclasses)
Qualitative	Isohaemagglutinins
	Response to vaccines

Phagocytes

Adhesion molecule expression	CD15s (LAD2), CD18 (LAD1)

Functional assays	Mobility and chemotaxis (rarely done)
Phagocytosis	Chemiluminescence
Phagocyte enzyme analysis	Cytochrome gp 92 phox, cytosolic proteins

Inherited immunodeficiencies

Classification of diseases in immunology is complex and changing, therefore they may appear elsewhere classified slightly differently. It is best to concentrate on differentiating the individual diseases rather than their classification.

PREDOMINANTLY B CELL DISORDERS

Bruton's X-linked agammaglobulinaemia
X-linked recessive. Presents at six months to two years.

Immune defect	Very low or absent B cells
	IgA, IgM, IgG, IgD, IgE *all* low
Underlying defect	Mutation in the *btk* gene at Xq22.3−22 causing absence of B-cells cytoplasmic tyrosine kinase
	Pre-B to B cell transformation is defective

Clinical features

- *Recurrent bacterial infections*
- *Unusual enterovirus infections (chronic meningoencephalitis)*
- *Tonsils, adenoids and lymph nodes small or absent*

Management
gamma-globulin (IVIG) infusions 3−4 weekly.

Common variable immunodeficiency (CVID)

Immune defect	Abnormal B cell function (normal or reduced B cell numbers)
	Low IgA, IgG ± IgM
	Abnormal T cell function in 1/3rd (thus the disease could be considered a combined defect)
Underlying defect	Unknown

Clinical features
Usually present later in life (in 2nd or 3rd decades).

Sinopulmonary infections	
Other infections	Gastrointestinal (giardia, campylobacter)
	Chronic enteroviral meningoencephalitis
Splenomegaly	(Diffuse lymphadenopathy may also occur)
GI tract	Follicular lymph node hyperplasia, malabsorption, weight loss, diarrhoea
Malignancies	Lymphomas, gestrointestinal malignancies
Autoimmune associations	Pernicious anaemia, haemolytic anaemia, thrombocytopenia, leucopenia

Management
Immunoglobulin replacement.

Selective IgA deficiency
Incidence 1:700 caucasians, variable inheritance.

Associations	HLA-B8, DR3
	Autoimmune disease eg. RA, SLE, coeliac disease, thyroiditis
Immune defect	Low or absent IgA
	Sometimes IgG_2 and IgG_4 subclass deficiency also (20%)
Underlying defect	Impaired switching or maturational failure of IgA-producing lymphocytes

Clinical features

- *Asymptomatic*
- *Respiratory infections (URTI, sinusitis, wheeze, polysaccharide infections)*
- *Chronic diarrhoea*
- ↑ *Type III hypersensitivity*

Management
Specific therapy for infections. NB. Transfusion reactions more common.

Transient hypogammaglobulinaemia of infancy

Immune defect	Slow maturation of antibody production
	Low IgG $\pm$ IgA before six months

Clinical features

- *More common in preterm infants*
- *Recurrent respiratory tract infections in infancy*
- *Spontaneous improvement with age*

Management
Usually none required.

Duncan's syndrome (X-linked lymphoproliferative syndrome)

Immune defect	Inadequate immune response to EBV, and other defects
Underlying defect	Unknown. Gene defect at Xq26

Clinical features

- *Susceptibility to EBV infection*
- *Abnormal immune response leading to liver necrosis, aplastic crisis and lymphoproliferative disease*
- *If they survive primary infection, they develop hypogammaglobulinaemia and B lymphomas*

Management

- *Intravenous immunoglobulin and antibiotics*
- *BMT*

IgG subclass deficiency

Immune defect	Low IgG subclasses (normal total levels of IgG)
	IgG$_2$ deficiency (most common type in children) often have low IgA levels
	IgG$_3$ most common in adults
Underlying defect	Defect of isotype differentiation

Clinical features

- *Variable, usually mild*
- *Frequent infections*
- *Increased allergy*
- *Encapsulated bacterial infections if IgG2 deficiency*

Management

- *Prophylactic antibiotics*
- *Intravenous immunoglobulin (occasionally)*

PREDOMINANTLY T CELL DISORDERS

DiGeorge anomaly

The autosomal dominant DiGeorge anomaly is one of several syndromes involving microdeletions of chromosome 22q. They are collectively known as *CATCH 22* (**C**ardiac, **A**bnormal facies, **T**hymic hypoplasia, **C**left palate and **H**ypocalcaemia). They include the velocardiofacial (Shprintzen) syndrome (see p. 12).

Immune defect	One or more of:
	Decreased numbers and function of T cells
	Reduced PHA
	Specific antibody deficiency
Underlying defect	4th branchial arch (3rd and 4th pharyngeal pouches) malformation
	Microdeletions of chromosome 22q11

Clinical features

Thymus	Aplasia or hypoplasia
Parathyroid	Hypoparathyroidism, Ca ↓, neonatal seizures, tetany, cataracts
Cardiac	Right-sided aortic arch defects, Fallot's tetralogy, PDA, VSD, truncus arteriosus, interrupted aortic arch
Oesophagus	Atresia
Dysmorphism	Short palpebral fissures, low-set notched ears, micrognathia, bifid uvula, short philtrum

Infections   Respiratory, diarrhoea, candida (severity varies, infections are not usually a presenting feature and immunodeficiency may correct over time)

Management
Thymus transplant and BMT if necessary.

Chronic mucocutaneous candidiasis
Immune defect   Impaired cell-mediated immunity to candida
                       Negative skin tests to candida
Underlying defect   Unknown

Clinical features
Chronic candidiasis Skin, nails and mucous membranes, not systemic infection
Others   Hypoparathyroidism, autoimmune disorders

Management
Antifungal therapy.

COMBINED IMMUNODEFICIENCIES

Severe combined immunodeficiency (SCID)
This comprises various syndromes, which have the following basic characteristics. The definition of SCID is based on the severity of the condition and presence of typical features. SCID is further distinguished on the basis of pathogenesis (where known).
    SCID must be differentiated from AIDS.

Immunological
Absence or impaired function of T and/or B cells from birth. There are two groups of SCID:

1. *T−B− SCID (lack T and B lymphocytes) − RAG-1 or RAG-2 gene mutations*
2. *T−B+ SCID (lack T cells, normal number of B cells) − profound lymphopenia, hypogammaglobulinaemia, very small thymus.*

Clinical features

- *Severe failure to thrive*
- *Absent lymphoid tissue*
- *Diarrhoea*
- *Infections − pneumonia, otitis media, sepsis, cutaneous infections, opportunistic*
- *GVH symptoms − features similar to graft versus host disease in the neonatal period*

Management
Death occurs <2 years unless given BMT.

Causes of SCID

X-linked (50%)	T− B+
	Defective γc-chain of IL-2, 4, 7, 9 and 15
Autosomal recessive	T− B+
	Jak 3 mutation (intracellular kinase)
Omenn syndrome	T cell infiltration of tissues
	Hypereosinophilia, erythroderma, picture of GVHD
RAG-1/-2 deficiency	T− B−
	NK cells normal or ↑
	Mutations in RAG-1 or RAG-2 genes
	Autosomal recessive
Adenosine deaminase	T− B−
deficiency (ADA) (20%)	Autosomal recessive, chromosome 20q13
	Gene therapy currently being developed
Purine nucleoside	T(reduced), B (less affected)
phosphorylase (PNP)	Autosomal recessive, chromosome 14q13
deficiency (4%)	Neurological abnormalities (2/3rds)
	Autoimmune disease (1/3rd)
MHC class II deficiency	Failure of antigen presentation
	Heterogeneous condition
	CD4 lymphocytes particularly impaired

Wiskott–Aldrich syndrome

X-linked recessive (boys only).

Immune defect	Impaired cell-mediated immunity, progressive T lymphocyte ↓
	Impaired antibody production (normal initially, then IgM ↓)
	Isohaemagglutinins ↓
Underlying defect	Abnormal microvilli on T cells
	WASp gene on Xp11

Clinical features

Platelets	Small size, thrombocytopaenia purpura over skin (normal megakaryocytes)
Eczema	Severe
Infections	Pneumonia, otitis media, meningitis
	HSV, VZV, PCP, encapsulated organisms eg. pneumococcus
Malignancies	Lymphoma
Autoimmune	JCA, haemolytic anaemia, vasculitis, glomerulonephritis

Management

These children will die <2 years without BMT.

Ataxia telangiectasia

Autosomal recessive.

Immune defect	Impaired cell-mediated immunity (T cell numbers and function ↓)

Impaired antibody production (IgA very low, IgE $\downarrow$, IgG$_2$$\downarrow$ and IgG$_4$)

Underlying defect   Abnormal DNA repair especially chs. 7 and 14

Mutations in ATM gene, chromosome 11q23.1

Additional   CEA $\uparrow$, α-FP $\uparrow$, fatty liver changes

Cells have an extreme hypersensitivity to ionising radiation (frequent somatic mutations)

Clinical features

Cerebellar ataxia   Progressive

Telangiectasia   Occulocutaneous, particularly on ear lobes and conjunctival sclera

Infections   Chronic sinopulmonary

Malignancy   Lymphomas, adenocarcinomas

Endocrine   Hypogonadism (ovaries or testes), glucose intolerance

Management

Supportive.

X-linked immunodeficiency with hyper IgM

Immune defect   Impaired antibody formation, low IgA and IgG

IgM normal or $\uparrow$, absent germinal centres

Recurrent neutropenia and thrombocytopenia

Underlying defect   Absent CD40 ligand on T cells (B cells need this to switch isotypes)

Clinical features

- *Recurrent respiratory infection (URTI, LTRI, PCP)*
- *Autoimmune features may be present*

Management

IV gammaglobulin

Hyper IgE (Job syndrome)

Immune defect   Possible immune dysregulation of IgE

Very high IgE (>1000), impaired neutrophil locomotion

T cell abnormalities

Underlying defect   Unknown

Clinical features

Eczema

Infections   Staphylococcal abscesses in lung, skin, joints

Management

1. *Antibiotic prophylaxis (penicillin)*
2. *Gammaglobulin infusions if deficient*
3. *Drainage of abscesses*

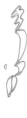

NEUTROPHIL DISORDERS

Chronic granulomatous disease (CGD)

Immune defect	Failure of superoxide production (therefore inability to kill)
Underlying defect	Defective cytochrome b558 (the enzymatic unit of NADPH oxidase) from a defect in one of its subunits
	Absent gp91phox (X-linked, 66%)
	Absence of p22phox (autosomal recessive, 33%)

Clinical features

Infections	Recurrent abscesses of bone, lung, liver, lymph nodes, gastrointestinal tract
	Aspergillus infection
Granulomas	GIT, liver, spleen, skin, lung, bone
Other	Gingival hyperplasia, cervical lymphadenopathy, hepatosplenomegaly

Diagnosis

- *NBT test (failure to reduce nitroblue tetrazolium)*
- *Biopsy granuloma*
- *Hypergammaglobulinaemia*
- *Radiology – liver/spleen CT scan, bone scan, CXR*

Management

- *Treat acute infection with antibiotics and neutrophil transfusions*
- *Long-term therapy with γ-interferon and prophylactic antibiotics*

Chediak–Higashi syndrome

Immune defect	Giant granules in all nucleated cells
	Neutropenia, granulocyte mobility and chemotaxis defects
	NK cell cytotoxicity defective
Underlying defect	Cytoskeletal microtubule defect
	Autosomal recessive

Clinical features

Infections	Recurrent, bacterial (skin, respiratory, abscesses)
Albinism	Partial occulocutaneous
	Photophobia, nystagmus
Neurological	CNS and peripheral nerve lesions

Accelerated phase of disease can occur with EB virus infection resembling familial lymphohistiocytosis (FLH) leading to pancytopenia, hepatosplenomegaly and death.

Diagnosis

- *Neutrophil analysis (giant granules)*
- *Giant melanosomes in melanocytes*
- *Bleeding time prolonged due to platelet aggregation defects*

Management

- *Treatment of acute infections*
- *BMT*

Schwachman–Diamond syndrome (see p. 160)

Immune defect   Cyclical neutropenia, defective neutrophil mobility and chemotaxis
Underlying defect   Unknown
                        Autosomal recessive

Clinical features

1. *Cyclical neutropenia*
2. *Exocrine pancreatic failure (steatorrhoea)*
3. *Metaphyseal dysostosis (short stature)*
4. *Anaemia, thrombocytopenia (variable)*

Management

Supportive, pancreatic exocrine supplements, GMCSF

Leucocyte adhesion defects (LAD)

Immune defect   Abnormal leucocyte adhesion
                        Peripheral neutrophils ↑
Underlying defect   Absence of CD18 (LAD1) resulting in LFA1, C3b or p150 deficiency
                        Autosomal recessive

Clinical features

Infections   Skin, necrotic ulcers, periodontal infections
Fistulas   Intestinal or perianal

Management

- *Aggressive use of antibiotics and antifungals*
- *BMT*

COMPLEMENT DEFICIENCIES

Congenital deficiencies of almost all the complement components have been found, and of complement control proteins.

Two major patterns of infection exist:

1. *encapsulated bacteria* – deficiencies of C2, C3, C4 and C1q *(complement components); deficiencies of factor H or I (complement control proteins)*
2. *neisserial infections* – deficiencies of the lytic pathway (C5–9) *(complement components).*

Hereditary angioedema

This is due to C1 esterase inhibitor deficiency or defectiveness. Activation of C1 leads to uncontrolled C1 activity, breakdown of C2 and C4 and release of kinin (vasoactive peptide) from C2. The disease manifests as episodes of non-pitting oedema (with no itch, urticaria or redness) lasting 2–3 days. Laryngeal involvement may cause respiratory obstruction, and intestinal wall swelling can cause abdominal pain, vomiting and diarrhoea. Stress, surgery or exercise may trigger attacks. Treatment is with hydrocortisone ± adrenaline, FFP or purified inhibitor in acute attack. Danazol for long-term. Autosomal dominant acquired form exists.

Acquired immunodeficiency

CAUSES

Immunoglobulin deficiency

- *Lymphoproliferative disease eg. CLL*
- *Bone marrow aplasia, hypersplenism*
- *Protein loss:*
    protein-losing enteropathy
    burns
    nephrotic syndrome
    malnutrition states

Cell-mediated immunodeficiency

- *Drugs eg. cyclosporin, cyclophosphamide, steroids, azathioprine, tacrolimus*
- *Lymphoproliferative disease eg. lymphoma*
- *Bone marrow aplasia, hypersplenism*
- *HIV infection*

HIV AND AIDS

HIV (human immunodeficiency virus) is in the lentivirus group of retroviruses. Retroviruses contain the enzyme reverse transcriptase, which enables viral RNA to be incorporated into host cell DNA. There are two main types: HIV-1 (widespread) and HIV-2 (West Africa).

The cellular receptor for the virus is the CD4 molecule, which is found on T helper cells (TH1 subset), the cells most affected by the disease. The CD4 cell numbers decline and the host develops a profound immunodeficiency, encouraging opportunistic infections.

Transmission
Mode of transmission:

- *via mucous membranes during sexual intercourse (NB. sexual abuse)*
- *Blood transmission directly into the circulation (eg. IV drug abusers)*
- *Vertical transmission (mother to child, the majority of childhood HIV)*

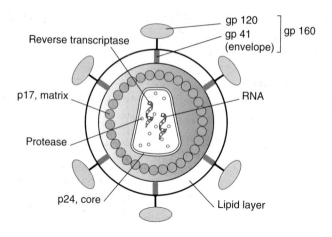

Figure 2.2 Structure of HIV

Vertical transmission may occur:

- *prenatally*
- *intrapartum*
- *postnatally through breastfeeding*

The overall vertical transmission rate estimates vary from 14% to 35% (see below).

Diagnosis
There are various techniques to detect HIV.

1. *Virus detection by PCR (rapid, sensitive, specific and expensive) or viral culture (slower)*
2. *Viral p24 antigen – present shortly after infection until 8–10 weeks. Can reappear as disease becomes worse*
3. *Detection of IgG antibody to envelope components (gp 120 and subunits). There is a window of <3 months after infection before this becomes positive. These antibodies cross the placenta, therefore all infants of HIV-positive mothers possess these, whether they are infected or not. The antibody disappears by around 12–18 months if infant is not infected*
4. *Detection of IgG antibody to p24, present early in infection only*

Repeat testing during the first few months should be done on all infants at risk (especially PCR) to be sure of not missing an infected infant. It is important also to *confirm* a positive test.

Clinical manifestations
Infants are generally asymptomatic in the neonatal period. There are two patterns of disease seen:

1. *AIDS-defining symptoms developing early (mean five months)*
2. *AIDS-defining symptoms developing later, any time from 1–12 years (mean 8.4 years).*

The disease develops more rapidly in children than in adults and opportunistic infections occur more frequently early in the disease.

The disease criteria were revised in 1994, as below.

CDC 1994 classification for HIV disease in children <13 years

This involves four clinical categories listed below and three immunological categories based on the CD4 T lymphocyte counts at different ages.

Clinical categories	
Category N: Asymptomatic	No symptoms or only one of those in category A
Category A: Mildly symptomatic	≥2 of the following symptoms: lymphadenopathy (>0.5 cm at >2 sites) hepatomegaly splenomegaly parotitis dermatitis recurrent or persistent URTIs (>3 episodes/year)
Category B: Moderately symptomatic	Symptomatic conditions not listed in category C attributed to HIV infection There are many listed examples, including: anaemia <8 g/dl or neutropenia <1000/m³ persisting >30 days oropharyngeal candidiasis for >2 months in a child >6 months of age chronic or recurrent diarrhoea herpes zoster, two episodes or >1 dermatome
Category C: Severely symptomatic	Any condition listed in the 1987 surveillance case definition of AIDS except LIP. Examples include: oesophageal or pulmonary candidiasis multiple or recurrent serious bacterial infections (any combination of at least two culture-proven infections within a two-year period, including: septicaemia, pneumonia, meningitis) *Pneumocystis carinii* pneumonia progressive multifocal leucoencephalopathy Kaposi's sarcoma

From Centres for Disease Control 1994 classification system for HIV infection in children less than 13 years old.

Failure to thrive

This may be apparent in the first few months of life and HIV with failure to thrive is a differential diagnosis of SCID. It occurs due to a combination of factors:

- *reduced intake (appetite poor, HIV encephalopathy)*
- *malabsorption (GI infections, HIV enteropathy)*
- *increased metabolic requirements (recurrent infections)*

Lymphocytic interstitial pneumonitis (LIP)

This is a chronic lung disease of uncertain aetiology (possibly EBV), seen in 40–50% of vertically infected children.

Clinical features are variable. Patients may be asymptomatic, diagnosed on CXR or have features of respiratory distress including dyspnoea and hypoxia.

CXR findings   Diffuse, interstitial reticulonodular infiltrate
Hilar or mediastinal lymphadenopathy may be present

Management is symptomatic only. Steroids may reduce oxygen dependency.

HIV encephalopathy

This is common in HIV-infected children. It presents as motor and language developmental delay and an acquired microcephaly may occur. Brain-imaging studies (CT/MRI) may demonstrate cortical atrophy, basal ganglia calcification, ventricular enlargement and white matter abnormalities.

Opportunistic infections

Protozoa

Pneumocystis carinii pneumonia (PCP) → fungi

Pnemocystis carinii is an extracellular protozoan which causes opportunistic infection in immunocompromised individuals. It is an AIDS-defining illness. It often presents at 3 months of age in severely affected infants.

Clinical features

- *hypoxia* often *more* severe than expected from chest examination findings
- *persistent non-productive cough*
- *dyspnoea*
- *high fever*

Investigations

CXR   Diffuse perihilar bilateral '*butterfly*' shadowing, ground glass appearance, cavities. May be normal
Bronchoalveolar lavage   Immunofluorescence staining with monoclonal antibodies

Management

Pneumonia   High-dose co-trimoxazole (Septrin) IV/orally or pentamidine IV for 21 days. Corticosteroids often used in severe pneumonia
Prophylaxis   Low-dose co-trimoxazole orally or pentamidine nebulisers monthly

Toxoplasmosis

Toxoplasma gondii   Cerebral abscesses, encephalitis (more common in adults)
                    Diagnosis   CT or MRI scan
                                     Positive IgG antibody to toxoplasmosis
                    Treatment   Long-term pyrimethamine + sulphonamide

Cryptosporidiosis

Cryptosporidium parvum Severe secretory diarrhoea, abdominal pain, bowel wall cysts, sclerosing cholangitis
Diagnosis Stool specimens (cysts), small bowel biopsy
Treatment Supportive, Paromamycin

Fungi

Candida

Candida albicans Oropharyngeal (>70% symptomatic children)
Oesophageal (dysphagia), vulvovaginal, disseminated (rare)
Treatment Chronic antifungal therapy eg. fluconazole
IV amphotericin B may be needed

Cryptococcus

Cryptococcus neoformans Meningitis (atypical presentation), pneumonia
Diagnosis CSF (India ink staining, antigen titres, culture)
Serum (organism culture)
Treatment Long-term fluconazole

Viruses

Many viruses can cause unusually severe disease in HIV-infected children. These include VZV (severe primary disease, recurrent zoster), RSV and adenovirus (severe pneumonitis), measles (pneumonitis and encephalitis), CMV and HSV (as below).

Cytomegalovirus (CMV)

Retinitis Decreased acuity, floaters, orbital pain
'Pizza-pie' appearance of haemorrhages and exudate on ophthalmoscopy
Treatment with gancyclovir IV
Colitis Bloody diarrhoea, fever, toxic dilatation, ulcers, hepatitis, sclerosing cholangitis
Diagnosis on colonoscopy and biopsy ('Owl's eye' cytoplasmic inclusion bodies)
Treatment with gancyclovir IV
Other Pneumonitis, hepatitis, pancreatitis, adrenal insufficiency

Herpes simplex virus (HSV)

HSV 1 and 2 Extensive oral and genital ulceration
Diagnosis Clinical, virus isolation from ulcers, serology
Treatment Acyclovir IV (NB. Resistance problems)

Bacteria

Recurrent serious bacterial infections are seen, as dysregulation of B cell function occurs in HIV. Of particular note is atypical mycobacterial infection (eg. *Mycobacterium avium intracellulare*).

Tumours

Less common in children than adults.

Kaposi's sarcoma

This is a tumour of vascular endothelial cells associated with HHV–8 and appears as purple lesions. It commonly involves skin, gut, lymphatics and lung. Treatment is with anti-retrovirals, radiotherapy (if local) or chemotherapy (if disseminated).

Lymphoma

Non-Hodgkin B cell lymphoma, primary CNS lymphoma. Poor response to therapy unless it occurs when immunosuppression is mild.

HIV therapy

The treatment recommendations frequently change. Currently in children, septrin prophylaxis is given until they are shown to be HIV negative. If they are HIV positive, the septrin is continued until 12 months of age and then treatment is given according to the CD4 count.

Combinations of two or three drugs are used (often including one protease inhibitor), using viral load and CD4 cell count as monitors of therapy.

Drug	Side-effect
Nucleoside analogues (reverse transcriptase inhibitors)	
Zidovudine (AZT, 3-Azido-3-deoxythymidine)	Nausea, abdominal pain, headache, insomnia. Bone marrow suppression, neutropenia, myopathy
Dideoxyinosine (DDI) and Dideoxycitidine (DDC)	Gastrointestinal disturbance, pancreatitis, peripheral neuropathy
Stavudine (D4T)	Peripheral neuropathy, elevation of liver transaminases. Neutropaenia, pancreatitis
Lamivudine (3TC)	Uncommon (pancreatitis, peripheral neuropathy)
Protease inhibitors (prevent viral maturation)	
Ritonavir	Gastrointestinal effects common in first 4 weeks. Paraesthesia (perioral, hands and feet), elevated liver enzymes
Indinavir	Gastrointestinal, headache, lethargy, rashes. Elevation of bilirubin or liver transaminases kidney stones
Saquinavir	Mouth ulcers, nausea, diarrhoea, abdominal pain
Nelfinavir	Diarrhoea

Reduction of vertical transmission

Pregnant women with HIV infection have a transmission risk (untreated) of approximately 14–39%. Measures to reduce transmission to <5% include:

- *antiretroviral therapy during pregnancy and delivery*
- *correct any maternal vitamin A deficiency (increased risk of transmission if deficient)*
- *elective caesarean section*
- *avoid invasive fetal procedures (eg. fetal scalp electrodes and blood sampling)*
- *avoid breastfeeding (this is not advised in developing countries by the WHO)*
- *oral AZT to infant for the first 4–6 weeks*

FURTHER READING

Roitt I, Brostoft J, Male D. *Immunology* 5th Ed, Mosby, Philadelphia, 1997
Primary Immunodeficiency Diseases, Report of a WHO Scientific Group. *Clinical and Experimental Immunology* 1997 **109**: Suppl 1:1–28

3

Infectious diseases

- *Vaccination*
- *The febrile child*
- *The seriously unwell child*
- *Viral infections*

- *Bacterial infections*
- *Protozoal infections*
- *Fungal infections*
- *Helminthic infections*

Vaccinaton

IMMUNISATION SCHEDULE

Age	Vaccination
Birth	BCG (in at risk individuals)
2 months	DTP, Polio, Hib, men C
3 months	DTP, Polio, Hib, men C
4 months	DTP, Polio, Hib, men C
12–18 months	MMR
3–5 years	DT, Polio, MMR
10–14 years	BCG (if tuberculin negative)
15 years	DT, Polio

Key: D = Diphtheria, P = Pertussis, T = Tetanus, MMR = Measles, mumps, rubella, men C = meningococcal C conjugate, Hib = Haemophilus influenze type b conjugate
NB: Premature infants are scheduled for age since *birth*, irrespective of their prematurity.

VACCINES

Live attenuated vaccines	Killed organism vaccines	Subunit vaccines	Egg protein vaccines
Measles	Cholera	Haemophilus influenzae	Measles
Mumps	Pertussis	Neisseria meningitidis	Influenza
Rubella	Typhoid	Streptococcus pneumoniae	Yellow fever
Polio (oral, Sabin)	Polio (Salk)	Hepatitis B	Mumps
Varicella zoster virus	Influenza	Pertussis acellular	
BCG	Rabies		
Yellow fever			
Cholera (live attenuated, oral)			
Typhoid (live, oral, attenuated)			

NB. Polio Salk vaccine is a killed vaccine.

Contraindications to vaccination

All vaccines

1. *Acute febrile illness. NB. Mild infection without fever or systemic upset is not a contraindication.*
2. *Definite history of general or severe local reaction to preceding dose:*

   Severe local reaction = *Extensive erythema and swelling involving most of the antero-lateral surface of the thigh or a large part of the upper arm circumference*

   General reaction = *Fever ≥39.5°C <48 hours of vaccination, anaphylaxis, bronchospasm, laryngeal oedema, collapse, prolonged unresponsiveness, inconsolable crying for >4 hours*
   Convulsions or encephalopathy <72 hours

Live vaccines

1. *Treatment for malignant disease with chemotherapy or radiotherapy within six months*
2. *On immunosuppressive therapy for organ transplant*
3. *Bone marrow transplant (BMT) within six months*
4. *On prednisolone (oral/rectal) 2 mg/kg/day for at least one week or 1 mg/kg/day for at least one month*
5. *Lower dose of prolonged steroids or in combination with immunosuppressives, to discuss with immunologist*
6. *Impaired cell-mediated immunity (Antibody deficiency is a contraindication to oral polio vaccine)*

HIV-positive children

These may receive all standard vaccines in the schedule except BCG. Inactivated polio vaccine may be used instead of live vaccine in symptomatic individuals.

Pertussis vaccine

In children with an *evolving* neurological problem immunisation is deferred until the condition is stable.

Ref: Immunisation against Infectious Diseases, HMSO

The febrile child

The majority of children with a fever will have a self-limiting viral infection; however, it is important to distinguish and treat those children with a more serious cause. Fevers can be divided into:

1. *fever with localising signs*
2. *fever without localising signs*
3. *fever of unknown origin (this term is generally applied to fevers lasting >1 week).*

Management of a febrile child includes a thorough history and examination to help elucidate the cause. There is no single clinical or laboratory finding that distinguishes viral from bacterial infection and thus the whole picture must be looked at.

IMPORTANT POINTS IN THE HISTORY

- *Contact with infectious diseases*
- *Travel*
- *Contact with animals and insects*
- *Dietary history*
- *Age (age-related infections)*
- *Immunisation status*
- *Season*
- *Immunocompromised state (eg. Chemotherapy patient, HIV patient, congenital immunodeficiency)*

IMPORTANT POINTS IN THE EXAMINATION

- *General clinical state (see below)*
- *Rash*
- *Trauma*
- *Localising signs (eg. tonsillar exudate, joint or bone tenderness)*
- *Features of immunodeficiency (see p. 31)*

INVESTIGATIONS AND TREATMENT

Fever with localising signs   Treat and investigate as appropriate for the condition

Fever without localising signs   It is important not to miss a bacteraemic illness

Some features to distinguish bacteraemic illness from viral illness are outlined (see below) however, these features overlap and none are diagnostic.

Those children who are clinically ill may be investigated (with FBC, blood, ± CSF, throat and urine cultures) and commenced empirically on antibiotics, or observed with antibiotics only given if exact cause of illness found, or sepsis is apparent. The management will depend on the clinician and the clinical state of the child.

Fever of unknown origin   If a fever persists > a few days with no cause found, despite basic investigations the more unusual causes of fever should be looked for (see below).

Features suggestive of bacteraemia

Symptom/Sign/Test	Observation
Temperature	Markedly elevated
Pulse rate	Tachycardia
Colour	Pale or mottled
Capillary refill time	Prolonged
Peripheries	Cool
Tone	Floppy
Responsiveness	Intermittent or unresponsive

WCC	$>15 \times 10^9/l$ or $<2.5 \times 10^9/l$, neutrophilia
ESR, CRP	Elevated

Causes of prolonged fever

Viral infections	CMV, EBV, Human herpes virus 6, HIV
Bacterial infections	TB, leptospirosis, brucellosis, spirochaetes, salmonella
	Bacterial endocarditis, osteomyelitis, abscesses
Other infections	Malaria, toxoplasmosis, chlamydia, rickettsia, fungal infections
Non-infectious causes	Kawasaki disease, collagen vascular disease, malignancies, drugs
	Inflammatory bowel disease, Familial Mediterranean Fever

The seriously unwell child

MENINGITIS

This is an acute infection with an inflammatory process involving the meninges and may be bacterial, viral, fungal or other microbial (the latter 3 are 'aseptic meningitis').

Causes of bacterial meningitis

<3 months	3 months–5 years	>5 years
Group B β-haemolytic streptococcus	*N.meningitidis* (meningococcus)	Meningococcus
Escherichia coli	*S. pneumoniae* (pneumococcus)	Pneumococcus
Listeria monocytogenes	*Haemophilus influenzae*	

Causes of viral meningitis

- *Enteroviruses (85%, especially coxsackie and echovirus)*
- *Adenovirus*
- *Mumps*
- *EB virus, CMV, VZV, HSV*
- *HIV*

Clinical features

Sudden onset and rapid deterioration seen in meningococcal meningitis.

Neonate	Non-specific features, apnoea, respiratory distress, lethargy, temperature instability, shock, high-pitched cry, irritability, seizures, bulging fontanelle.
Infant	Fever, lethargy, irritability, poor feeding, vomiting
	Bulging fontanelle, shock, seizures, coma
Older child	Fever, headache, drowsiness, shock, seizures (late), papilloedema (rare)
(>18 months)	Meningeal irritation: Headache, neck stiffness, photophobia
	Kernig sign (pain on lower leg extension, with hip flexed)
	Brudzinski sign (involuntary flexion of knees and hips with neck flexion)

Rash	Petechial rash seen classically in meningococcal infection (can also be seen in pneumococcal haemophilus and influenzae infections)

Investigations

Blood	Glucose, blood gases, FBC, APTT, PT, TT, U&E, CRP
	Bacterial cultures
	Bacterial PCR
	Viral (PCR)
	Viral serology, Bacterial serology (eg. meningitides.)
CSF	Microscopy, culture, protein, glucose, bacterial antigens, viral and bacterial PCR
Throat and stool	M, C + S and viral culture
Urine	Rapid antigen tests

Contraindications to lumbar puncture

1. *Focal or prolonged seizures, impaired consciousness, papilloedema, focal neurological signs*
2. *Cardiopulmonary compromise*
3. *Local skin infection overlying LP site*
4. *Coagulopathy*

Lumbar puncture findings

	Normal	Bacterial	Viral	TB
Appearance	Clear	Turbid	Clear	Viscous or clear
Lymphocytes/mm^3	<5	<50	10–100	100–300
Polymorphs/mm^3	Nil	>200	Nil	0–200
Protein g/l	0.2–0.4	0.5–3↑	0.4–1.0↑	0.5–6.0↑↑
Glucose	> ½ serum	< ½ serum (↓)	> ½ serum (N)	< ⅓rd serum (↓↓)

NB. Neonates have different normal ranges, with higher CSF protein levels.

Management
Bacterial meningitis

Antibiotics	IV therapy to commence immediately. Do not delay for LP
	Choice depends on likely pathogen, generally: 3rd-generation cephalosporin (eg. ceftriaxone) for 7-10 days.
	Add ampicillin if <3 months to cover Listeria.
	Rifampicin two days following treatment of meningococcal disease (if used antibiotic other than ceftriaxone).
Dexamethasone	If given, it is better given with or before antibiotics commenced (only of proven benefit in *H.influenzae* meningitis)
Supportive measures	Initial resuscitation with oxygen and fluids
	Monitoring of neurological status
	Intubation and ventilation if necessary and circulatory support (fluids, inotropes, CVP) as needed

Complications

SIADH	Common complication, monitor plasma and urine electrolytes and osmolality. Maintenance fluids usually at ⅔rds normal
Cerebral	Abscess, infarction, subdural effusion, hydrocephalus
Deafness	Due to VIII nerve vasculitis
Meningococcal disease	This may present as septicaemia (worse prognosis) or meningitis, with rapid deterioration
	Due to Group B in 60% and in C 30–40%
	Purpuric rash, may lead to necrotic areas
Haemophilus influenzae	Reduced incidence due to *H. influenzae* (Hib) vaccine. Subdurals common
Pneumococcal meningitis	High mortality (10%) and morbidity (30% neurological sequelae)

Viral meningitis

Less severe infection, full recovery usual, enterovirus in the majority. Treat as bacterial if in doubt until culture results at 48 hours.

TB meningitis (see p. 145)

Unusual features	Chronic presentation, vague headache, anorexia, vomiting
	Focal neurological signs, seizures, cortical blindness
Investigations	Mantoux test (NB. May be negative)
	CXR (changes commonly seen)
	CT brain (oedema, infarction, hydrocephalus, abscess, tuberculoma)
	CSF, gastric aspirate and early morning urine for microscopy, PCR and TB culture
Management	Commence on suspicion, 12 months of antituberculous therapy (Rifampicin, Isoniazid, Pyrazinamide). Consider steroids.

Partially treated bacterial meningitis

The picture may be confused, with culture negative CSF but leucocytosis. Rapid antigen tests ± PCR may be useful. If concerned, treat as bacterial.

Prevention for contacts

Contacts	Meningococcal	All close contacts given two days oral Rifampicin
	H. influenzae	All close family contacts given 4 days oral Rifampicin if there is a child <4 years unvaccinated
Vaccination	Hib vaccine all children	
	Meningococcal vaccine currently available to groups A, C, Y and W135 only.	

Prognosis

- *Mortality of bacterial meningitis 5–10% with treatment*
- *Neurological impairment in survivors >10%*

ENCEPHALITIS

An inflammation of the brain parenchyma, which may be due to:

- *Direct viral invasion*
- *Post-infectious due to immune response*
- *Slow virus infection eg. SSPE*

Viral encephalitis and meningitis are caused by the same organisms and form a continuum.

Viral encephalitis

Cause	Specific features
HSV 1 and 2	Temporal lobe abnormalities on EEG and MRI
	70% mortality untreated
	Acyclovir treatment
VZV	Post-infectious cerebellar ataxia
Mumps	VIII nerve damage, with deafness
Enteroviruses	Echovirus, coxsackie virus
Measles	
Rubella	
HIV-I	
Rabies	

Clinical features

- *Fever, headache, meningeal irritation (uncommon in young infants), decreased consciousness, seizures*
- *Focal neurology, features of ICP ↑*

Investigations

Serum	Glucose, FBC, blood cultures
	Bacterial rapid antigen tests
	Serology (incl. viral, mycoplasma raised specific IgM, or increase in IgG in paired sera)
Urine and stool	Microscopy and culture (viral and bacterial)
Throat swab	Microscopy and culture (viral and bacterial)
CSF	Glucose, protein, viral PCR, microscopy and culture (viral and bacterial)
Imaging	CT or MRI
Other	EEG

Management

- *Supportive care (shock, ICP ↑ treatment)*
- *Antiviral agents (intravenous)*
- *Treat with antibiotics as for bacterial meningitis until viral aetiology confirmed/bacterial cultures negative*

Viral infections

DNA VIRUSES

Family	Virus	Disease
Adenoviridae	Adenovirus	Croup, pharyngitis, mesenteric adenitis
Herpesviridae	HSV	HSV-1 and 2 infections
	VZV	Chicken pox, shingles
	CMV	CMV infection
	EBV	Mononucleosis
	HHV6, HHV7	Roseola infantum (exanthum subitum, 6th disease)
Hepadnaviridae	HBV	Hepatitis (see p. 201)
Papovaviridae	Human papillomavirus	Warts (see p. 310)
Parvoviridae	Parvovirus B19	Fifth disease, (erythema infectiosum)
Poxviridae	Variola virus	Smallpox
	Orf	Hard skin lesions (from sheep)
	Molluscum contagiosum	Molluscum (see p. 311)

Herpes Simplex Virus (HSV)

Transmission   Direct contact
Incubation   2–20 days

Two types of HSV exist

HSV-1 Herpetic gingivostomatitis (primary infection), keratoconjunctivitis. Fever for 2–3 days, then ulceration, healing in 5–6 days. Peak age 1–3 years. Dormancy in trigeminal ganglia. NB. Primary infection may be asymptomatic
   Herpetic whitlow (finger infection)
   Herpes labialis (cold sore, recurrent form of disease, triggered by stress, illness, sun exposure)
   CNS   Encephalitis (temporal lobe damage, 70% mortality untreated)
         Aseptic meningitis
HSV-2   Genital herpes. Dormancy in sacral ganglia.
(NB. The two forms of HSV infections overlap.)

Systemic infection in immunocompromised individuals. Neonatal infection (from maternal genital tract active lesions during delivery; high morbidity and mortality).

Eczema herpeticum is (widespread infection seen in children with atopic eczema).

Diagnosis

Usually clinical
Vesicle fluid   Electron microscopy (EM), immunofluorescence or viral culture
Blood   Serology
CSF   PCR

Treatment

Acyclovir   IV in severe disease (neonates, immunocompromised, eczema herpeticum, encephalitis, ophthalmic disease)

Oral treatment considered in some cases

Topical to cold sores

Eye drops (ocular infection)

Varicella Zoster Virus (VZV)

This produces two diseases

Varicella (Chicken pox)

Transmission	Airborne or contact
Incubation	14–21 days, infectious 48 hours pre-rash and five days after rash appearance
Clinical features	Mild prodromal illness with fever 2–3 days (not in young children). Rash: face, scalp and trunk, spreads centrifugally Macules → papules → vesicles → pustules → crusts. *All stages are seen at once* on the skin
Complications	Encephalitis – Acute truncal cerebellar ataxia (*post*-infectious) Pneumonia – Common in adults (30%), CXR dramatic. Superinfection – Bullous lesions (*Staphylococcus aureus*) Other – Thrombocytopenia, hepatitis, arthritis, pancreatitis, nephritis. Immunocompromised – severe disseminated haemorrhagic disease
Congenital infection	This can produce severe malformations, with limb deformities (see p.465)

Zoster (Shingles)

This occurs from reactivation of dormant VZV, from the dorsal root or cranial ganglia. Triggered by immunocompromise, though seen in normal children. Lesions identical to varicella, itchy and less painful in children, and usually restricted to <3 dermatomes. Infection of the geniculate ganglion causes ear pinna vesicles (= Ramsay-Hunt syndrome).

Diagnosis		
	Clinical diagnosis	
	Vesicle fluid	Electron microscopy, immunofluorescence, viral culture (difficult)
	Serology	
	CSF	PCR
Treatment	None required in healthy children, except for ophthalmic herpes.	
	Immunocompromised	Acyclovir IV
	Neonatal	Maternal infection five days predelivery to two days post: Give ZIG to infant If infant develops vesicles, treat with IV acyclovir

Prophylaxis

VZV vaccine exists for those at risk (in the UK). Zoster immunoglobulin (ZIG), a specific immunoglobulin, (ie passive immunisation) is given to immunocompromised children exposed to VZV and neonates (as above).

Cytomegalovirus (CMV)

Transmission   Close contact, blood (organ transplant)

Clinical features

Healthy individuals	Asymptomatic (usually)
	Similar clinical picture to EBV
Immunocompromised	Severe infection including encephalitis, retinitis, pneumonitis, gastrointestinal infection, hepatitis
	NB. An important pathogen in organ transplant
Congenital infection	See p. 465

Investigations

Serology   Primary infection (IgM), latent infection (IgG)

Tissues   Intranuclear 'owl's eye' inclusions, direct immunofluorescence, viral culture

Treatment

None in healthy individuals. Ganciclovir IV if immunocompromised.

Epstein–Barr Virus (EBV)

This produces infectious mononucleosis (glandular fever).

Transmission   Aerosol, saliva

Clinical features

- *Fever, headache, sore throat, palatal petechiae, generalised lymphadenopathy*
- *Rash if ampicillin given in 90%*
- *Splenomegaly (tender), hepatitis, arthropathy, thrombocytopenia, haemolytic anaemia*
- *May produce depression and malaise for months*

Complications

- *Meningitis, encephalitis*
- *Myocarditis*
- *Mesenteric adenitis*
- *Splenic rupture*

Burkitt lymphoma and nasopharyngeal carcinoma are thought to be caused by EBV infection (see p. 455).

Diagnosis

- *Atypical mononuclear cells in the blood*
- *Monospot test*

- *Positive Paul-Bunnell reaction* (*IgM antibodies that agglutinate sheep RBCs-often negative in young children*)
  False positives: Leukaemia, non-Hodgkin lymphoma, hepatitis
- *EBV IgM and other antibodies may be detected*

Treatment
None specific.

Parvovirus B19
This virus attacks the erythroid cell line, and leads to transient arrest of erythropioesis.
Transmission: Respiratory route, blood.
Incubation: Variable.
It produces various clinical features:

1. *Fifth disease (Slapped cheek disease, erythema infectiosum): Incubation 4–21 days. Seen in school-age children.*
   A well child with erythematous cheeks, macular erythema over the trunk and limbs with central clearing of the lesions resulting in a lacy pattern which may recur over weeks.
2. *Asymptomatic infection*
3. *Arthropathy*   *Usually transient, older children, may develop arthritis.*
4. *Immunocompromised*   *Chronic infection with anaemia.*
5. *Chronic haemolytic state*   *Transient aplastic crisis.*
   Eg. In Sickle cell disease, thalassaemia, spherocytosis.
6. *Congenital infection*   *Severe anaemia with hydrops fetalis.*

RNA VIRUSES

Family	Virus species	Disease
Picornaviridae	Polio virus	Poliomyelitis (see p. 392)
	Coxsackie A virus (A1–A24)	Herpangina, Hand, Foot and Mouth disease (HFM), Encephalitis
	Coxsackie B virus (B1–B6)	Myocarditis (B5), Bornholm disease, HFM disease
	Echovirus (types 1–33)	Herpangina, encephalitis, myocarditis (type 6)
	Enterovirus (types 68–72)	HFM disease, encephalitis
	Rhinovirus (many)	Common cold
	HAV	Hepatitis (see p. 201)
Reoviridae	Reovirus (many)	URTI, diarrhoea
	Rotavirus (many)	Diarrhoea
Togaviridae	Rubella virus	Rubella
	Alphavirses	Ross river fever etc
Flaviviridae	HCV	Hepatitis (see p. 204)
		Yellow fever, Dengue fever, Japanese encephalitis
Orthomyxoviridae	Influenza virus A,B,C	A-Pandemic, epidemics B-Small outbreaks

Paramyxoviridae	Parainfluenza virus	Common cold, croup
	Measles virus	Measles
	Mumps virus	Mumps
	Respiratory syncytial virus	Bronchiolitis (see p. 134)
Rhabdoviridae	Rabies virus	Rabies
Retroviridae	Human immunodeficiency virus	HIV and AIDS (see p. 41)
Calciviridae	Hepatitis E virus	Hepatitis
Arenavirus	Lassa virus	Lassa fever

NB. Poliovirus, Coxackie A and B, Echovirus and enterovirus are all in the Genus Enteroviruses.

Hand, foot and mouth disease

Organisms　　　Coxsackie A (A16) and B, enterovirus (71)
Transmission　　Faecal-oral, droplet, direct contact.
Clinical features　Mild disease lasting a week, mostly in pre-school children
　　　　　　　Fever with vesicles in the oropharynx, palms and soles. Maculopapular rash also on palms, soles and buttocks

Rubella (German measles)

Transmission　　Droplet, Winter and Spring
Incubation　　　14–21 days

Clinical features

<5 years　　Usually asymptomatic
>5 years　　Prodrome of conjunctivitis, fever, cervical lymphadenopathy (suboccipital, post-auricular)
　　　　　Forcheimer spots (palatal petechiae), splenomegaly
　　　　　Maculopapular rash within seven days on face, then body, lasting 3–5 days
　　　　　Infectious for <7 days from onset of rash.

Complications

- *Arthritis, myocarditis*
- *Secondary bacterial infection*
- *Thrombocytopenia*
- *Encephalitis*
- *Congenital rubella syndrome (see p. 465)*

Diagnosis

Viral culture　Throat swab, urine
Serology　　　Rubella-specific IgM levels and rising antibody titre (acute and convalescent samples)

Management

- *No treatment usually necessary*
- *Vaccination (contraindicated during pregnancy)*

Measles

Transmission	Droplet
Incubation	7–14 days

Clinical features

Infectious pre-eruptive stage	Unwell, fever, cough, conjunctival suffusion, rhinorrhoea Koplik spots – *pathognomonic* (small white lesions on gums next to 2nd molar tooth or labial mucosa). 2–3 days later:
Non-infectious eruptive stage	Maculopapular rash behind ears and on face, progressing to whole body. (Infectious up to 4 days after onset of rash). NB. EEG abnormalities seen in 50%.

Complications

- *Common in malnourished children*
- *Otitis media, bronchitis, secondary bacterial pneumonia*
- *Hepatitis, myocarditis, diarrhoea*
- *Encephalomyelitis (post-infectious)*
- *SSPE (see neurology p. 386)*

Investigations

Viral isolation	Immunofluorescence (CSF, serum, nasal secretions)
Viral culture	Throat swab
Serology	Serum, CSF, saliva (anti-measles IgM)

Treatment

- *Symptomatic only*
- *Human pooled immunoglobulin can be given <6 days of exposure (immunocompromised, <3 years)*
- *Immunisation available*

Mumps

Transmission	Droplet, direct contact, Winter and Spring
Incubation	14–21 days, infectious for one week after parotid swelling appears

Clinical features

- *Prodrome of fever, anorexia, headache, earache*
- *Painful salivary gland swelling in 2/3rds -bilateral (usually) or unilateral, parotid 60%, parotid and submandibular 10%.*
- *Trismus*
- *Infectious 6 days pre-9 days post gland swelling*

Complications

- *Meningeal signs (10%), encephalitis (one in 5,000), transient hearing loss*
- *Epididymo-orchitis (30% after puberty), pancreatitis, oophoritis, myocarditis, arthritis, mastitis, hepatitis*

Investigations
Viral isolation/culture Urine, saliva, throat swab, CSF (meningism)
Serology Rise in antibody titre ('S' antigen early, and 'V' antigen later, for life).

Rabies
Transmission Saliva (animal bite)
Incubation 1–3 months (average 10 days)

The rabies virus enters through the bite wound, replicates in local muscle, travels up the peripheral nerves to the brain and replicates further. Then it travels via autonomic nerves to the salivary glands, lungs, kidneys, etc.

Clinical features
Initial Pain at site of wound, fever, headache
Furious rabies Anxiety, hallucinations, hyperexcitability with visual and auditory stimuli
Hydrophobia (50%), Aerophobia (*pathognomonic*)
Sympathetic overactivity, cardiac arrhythmias, convulsions
Death <10–14 days
Dumb rabies Symmetrical ascending paralysis with areflexia

Diagnosis
Rabies antigen Salivary secretion, corneal impressions or skin sections (using fluorescent antibodies)
Postmortem Negri bodies in cerebellum and hippocampus

Treatment
1. *Clean the wound*
2. *Local anti-serum (rabies immunoglobulin) around wound*
3. *Postexposure vaccine, human diploid cell strain vaccine (HDCSV) IM on days 0, 3, 7, 14 and 28*
4. *Symptomatic treatment with quiet, dark environment, sedation and analgesia*

Prophylaxis
Rabies vaccine HDCSV IM two or three doses

Bacterial infections

GRAM POSITIVE AND GRAM NEGATIVE COCCI

Group	Organism		Disease
Gram-positive cocci			
Staphylococci	Coagulase positive	Staph. aureus	25% population carriers
	Coagulase negative	Staph. Epidermidis	
		Staph. Saprophyticus	

Streptococci	Group A β-haemolytic Strep. (*Strep. Pyogenes*)	95% infections
	Group B β-haemolytic Strep.	Neonatal sepsis
	Strep.pneumoniae	Pneumonia, meningitis
		Otitis media
	α-haemolytic Strep. (*Strep. Viridans*)	SBE
Gram-negative cocci		
Neisseria	*N. meningitidis*	Meningitis, septicaemia (see p. 52)
	N. gonorrhoea	Gonorrhoea

STAPHYLOCOCCAL INFECTIONS

Staphylococci are part of the normal flora of skin, upper respiratory tract and gastrointestinal tract.

Infections due to bacterial invasion		Infections due to toxins
Skin	Impetigo (see p. 309), cellulitis	SSSS (see p. 309)
Lungs	Pneumonia, lung abscess (see p. 143)	Bullous impetigo
CNS	Meningitis (see p. 52)	Staphylococcal scarlet fever
Cardiac	Acute endocarditis (see p. 117)	Toxic shock syndrome
General	Septicaemia	Food poisoning (toxins A–E, heat
Gut	Enterocolitis	stable,onset six hours from ingestion)
Bones	Osteomyelitis; septic arthritis (p. 333)	
Eyes	Orbital cellulitis (see p. 129)	

Toxic Shock Syndrome (TSS)

This is due to *Staph.aureus* (phage group I) exotoxins; toxic shock syndrome toxin-1 (TSST-1) or others, which trigger the cytokine cascade. The focus of infection is usually minor, and there is an association with tampon use.

Diagnostic features
- *Fever $>= 38.9°C$*
- *Hypotension*
- *Patchy then diffuse erythema followed by desquamation*
- *Vomiting and diarrhoea*
- *Toxic actions in other systems: eg. myalgia, renal impairment, thrombocytopenia drowsiness*

Anti-TSST-1 antibodies are positive. Management is mostly supportive, with IV antibiotics, cardiovascular support, IPPV and renal dialysis as necessary. IVIG may be considered.

Methicillin-resistant Staph. aureus (MRSA)

MRSA is a cause of outbreaks of infections, particularly among seriously ill patients, and those with chronic skin diseases (eg. eczema), usually acquired within hospitals. The patient must be isolated and treatment if given is with IV vancomycin. Topical antibiotics are used to reduce nasal carriage.

STREPTOCOCCAL INFECTIONS

Infections due to bacterial invasion		Infections due to toxins	Post-infectious
Skin	Impetigo, Bullous impetigo Cellulitis, erysipelas	Scarlet fever Streptococcal scalded skin syndrome	Erythema nodosum Glomerulonephritis
Respiratory otitis media			
	Tonsillitis, pneumonia	Streptococcal toxic shock	Rheumatic fever
Bone	Osteomyelitis	syndrome (invasive group A	Arthritis
CNS	Meningitis	strep. disease)	
General	Septicaemia		

Scarlet fever

This is due to Group A β-haemolytic Streptococci producing an erythrogenic exo-toxin in individuals with no neutralising antibodies.

Transmission	Contact, droplets.
Incubation	2–4 days poststreptococcal pharyngitis
Clinical features	Fever, headache, sore throat, rigors, vomiting.
	'White strawberry tongue' (white coating, red papillae), then 'Strawberry tongue' (bright red)
	Flushed cheeks with circumoral pallor. Erythematous, coarse rash (feels like sandpaper) commencing on the neck, spreading to the rest of the body (face, palms and soles usually involved), desquamation after five days.
	School age children.
Diagnosis	Throat swab (positive culture)
	ASOT (antistreptolysin O toxin) and anti-DNAse B present
Management	Penicillin for 10 days (erythromycin if penicillin allergic)

GRAM POSITIVE AND GRAM NEGATIVE BACILLI

	Bacteria		Disease
Gram positive bacilli	Corynebacteria	C.diphtheriae	Diphtheria
	Listeria	L.monocytogenes	Meningitis, sepsis
	Clostridium	C. tetani	Tetanus
		C. botulinum	Botulism
		C. perfringens	Gas gangrene
		C. difficile	Pseudomembranous colitis
	Bacillus	B. anthracis	Anthrax
		B. cereus	Food poisoning, wound sepsis
Gram negative bacilli	Brucella	B. abortus	Brucellosis
		B. melitensis, B. suis	
	Bordatella	B. pertussis	Whooping cough
		B. parapertussis	(see p. 139)
	Haemophilus	H. influenzae type B	Meningitis, epiglottitis
		Non-capsulated H. influenzae	Otitis media, pneumonia

Legionella	*L. pneumophilia*	Legionnaire's disease
Pseudomonas	*P. aeruginosa*	Opportunistic infections (usually)
	P. cepacia	End-stage cystic fibrosis
Vibrio	*V. cholerae*	Cholera
Escherichia coli		Gastroenteritis
Salmonella	*S. enteritidis*	Enterocolitis, food poisoning
	S. typhi	Typhoid/paratyphoid fever
	S. paratyphi	Osteomyelitis
Shigella	*Sh. boydii*	Gastroenteritis
		Gastritis (see p. 161)
Yersinia	*Y. enterocolotica*	Enterocolitis
	Y. pseudotuberculosis	Mesenteric adenitis
Klebsiella	*K. pneumoniae*	
Campylobacter	*C. coli, C. jejuni*	Gastroenteritis
Helicobacter pylori		Gastritis (see. p. 166 gastro)

DIPHTHERIA

Organisms: *Corynebacterium diphtheriae*, types mitis (mild disease), intermedius and gravis

Exposure of the bacteria to bacteriophage β results in toxin production and disease. The toxin has:
- *Subunit A* *Produces clinical disease*
- *Subunit B* *Transports the toxin to target receptors*

Transmission Droplets, fomites
Incubation 2–7 days

Clinical features

Local Thick grey membrane over tonsils, progressing to husky voice, dyspnoea and respiratory obstruction

Systemic Fever, tachycardia, irritability
'bull-neck' from lymphadenopathy

Other Day 10 acute myocarditis (usually fatal)
Myocarditis weeks later
Neurological (eg. palatal paralysis, cranial nerve palsies, peripheral neuropathy. Recovery usual.)

Cutaneous diphtheria (ulcers with covering membrane) seen in burns patients.

Diagnosis

Clinical diagnosis and organism culture.

Management

- *Antitoxin IV (NB. Only neutralises unfixed toxin, anaphylaxis risk)*
- *Antibiotics IV (eg. penicillin)*
- *Supportive therapy as needed*

LISTERIOSIS

Listeriosis (due to *Listeria monocytogenes*) can be severe in pregnant mothers, neonates and immunocompromised individuals.

Transmission	Ingestion of unpasteurised soft cheese, pâté, raw vegetables and chicken.
Diseases seen	Neonates – Pneumonia, Meningitis, septicaemia (see p. 466)
	Pregnancy – Abortions
	Immunocompromised – Meningitis, septicaemia
Diagnosis	Blood or CSF culture
Treatment	Antibiotics eg. Ampicillin and gentamicin

TETANUS

Clostridium tetani produces disease via tetanospasmin (neurotoxin).

Transmission	Direct contact onto open wound
Incubation	4–21 days

Clinical features

Generalised tetanus	Malaise, trismus, *risus sardonicus* (fixed smile)
	within 42–72 hours spasms, opisthotonus, autonomic dysfunction
Localised tetanus	Wound site pain and stiffness
Cephalic tetanus	This occurs from entry via the middle ear, mortality nearly 100%
Tetanus neonatorum	Features as for generalised disease, entry via umbilical stump, mortality nearly 100%

Diagnosis
Clinical

Management
- *Wound debridement, IV penicillin, antitetanus immunoglobulin IM,*
- *Control of spasms (eg. diazepam) and systemic support as necessary*

Tetanus immunisation recommendations

Immunisation status	Clean wound	Tetanus prone wound
3 dose course given, or reinforcing dose <10 years	Nil	Nil or adsorbed vaccine dose
Course or reinforcing dose >10 years	Reinforcing dose of adsorbed vaccine	Human anti-tetanus immunoglobulin + reinforcing dose adsorbed vaccine
Not immunised Or status uncertain	Full 3 course dose of adsorbed vaccine	Human anti-tetanus immunoglobulin + full 3 dose course of adsorbed vaccine

Tetanus prone wound:
1. Wound or burn > 6 hours prior to surgery
2. Wound or burn of: Puncture type
   Significant degree of devitalised tissue
   Soil or manure contact
   Sepsis present

GRAM-NEGATIVE BACILLI

Brucellosis
Brucella endotoxin produces disease symptoms. Organism: *Brucella melitensis*.

Transmission	Ingestion of raw milk from cattle or goats
	Also abraded skin, respiratory tract and genital tract entry
Incubation	1–3 weeks

Clinical features

Acute brucellosis	Fever, headache, malaise, night sweats
	Hepatomegaly, lymphadenopathy, splenomegaly (if severe), arthritis (33%, large joints, oligoarticular), endocarditis, osteomyelitis, epididymitis, meningoencephalitis.
Chronic brucellosis	Tiredness, episodes of fever, depression, splenomegaly

Diagnosis
- *Blood cultures (50% positive during acute phase)*
- *Serological tests (titre rise over four weeks, raised IgG)*

Treatment: Cotrimoxazole high dose.

Typhoid fever

Organism	*Salmonella typhi*
Transmission	Ingestion of contaminated foods (humans only reservoir). Common in Asia, Africa, S.America.
Incubation	10–14 days

Clinical features

Week 1	Fever, headache, malaise, sore throat, abdominal pain, altered behaviour Toxic with *relative bradycardia*.
Week 2	'Rose spots' (erythematous maculopapular rash) on thorax and upper abdomen, splenomegaly (75%), toxic, confused, hepatomegaly (30%)
Week 3	Complications: seizures, gastrointestinal haemorrhage and perforation, pneumonia, meningitis, peripheral neuropathy, haemolytic anaemia, osteomyelitis, cholecystitis
Week 4	Recovery

Diagnosis
- *Blood cultures positive (80% during week 1, 30% during week 3)*
- *Widal test (serum agglutinins to O and H antigens rise)*
- *Leucopenia*

Treatment
This depends on age and clinical severity. If unwell, IV antibiotics are given eg. Cephalosporin, or oral ciprofloxacin if appropriate.

Carrier state Chronic carriers excrete salmonella for >1year (gall bladder often the focus) and may be treated with four weeks of antibiotic and if ineffective, cholecystectomy.

Paratyphoid fever is a similar, milder illness caused by *S.paratyphi A, B* or *C*. Treatment is co-trimoxazole for two weeks.

OTHER BACTERIA

Group	Bacteria	Disease
Mycobacterium	*M. tuberculosis*	TB (see p. 144)
	M. leprae	Leprosy
Mycoplasma	*M.pneumoniae*	Pneumonia in children and adolescents
Spirochaetes	*Treponema pallidum*	Syphilis, Bejel, Yaws, Pinta
	Leptospira interrogans	Leptospirosis
	Borrelia burgdorferi	Lyme disease
Rickettsiae	*R.prowasekii*	Epidemic typhus
	R.typhi, R.conorii	Endemic, tick and scrub typhus
	R. rickettsii	Rocky mountain spotted fever
	Coxiella burnetii	Q fever
Chlamydiae	*C.trachomatis*	Trachoma, urethritis, cervicitis
	C.psittaci	Psittacosis
	C.pneumoniae	Pneumonia (see p. 466)

Mycoplasma

Mycoplasma pneumoniae is unusual in that it is the smallest organism that can survive outside a host cell and has no cell wall.

Transmission Droplet
Incubation 10–14 days

Clinical features
Bronchopneumonia Gradual onset mild URTI, then persistent cough, fever, malaise, headache, wheeze.
Young school age children. Resolves within 3–4 weeks.
Other features Skin rashes (maculopapular erythematous, vesicular) common,
Vomiting, diarrhoea, arthralgia, myalgia (common)
Bullous myringitis, haemolytic anaemia, Stevens-Johnson syndrome
Hepatitis, pancreatitis, splenomegaly,
Asceptic meningitis, encephalitis, cerebellar ataxia,
Guillain-Barré syndrome

Investigations
Blood Serology (specific IgM antibody)
Cold agglutinins (in 50%)
CXR Diffuse patchy shadowing, often looks unexpectedly severe.

Treatment
Erythromycin 2 weeks.

Leprosy
Organism   *Mycobacterium leprae.* Acid and alcohol – fast, weekly gram positive bacilli.
Transmission   Uncertain
Incubation   Months – years

Found in Asia, Africa, USA, former Russia. The clinical disease is dependent on the immune status of the individual.

Clinical features
Tuberculoid leprosy (TL)	Good immune response mounted
	A single hypopigmented skin lesion with decreased sensation, central atrophy and a thickened, tender nerve
Lepromatous leprosy (LL)	Poor cell-mediated immunity
	Many florid skin lesions
	All internal organs may be involved
	Nasal snuffles, saddle nose deformity, *leonine facies*, hoarse voice, fingers disappear, peripheral neuropathy
Intermediate forms	Borderline leprosy, indeterminate leprosy, neuritic leprosy (nerve lesion only)

Investigations
Clinical diagnosis
Organism isolation   Acid-fast bacilli found in skin or nasal mucosa smears
                       NB. Organism cannot be cultured in artificial media
Culture   In mouse foot pad
Lepromin test This is a measure of *host resistance* to disease. Dead bacilli are injected intradermally

Treatment
Multidrug regimes (eg. dapsone, rifampicin and clofazimine) for at least two years

Syphilis
Organism   *Treponema pallidum*
Transmission   Sexual contact, transplacentally (congenital syphillis)
Incubation   10–90 days

Clinical features
Early stages	Primary (3 weeks)	Painless hard chancre, regional lymphadenopathy
	Secondary (4–10 weeks)	Fever, malaise, sore throat, arthralgia, myalgia
		Maculopapular, itchy rash, mucosal ulcers
		Condylomata lata (perianal plaque warts)

Late stages	Tertiary (years)	Gummas (granulomatous ulcers) in bones, liver, testes
		CNS disease (meningovascular involvement
		General paralysis of the insane, tabes dorsalis)
		Cardiac disease (aortitis, aortic regurgitation)

Diagnosis

Dark ground microscopy	From chancres or mucous ulcers
Serology	
VDRL	(Venereal Disease Reference Laboratory)
	Positive <3 weeks of infection, negative >6 months after treatment
	False positive: EBV, hepatitis, mycoplasma, malignancy, autoimmune disease
TPHA	(*T. pallidum* haemagglutination assay). Specific for Treponema, remains positive
FTA-ABS	(Fluorescent treponema antibodies). Specific for Treponema

Treatment

This is dependent on the stage. Penicillin is given via the IM route (long-acting) for some stages or IV route (eg. for CNS disease).

Congenital syphilis

High transmission rate, 40% mortality untreated.

Clinical features

Infancy	Snuffles, congenital nephrotic syndrome, glaucoma, chorioretinitis
	Hepatosplenomegaly, lymphadenopathy, osteochondritis, periostitis
	Rash (desquamation hands and feet, maculopapular, bullous, condylomata)
Childhood (>2 years)	*Hutchinson teeth* (peg-shaped incisors with central notch)
	Sabre tibia, saddle nose deformity, frontal bossing
	Meningovascular involvement
	Optic atrophy, corneal calcification (blindness), photophobia
	Vertigo and deafness (VIII nerve involvement)
	Paroxysmal nocturnal haemoglobinuria

Lyme disease

Organism	*Borellia burgdorferi*
Transmission	Ixodid ticks on deer and sheep, Europe, USA, Australia, Asia.
Incubation	7–10 days

Clinical features

| *Within days* | *Erythema chronicum migrans* (painless, red lesion with spreading edge, *not* always seen) |
| | Headache, fever, arthralgia, myalgia, lymphadenopathy |

Weeks to months later	CNS 15% (meningoencephalitis, cranial and peripheral nerve palsies)
	Cardiac 10% (myocarditis, heart block)
	Arthritis (oligoarticular, episodic, knee common)
	Other (myelitis, hepatitis, conjunctivitis, pharyngitis)
Years	Recurrent arthritis with erosion of bone and cartilage

Diagnosis

Clinical diagnosis	
Organism isolation	Serum, CSF, skin (difficult)
Serology	IgM antibodies (early) in CSF and serum

Treatment   Amoxicillin or erythromycin (if <9 years)
Doxycycline (if >9 years).

Typhus

Organism	Rikettsiae (Small bacteria that multiply intracellularly and cause a *vasculitis*)
Transmission	Human lice (epidemic), rat flea (endemic) in tropical areas.
Incubation	1–3 weeks

Clinical features

Epidemic typhus:

Week 1	Profound malaise, high fever, severe headache, orbital pain, conjunctivitis Measles-type rash on day 5, *becoming purpuric*
Week 2	Meningoencephalitis, myocarditis, pneumonia, splenomegaly, gangrene of peripheries, renal failure; death may occur
Week 3	Slow recovery

NB. Recurrence years later = Brill–Zinsser disease (from lymph node storage).

Endemic typhus	Similar but milder disease
Diagnosis	Serology
Treatment	Oral tetracycline

Rocky mountain spotted fever

Organism	*Rikettsia rikettsii*
Transmission	Tick on dogs and rodents in America
Incubation	1-2 weeks
Clinical features	As for epidemic typhus. NB. Crusted papule at bite site.
Diagnosis	Serology
Treatment	Tetracycline

Protozoal infections

Group	Organism	Vector/Reservoir	Disease
Plasmodium	*P.falciparum, P.malariae, P.vivax, P.ovale*	Mosquito	Malaria
Leishmania	*L.donovani. L.mexicana, L.braziliensis*	Sandfly	Leishmaniasis
Trypanosoma brucei	*T.b.gambiense, T.b.rhodesiense*	Tsetse fly	Trypanosomiasis
Toxoplasma	*T.gondii*	Cats, sheep, pigs	Toxoplasmosis
Entamoeba	*E.histolytica*	Water	Amoebiasis
Giardia	*G.lamblia*	Humans	Giardiasis
Cryptosporidium	*C.parvum*	Cattle	Cryptosporidiosis
Trichomonas	*T.vaginalis*	Humans	Trichomoniasis

MALARIA

Malaria is found in all countries between latitude 40°N and 30°S, and there are four types: *Plasmodium vivax, P. ovale, P. malariae, P. falciparum.*

Transmission	Anopheles mosquitos
Incubation	18 days–6 weeks *Pl.malariae*
	10–14 days All others

The malaria parasite lifecycle

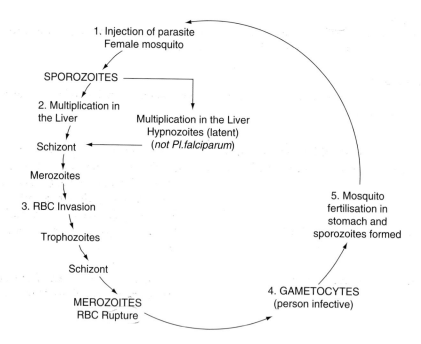

Figure 3.1 A malaria parasite lifecycle

Clinical features

General

Fevers	Due to schizont rupture
	Cold stage (½–1 hour, vasoconstriction, rapid temperature rise, patient feels cold)
	Hot stage (2–6 hours, patient feels hot, delirium)
	Sweating stage (profuse sweating, patient sleeps)
Other	Anaemia, splenomegaly, hepatomegaly
P. vivax and P. ovale	Mild disease, young RBCs and reticulocytes only affected. NB. Relapses and difficult to erradicate due to *latent phase*.
P. malariae	Mild, chronic course, growth retardation, massive splenomegaly, old RBCs only affected. *Nephrotic syndrome* may occur.
P. falciparum	Most severe form, all RBCs affected and become sticky to endothelium, causing vascular occlusion and ischaemic organ damage (brain, kidneys, liver, gastrointestinal tract). Worse if high parasitaemia (>2%).

Complications
- *Cerebral malaria*
- *Blackwater fever (acute renal failure)*
- *DIC, ARDS, metabolic acidosis, shock, jaundice*
- *Hypoglycaemia, splenic rupture, hyperpyrexia*

Diagnosis

Thin and thick peripheral blood smears (parasites seen with staining). Three smears on three successive days required to declare malaria-free.

Treatment

Advice should be obtained for up-to-date regimes as resistance is developing and the following may be altered.

Acute attack

Chloroquine-sensitive benign malaria:	Choroquine (oral) for three days
Chloroquine-resistant malaria, falciparum:	Quinine (oral) for seven days then fansidar if quinine resistance suspected (tetracycline if fansidar-resistant). Or Mefloquine (resistance common)
Severe disease (>1% RBCs)	IV quinine infusion, intensive care as necessary.

Eradication

(For *P. vivax* and *P. ovale*)	Primaquine for two weeks after acute treatment (NB. Not if G6PD present).

Prevention

Prophylaxis

- *Drugs taken two weeks prior to entering malaria area and for six weeks after return. Resistance affects choice of drugs, so up-to-date advice should be obtained. Drugs used (sometimes in combination) are: Chloroquine (weekly), Proguanil (daily), Maloprim (weekly), Mefloquine (weekly), Doxycycline (daily, not if < 12 years old)*

Natural protection

This is present in people with: Duffy-negative blood group (P. vivax)
  HbS and G6PD, thalassaemia, PK deficiency
  (*P. falciparum*)

AMOEBIASIS

Organism Entamoeba histolytica
Transmission Faecal-oral (cysts transferred). Tropics and sub-tropics.

Clinical features

In the intestine, trophozoites emerge from the cysts and multiply in the colon producing symptoms:

Amoebic colitis Colonic mucosa invaded, ulcers, bloody diarrhoea, amoebic granulomas (10%). Acute amoebic dysentery may occur
Hepatitis Travel of trophozoites via portal vein. Amoebic 'anchovy sauce' liver abscesses, high mortality
Asymptomatic cyst carrier

Diagnosis

'Hot' stools Trophozoites and cysts seen
Serology Amoebic fluorescent antibody titre (FAT) positive in symptomatic disease
Liver USS Abscess
Liver function Alkaline phosphatase ↑ (in liver abscess)

Treatment

Metronidazole orally. Drainage of liver abscesses.

GIARDIASIS

Organism Giardia lamblia
Transmission Faecal-oral, spreads easily in nurseries and institutions

Clinical features

Asymptomatic carrier
Gastroenteritis Abdominal pain, watery diarrhoea, vomiting
  Malabsorption, steatorrhoea, weight loss, growth retardation

Diagnosis

Isolation 'Hot' stool (trophozoites and cysts) (20% pick up rate only)

Treatment

Metronidazole orally for 7 days.

LEISHMANIASIS

Leishmania is spread by the **sandfly** and causes three diseases

Kala-azar (Visceral leishmaniasis)

Organism	*L. donovani* (Mediterranean, Africa, Asia and South America)
Incubation	Months to years
Clinical features	Fever, cough, vomiting, diarrhoea, *massive splenomegaly*, pancytopenia, death <3 years
Diagnosis	**Leishman-Donovan bodies** in macrophages and RE cells in the blood, liver, spleen and bone marrow
	Culture and serology tests available
Treatment	Sodium stibogluconate or amphotericin if severe

Cutaneous Leishmaniasis of the New World

This occurs in South America and presents as various skin lesions

1. *Chiclero's ulcer – L. mexicana, a skin ulcer that usually spontaneously resolves after six months*
2. *Mucocutaneous leishmaniasis – L. braziliensis, itchy skin nodules that resolve with nasal destruction due to secondary lesions years later*
3. *Diffuse cutaneous leishmaniasis – L. amazonensis, a chronic form of diffuse skin infiltration*

Cutaneous Leishmaniasis of the Old World

Organisms	*L. major* and *L. tropica* (Middle East, Mediterranean, Africa, former Soviet States)
	L. aethiopica (Ethiopia and Kenya)
Clinical features	Papules that ulcerate and heal with scarring

Diagnosis of cutaneous Leishmaniasis is best on skin biopsy, and treatment is as for Kala-Azar.

TOXOPLASMOSIS

Organism	*Toxoplasma gondii* (intracellular protozoan)
Transmission	Faecal-oral from cat faeces, sheep, pigs or goats

Clinical features

This may present as:

1. *Lymphadenopathy*
2. *Acute febrile illness with lymphadenopathy*

3. *Immunocompromised – Headache, neck stiffness (ICP ↑), intracerebral lesions, acute febrile illness, hepatosplenomegaly, chorioretinitis, sore throat*
4. *Congenital infection – Classical triad of choreoretinitis, hydrocephalus and cerebral calcification (see p. 465)*

Diagnosis
Serology   Rising antibody titre, IgM

Treatment
None if mild disease. Pyrimethamine and sulphadiazine in severe disease and pregnancy.

Fungal infections

Fungus	Disease
Histoplasma capsulatum	Histoplasmosis
Aspergillus fumigatus	Aspergillosis
Cryptococcus neoformans	Cryptococcosis
Coccidioides immitis	Coccidioidomycosis
Blastomyces dermatitidis	Blastomycosis
Candida albicans	Candidiasis (systemic, oral, perianal)
Dermatophytoses	Tinea (see p. 309)

Helminthic infections

Group	Organism	Disease
Nematodes (Round worms)	*Ascaris lumbricoides* (roundworm)	Intestinal infection
	Trichuris trichuria (whipworm)	Intestinal infection
	Enterobius vermicularis (thread worm)	Intestinal infection
	Strongyloides stercoralis	Strongyloidiasis
	Ankylostoma duodenale	} Hookworm infection and
	Necator americanus (hookworms)	} Cutaneous lava migrans
	Toxocara canis and *cati*	Toxocariasis
	Wucheria bancrofti	Filariasis, elephantiasis
	Loa loa	Loiasis
	Onchocerca volvulus	Onchocerciasis, elephantiasis
	Brugia malayi	Filariasis, elephantiasis
	Dracunculus medinensis (guinea worm)	Dracunculiasis
Trematodes (flukes)	Schistosoma	Schistosomiasis (Bilharzia)
	Fasciola hepaticus	Fascioliasis
	Clonorchis sinensis	Clonorchiasis
Cestodes (tapeworms)	*Taenia saginata* (beef tapeworm)	Intestinal infection
	Taenia solium (pork tapeworm)	Intestinal infection
	Echinococcus	Hydatid disease

INTESTINAL NEMATODE INFECTIONS

Organism	Clinical features	Diagnosis	Treatment
Roundworm *Ascaris lumbricoides* Worldwide	Asymptomatic Abdominal pain and distension Ileo-caecal valve obstruction, appendicitis, bile duct obstruction. Pneumonitis, pulmonary ascariasis, eosinophilia and dyspnoea (Loeffler syndrome)	Ova in stool	Mebendazole or piperazine
Threadworm *Enterobius vermicuarlis* Worldwide	Asymptomatic Pruritis ani, worse at night (the female lays her eggs perianally)	Sticky tape test	Mebendazole or piperazine
Whipworm *Trichuris trichuria* Worldwide	Asymptomatic Intestinal ulcers, blood and mucus loss, rectal prolapse, appendicitis	Ova in stool	Mebendazole
Hookworm *Ankylostoma duodenale* (Europe, Middle East, N. Africa) *Necator americanus* Temperate, Sub-tropical and Tropical areas.	Local irritation Intestinal ulcer-like symptoms Anaemia (0.2mls blood loss/day) Mild pulmonary symptoms	Ova in stool	Mebendazole
Strongyloidiasis *Strongyloides stercoralis* Worldwide	Local reaction Cough, pneumonitis Abdominal pain, diarrhoea, malabsorption, steatorrhoea (in heavy infection) Disseminated infection if immunocompromised	Larvae in stool or duodenal aspirates	Thiabendazole or albendazole

SCHISTOSOMIASIS

Organisms Schistosoma mansoni (Africa, Middle East, S. America), *S. japonicum* (Asia) and *S. haematobium* (Africa, Middle East).

Transmission Skin penetration of cercariae (the infective form) in water (from snail intermediate host)

The cercariae migrate via the circulation as schistosomules to the liver where they mature. They produce eggs in the mesenteric venules, which exit via the bladder or intestine.

Clinical features

Initial phase

- *Itch at entry site 'swimmer's itch'*
- *General malaise with fever, nausea, vomiting, diarrhoea, cough and hepatosplenomegaly (Katayama fever)*

Chronic phase

S.mansoni and S.japonicum   Colonic ulceration and granulomas, polyposis, fibrosis, pseudotumour (Bilharzioma), hepatomegaly, fibrotic liver disease, portal hypertension

S.haematobium   Urinary tract affected with chronic inflammation, obstructive uropathy, haematuria, dysuria, renal failure, bladder cancer, rectal inflammation

Diagnosis
Ova in stools or urine.
Serology.

Treatment
Medical therapy eg. praziquantel

HYDATID DISEASE

Organism   *Echinoccocus granulosus* (dog, sheep, cattle tapeworm). Africa, Australia, Mediterranean countries, Alaska, China.

Echinoccocus multilocularis (foxes and rodents). Northern Europe, China, Canada.

NB. Can occur in the UK.

Transmission   Faecal-oral (commonly from dog faeces)

The embryos hatch in the intestine and migrate via the portal system to the liver where they remain in cysts. They may spread to all organs, particularly the lungs, kidneys and brain.

Clinical features
1. *Pressure symptoms related to cyst position (eg. jaundice)*
2. *Cyst rupture (into biliary tree, peritoneal or pleural cavity) with fever, eosinophilia and symptoms related to position (eg. abdominal pain).*

Diagnosis
Serum   Hydatid complement-fixation tests positive
AXR   Calcified cysts
USS   Cysts

Treatment
Surgical   Fine needle aspiration of cyst with chemotherapy, or surgical removal.
Medical   Albendazole
Calcified cysts may be left.

FURTHER READING

Feigin RD, Cherry JD *Textbook of Paediatric Infectious Diseases*, 4th Ed, WB Saunders, Philadelphia 1997

Mandel GL, Bennett JE, Dolan L *Principles and Practice of Paediatric Infectious Diseases*, Churchill Livingstone

Isaacs D, Moxon RE *A Practical Approach to Paediatric Infectious Diseases*, Churchill Livingstone, 1996

Department of Health. Immunisation Against Infectious Disease. HMSO, London, Manual on Immunisation Practices in the UK 1997

4

Cardiology

- *Physiology*
- *The ECG*
- *Cardiac positions*
- *Innocent murmurs*
- *Heart failure*
- *Eisenmenger reaction*
- *Peripheral pulmonary stenosis*
- *Teratogens and maternal disorders associated with CHD*
- *Inherited conditions associated with CHD*
- *Structural congenital heart disease*
- *Duct-dependent circulations*
- *Arrhythmias*
- *Rheumatic fever*
- *Infective endocarditis*
- *Myocarditis*
- *Cardiomyopathy*
- *Pericarditis*

Physiology

NORMAL CORONARY ARTERY ANATOMY

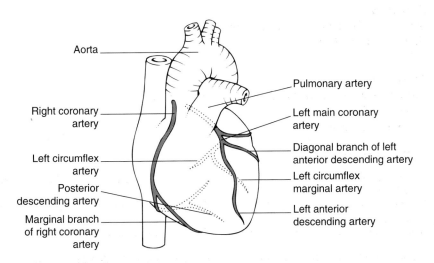

Aorta

Right coronary artery

Left circumflex artery

Posterior descending artery

Marginal branch of right coronary artery

Pulmonary artery

Left main coronary artery

Diagonal branch of left anterior descending artery

Left circumflex marginal artery

Left anterior descending artery

Figure 4.1 Normal coronary artery anatomy

THE FETAL CIRCULATION

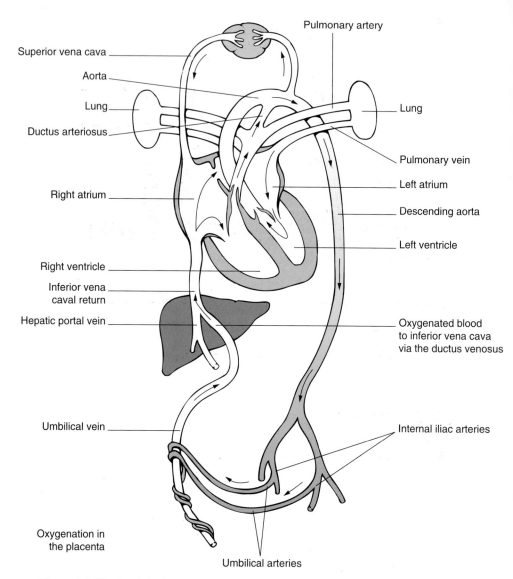

Figure 4.2 The foetal circulation

THE CARDIAC CYCLE

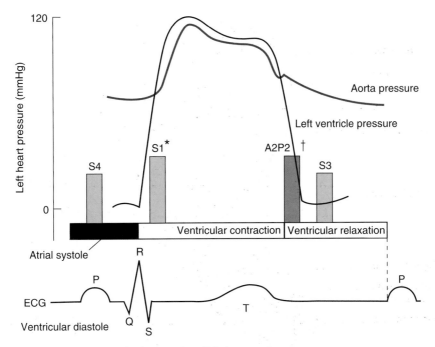

Figure 4.3 The cardiac cycle: ★ = ejection click; † = opening snap

THE HEART SOUNDS

First heart sound (S1)

Loud **S1** seen with: high cardiac output state, eg. anxiety

exercise
fever
thin chest
thyrotoxicosis
vasodilatation

                               mitral stenosis

Soft **S1** seen with: obesity
                                   emphysema
                                   impaired left ventricular function

Second heart sound (A2 P2)

Soft **P2** (Fig. 4.4B):   stenotic pulmonary valve eg. Fallot
Loud **P2** (Fig. 4.4C):   pulmonary hypertension
Normal splitting (Fig. 4.4D):   children
                                    young adults

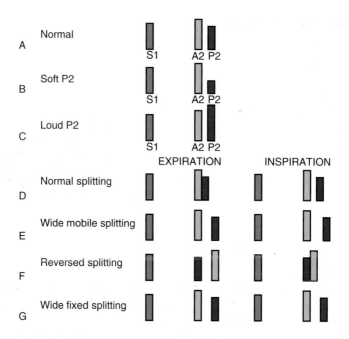

Figure 4.4 Heart sounds

Wide mobile splitting (Fig. 4.4E):	pulmonary stenosis
	pulmonary hypertension
	RBBB
Reversed splitting (Fig. 4.4F):	aortic stenosis
	LBBB
	HOCM
Wide fixed splitting (Fig. 4.4G):	ASD

Third heart sound (S3)

Due to rapid ventricular filling.

Causes Normal (in children, athletes and pregnancy)

Increased left ventricular stroke volume (aortic regurgitation, mitral regurgitation)

Restrictive ventricular filling (constrictive pericarditis, restrictive cardiomyopathy)

Ischaemic heart disease

Fourth heart sound (S4)

Due to forceful atrial contraction.

Causes HOCM

Long-standing hypertension

Ischaemic heart disease

JUGULAR VENOUS PULSE (JVP)

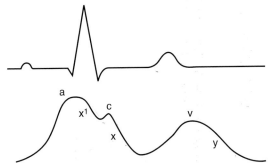

a = atrial systole
x¹ = atrium begins to relax
c = onset of ventricular contraction
v = atrial filling in ventricular systole
x = atrial relaxation commencing
y = tricuspid valve opens and ventricle relaxes

Figure 4.5 Jugular venous pulse

Changes in the JVP

	Seen in	Cause
Giant a waves (large a waves) Tricuspid stenosis	Pulmonary hypertension Pulmonary stenosis	↑ resistance to ventricular filling
Cannon a waves (very large a waves)	Complete heart block VT	Atrial contraction against closed tricuspid valve
Large v waves	Tricuspid regurgitation	
Steep y descent Tricuspid regurgitation	Constrictive pericarditis	

NORMAL VITAL SIGNS – AGE RELATED

Age	HR	RR	SBP	DBP
<1 year	120–160	30–60	60–95	35–69
1–3	90–140	24–40	95–105	50–65
3–5	75–110	18–30	95–110	50–65
8–12	75–100	18–30	90–110	57–71
12–16	60–90	12–16	112–130	60–80

Ref: Anaesthesia secrets by Duke J and Rosenberg SG, Hanley & Belfus, Mosby 1996.

CARDIAC CATHETERISATION DATA

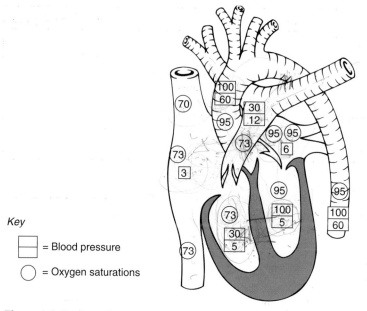

Figure 4.6 Cardiac catheterisation data

CXR SILHOUETTE

Right sided aortic arch	Big heart
Fallot tetralogy	Heart failure
Truncus arteriosus	Significant left-to-right shunts
Pulmonary atresia	HOCM/DCM
Congenital vascular ring	Pericardial effusion
	Ebstein anomaly

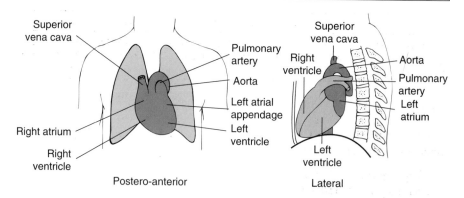

Figure 4.7 CXR silhouette

CARDIAC SCARS

Scar	Cause	Left brachial pulse
Left thoracotomy (only)	PDA ligation	N
	Blalock-Taussig shunt	↓ or N
	Coarctation repair (left subclavian flap)	↓ or N
	Pulmonary artery banding	N
	Non-cardiac	N
Right thoracotomy (only)	Right Blalock-Taussig shunt	N
	Non-cardiac	N
Median sternotomy	Any correction	N

The ECG

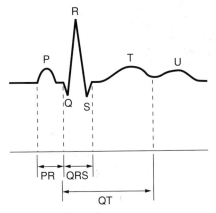

Figure 4.8 The ECG

	Birth–1 year	1–10 years	10–15 years	>15 years
PR interval (s)	0.08–0.15 (**0.10**)	0.08–0.15 (**0.12**)	0.09–0.18 (**0.14**)	0.10–0.22 (**0.16**)
QRS duration (s)	0.03–0.07 (**0.05**)	0.04–0.08 (**0.06**)	0.04–0.09 (**0.07**)	0.06–0.1 (**<0.1**)
Maximum QTc (s)	0.45	0.44	0.44	0.44

RATE

The heart rate varies with age (outlined above p. 83). It is calculated by noting the number of large squares between QRS complexes:

1 large square = 300/min
2 large squares = 150/min
3 large squares = 100/min
4 large squares = 75/min

5 large squares = 60/min

NB. 5 large squares = 1 second, 1 large square = 0.2 seconds

AXIS

The cardiac axis is the average direction of spread of the depolarisation wave through the ventricles (as seen from the front) and it changes from right and anterior in infants to left and posterior in adults.

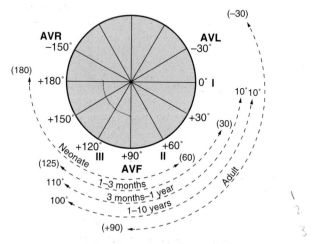

Figure 4.9 Cardiac axis

The axis can be derived by noting the direction of the QRS complexes in leads I, II and III. It can also be estimated by observing the direction in leads I and AVF (though this is less accurate).

The axis may be normal, left axis deviation (LAD) or right axis deviation (RAD). A superior axis is seen when the S wave > R wave in AVF.

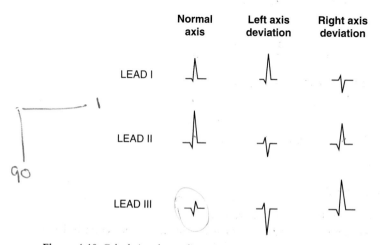

Figure 4.10 Calculating the cardiac axis

Axis deviation		
RAD	**LAD**	**Superior axis**
Normal in children	Primum ASD	Primum ASD
RVH	LVH	AVSD
RBBB	LBBB	Tricuspid atresia
Secundum ASD	AVSD	Noonan syndrome
		Double inlet left ventricle
		Familial
		Myocarditis

HEART BLOCK

FIRST DEGREE BLOCK

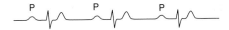

SECOND DEGREE BLOCK
1. Mobitz type I (Wenkebach)

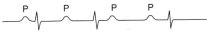

The PR interval gradually increases until
it does not conduct to the ventricles

2. Mobitz type II

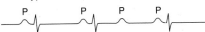

The P waves that do not conduct to the
ventricles are *not* preceeded by a gradual
PR prolongation

3. 2:1 AV block

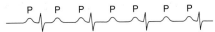

THIRD DEGREE (COMPLETE) BLOCK

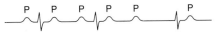

No relation between P waves and QRS complexes

Figure 4.11 Heart block

BUNDLE BRANCH BLOCK

Right bundle branch block (RBBB) (Fig. 4.12A)

The left ventricle and septum are activated normally and the right ventricle has a
slower conduction spreading from left to right. ECG features include:

A. RBBB

B. LBBB

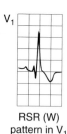

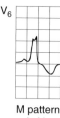

RSR (W)
pattern in V₁

M pattern
in V₆

Figure 4.12 (A) Right bundle branch block. (B) Left bundle branch block

- *QRS complex is prolonged*
- *an RSR pattern in the right precordial leads*

Left bundle branch block (LBBB) (Fig. 4.12B)

The septum depolarises from right to left and the left ventricle relies on late transmission of the activation wave. ECG features include:

- *QRS complex prolonged*
- *lead V1 negative and V5–V6 mostly positive with an M pattern*

NB. With complete LBBB or RBBB, ventricular hypertrophy and ischaemia changes *cannot* be interpreted from the ECG.

VENTRICULAR HYPERTROPHY

Left ventricular hypertrophy (LVH) (Fig. 4.13A)

This is difficult to predict accurately from the ECG and so it is best to have a combination of criteria, which include:

- *R wave amplitude in V5–V6 higher than the 98th centile for age (NB. voltage criteria for LVH are not very exact)*
- *S wave in V1*
- *lateral t wave inversion (strain pattern, in V5–V6 and II, III and AVF)*
- *LAD*

Right ventricular hypertrophy (RVH) (Fig. 4.13B)

ECG features include:

- *R wave amplitude in V1 >98th centile for age*
- *abnormal T wave direction in V1 (NB. the T wave direction changes with age: it is upright in newborns, negative >7 days of age, then becomes positive again in adolescents and adults)*
- *S wave depth in V6 is lower than the 98th centile for age*
- *in marked RVH the R wave is big and the T wave inverted (a strain pattern)*

A. LVH

V_5 V_6

(a) In V_5 or V_6 there is a tall R wave
(>25 mm in adults)

V_1 V_2

(b) In V_1 or V_2 there is a deep S wave

B. RVH

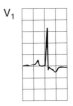

V_1

(a) In V_1 the height of the R wave
is > the depth of the S wave

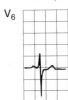

V_6

(b) In V_6 there is a deep S wave

Figure 4.13 (A) Left ventricular hypertrophy. (B) Right ventricular hypertrophy

EFFECTS OF HYPER- AND HYPOKALAEMIA ON THE ECG

$K^+ \uparrow$	$K^+ \downarrow$
Peaked T waves	Flat T waves
Wide QRS complexes	QRS axis rotates
Long PR interval	Long PR interval
Flat P waves	Long QT interval – *torsades de pointes*
Bradycardia/asystole	U waves
	ST depression

$K^+ \uparrow$

$K^+ \downarrow$

Figure 4.14 Effects of hyper- and hypokalaemia on the ECG

Cardiac positions

The classification of the normal and abnormal cardiac positions involves looking at the *visceroatrial situs* and the *apex* of the heart.

VISCEROATRIAL SITUS

Situs solitus	Viscera normal, lungs normal, atria normal
Situs inversus	Viscera reversed, lungs reversed, atria reversed
Situs ambiguous (isomerism)	**Asplenia syndrome** (right isomerism)
	No spleen, central liver, two right lungs
	Polysplenia syndrome (left isomerism)
	Multiple small spleens, no intrahepatic portion of IVC
	Bilateral left lungs

NB. Isomerism (right worse than left) is usually associated with severe congenital heart disease.

APEX OF THE HEART

Laevocardia	Normal (apex points to the left)
Dextrocardia	Apex points to the right

The following combinations are associated with severe congenital heart disease:

- *Situs solitus + dextrocardia*
- *Situs inversus + laevocardia*

The ECG in dextrocardia

The P waves are negative in lead I and reflect the position of the atria. The chest leads V1 to V6 show right ventricular complexes (Fig. 4.15).

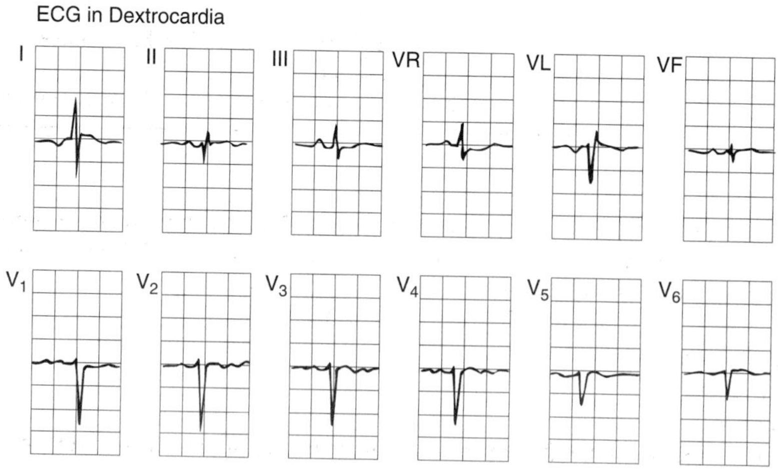

ECG in Dextrocardia

Figure 4.15 ECG in dextrocardia

Innocent murmurs

These are heard in 30% of children. There are two types:

Ejection murmur	Due to turbulent flow in the outflow tracts from the heart. A buzzing or blowing quality in the 2nd to 4th left intercostal space
Venous hum	Due to turbulent flow in the head and neck veins
	A continuous low-pitched rumble heard beneath the clavicles
	Disappears with compression of ipsilateral jugular veins or on lying down

Specific features

- *Systolic only (except venous hum)*
- *Soft*
- *Normal heart sounds*
- *No thrill or radiation*
- *Change with altered patient position*
- *Normal pulses*
- *Patient asymptomatic*
- *Normal CXR and ECG*

Heart failure

Symptoms	Signs
Shortness of breath (SOB)	Tachypnoea
Sweating	Tachycardia
Poor feeding	Cool peripheries
Failure to thrive	Cardiomegaly
Recurrent chest infections	Hepatomegaly
Abdominal pain (big liver)	Gallop rhythm/murmur/muffled heart sounds
Collapse/shock	Central cyanosis
	(NB. Lungs often sound clear in children/neonates)

CXR

Prominent pulmonary markings and cardiomegaly. NB. An important exception is with infradiaphragmatic TAPVD where the heart size is normal and therefore this can appear like primary lung disease.

Management

Sit patient up

Give oxygen

Diuretics	eg. frusemide (with potassium supplements), spironolactone (reduce pre-load and afterload)

Inotropes   Acute heart failure use IV dobutamine (peripherally)
               or dopamine (centrally)
               If less severe, oral digoxin may be used
Vasodilators eg. captopril and hydralazine (reduce afterload)

Eisenmenger reaction

This is when persistently increased pulmonary blood flow leads to increased pulmonary artery vascular resistance, pulmonary hypertension and eventually reversal of a previous left-to-right shunt. When this is due specifically to a VSD it is called *Eisenmenger syndrome*.

The Eisenmenger reaction is becoming rarer as the diagnosis of CHD improves and there is earlier management.

Causes

VSD, AVSD, PDA, ASD (rare) and any other condition with a communication between PA and the aorta.

Clinical features

- *Progressively worsening cyanosis, malaise, dyspnoea and haemoptysis*
- *Right ventricular heave*
- *Loud P2*

ECG

- *RVH*
- *P wave tall and spiked*

CXR

- *Prominent pulmonary artery with peripheral tapering of pulmonary vessels*
- *Cardiomegaly*
- *May be normal*

Management

Medical   Symptomatic treatment (oxygen, calcium channel blockers)
Surgical Heart–lung transplant or bilateral lung transplant with repair of the cardiac defect

Causes of peripheral pulmonary stenosis

Williams syndrome	Supravalvular AS, hypercalcaemia, mental retardation, elfin facies
Congenital rubella syndrome	
Alagille syndrome	Progressive bile duct destruction, TOF, butterfly vertebrae, nephritis, facial features, posterior embryotoxon (see p. 195)
CHD	ASD, VSD, PDA, TOF, supravalvular AS

Teratogens and maternal disorders associated with CHD

Drugs	Cardiac lesion
Sodium valproate	Coarctation of aorta, hypoplastic left heart, AS, interrupted aortic arch, secundum ASD, pulmonary atresia with no VSD, VSD
Lithium	Ebstein anomaly
Alcohol	ASD, VSD, TOF, coarctation of aorta
Phenytoin	AS, PS, coarctation of aorta, PDA

Maternal disorder	Cardiac lesion
Rubella	PDA, peripheral pulmonary stenosis
SLE, Sjögren's	Complete heart block
Diabetes	All types of CHD increase

Inherited conditions associated with CHD

Condition	Cardiac lesion
Down syndrome	AVSD, VSD, PDA, ASD, aberrant subclavian artery
Edwards syndrome	VSD, ASD, PDA, coarctation of aorta
Patau syndrome	VSD, PDA, ASD, coarctation of aorta
Turner syndrome	Bicuspid aortic valve, coarctation of aorta, AS
Chromosome 22 microdeletion	Aortic arch anomalies, truncus arteriosus, PDA, TOF
Holt-Oram	Secundum ASD, VSD
Marfan syndrome	Dissecting aortic aneurysm, AR, mitral valve prolapse
Neurofibromatosis	PS, coarctation of aorta
Noonan syndrome	PS, peripheral pulmonary stenosis, ASD, VSD, PDA, HOCM
Williams syndrome	Supravalvular aortic stenosis, PS, peripheral pulmonary stenosis, VSD, ASD

Tuberous Sclerosis	Cardiac rhabdomyoma
Ehlers–Danlos	Mitral valve prolapse, tricuspid valve prolapse, dilated aortic root
Hunter syndrome	AR, MR
Pompe disease	Hypertrophic cardiomyopathy
CHARGE syndrome	TOF, PDA, double outlet right ventricle, VSD, ASD, right-sided aortic arch

Structural congenital heart disease

The incidence of structural congenital heart disease is 8 in 1000. Recurrence risk is 3% if one child affected, 10% if two children affected and 25% if three children affected.

It can be divided into acyanotic conditions and cyanotic conditions. If CHD is suspected the child should be investigated with a CXR and ECG initially, then an echocardiogram with Doppler ultrasound to outline the defect(s). Cardiac catheterisation may be used for presurgical evaluation, evaluation of pulmonary vascular resistance, to monitor progress after surgical intervention and as a therapeutic tool in interventional cardiac catheterisation (eg. balloon dilatation, embolisation and closure of intracardiac defects).

ACYANOTIC CONGENITAL HEART DISEASE

Ventricular septal defect (VSD) (Fig. 4.16)
This comprises 32% of CHD, being the most common form. There are several types of VSD that may be classified as:

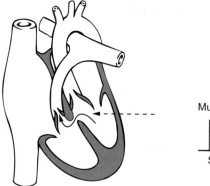
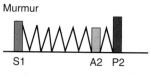

Figure 4.16 Ventricular septal defect

- *inlet*
- *muscular*
- *perimembranous*
- *outlet*
- *doubly committed*

The symptoms and signs depend on the size of the hole and any other cardiac defects present. Large ones and outlet VSDs are less likely to close spontaneously.

Clinical features

1. *Asymptomatic murmur*
2. *Features of cardiac failure*
3. *Recurrent chest infections*
4. *Endocarditis*
5. *Cyanosis (Eisenmenger syndrome) may develop at 10–20 years (only in untreated large VSDs).*

Signs

Murmur   Loud *pansystolic* murmur
Lower left sternal edge (LSE)
Parasternal thrill
± Mid-diastolic apical murmur (due to increased mitral flow) if large defect (smaller holes have shorter, louder murmurs)
Heart sounds   Loud P2 if pulmonary hypertension

ECG

Normal or LVH (RVH if pulmonary hypertension)

CXR

- *Cardiomegaly and increased pulmonary vascular markings*
- *May be normal*

NB. Important findings in **pulmonary hypertension**:

- *RVH on the ECG*
- *loud P2*

Management

Treat cardiac failure if present: oxygen, sitting up, diuretics (frusemide, spironolactone, ACE inhibitors, thiazides), digoxin.

Surgical repair is required in less than 10%, as most will close spontaneously during the first few years of life. Repair is needed if:

1. *severe symptoms with failure to thrive*
2. *pulmonary hypertension develops*
3. *aortic regurgitation develops*
4. *persistent significant shunting >10 years of age*

Atrial septal defect (ASD) (Fig. 4.17)

There are two types of ASD: ostium secundum and ostium primum.

Ostium secundum

This is the most common form of ASD and involves a defect(s) in the atrial septum. The defects may be single or multiple.

Associations   Holt–Oram syndrome

Clinical features

- *Asymptomatic (commonly)*
- *Heart failure (rare until adult life)*
- *Atrial arrhythmias (onset at 30–40 years)*

Signs

Murmur   Ejection systolic

Upper LSE (due to increased RV outflow)

± Mid-diastolic tricuspid flow murmur at the lower LSE (due to increased tricuspid flow)

Heart sounds   Fixed wide splitting of the 2nd heart sound

ECG

- *RAD*
- *Partial RBBB (in 90%)*   } NB. All *right*
- *RVH*

CXR

Cardiomegaly, large pulmonary artery, straight left heart border and increased pulmonary vascular markings.

Ostium secundum atrial septum defect

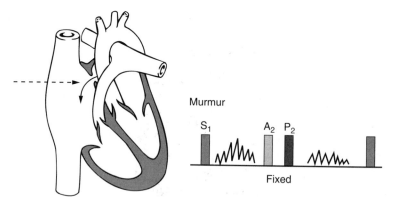

Figure 4.17 Atrial septal defect

Management
Catheter device closure to prevent problems in adult life. Elective repair performed at 4–5 years if:

1. *symptomatic (may be closed earlier if necessary)*
2. *evidence of ventricular overload.*

Ostium primum
Here there is failure of development of the septum primum (which divides the mitral and tricuspid valves) and usually also a cleft in the anterior leaflet of the mitral valve.

Associations   Down syndrome and Ellis–van Crevald syndrome

Clinical features
- *Many asymptomatic (if small defect)*
- *Heart failure and recurrent pneumonias (severity depending on A-V valve regurgitation)*

Signs
As for ostium secundum with a mitral regurgitation murmur (apical, pansystolic).

ECG
- *LAD or superior axis*
- *Partial RBBB*
- *RVH*

Management
Surgical repair is required.

Atrioventicular septal defect (AVSD) (Fig. 4.18)
Association   Common in Down syndrome

Atrioventricular septal defect (also known as A-V canal defect or endocardial cushion defect) is a severe form of CHD where there is a contiguous atrial and ventricular

Atrioventricular defect

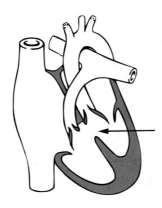

Figure 4.18 Atrioventricular septal defect

septal defect and defects of the mitral and tricuspid valves. (There are variable degrees of severity of AVSD.)

The clinical features are usually severe with early development of heart failure, recurrent pneumonias, failure to thrive and pulmonary hypertension due to the large left-to-right shunt across both the atria and the ventricles. Some right-to-left shunting may also occur. The ECG shows LAD or superior axis and biventricular hypertrophy and the CXR shows a large heart with pulmonary plethora.

Repair is usually needed within six months to prevent the development of pulmonary hypertension.

Patent ductus arteriosus (PDA) (Fig. 4.19)

Associations   Sick premature neonates
Congenital rubella
Maternal warfarin therapy
Commoner in girls

Clinical features and signs

Preterm infants   Systolic murmur at the left sternal edge
Collapsing pulse (visible brachial artery)
Heart failure

Older children   Continuous murmur beneath the left clavicle, '*machinery murmur*' (continuous because the PA pressure is always lower than the aortic pressure)
Collapsing pulse, '*waterhammer pulse*' (systolic pressure = twice the diastolic pressure)
If severe there is heart failure and eventually pulmonary hypertension

ECG

- *Usually normal*
- *May show LVH (or RVH if pulmonary hypertension)*
- *Indistinguishable from VSD*

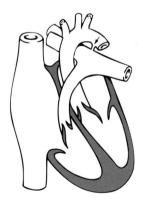
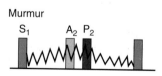

Murmur

S_1 A_2 P_2

Figure 4.19 Patent ductus arteriosus

CXR

- *Increased pulmonary vascular markings*
- *May be normal*

Management

Neonate   Fluid restrict
            Indomethacin if <34 weeks gestation and within three weeks of birth
            (check renal function, platelets and predisposition to NEC)
            Surgical ligation if failure of medical management

Older child Transvenous umbrella/coil occlusion
            Surgical correction

NB. PDA must be closed even if asymptomatic because of the risk of endocarditis.

Pulmonary stenosis (PS) (Fig. 4.20)

Associations   Noonan syndrome
               Maternal warfarin therapy

Clinical features

- *Usually asymptomatic*
- *Right heart failure*
- *Arrhythmias (later in life)*

NB. In neonates critical pulmonary stenosis presents as a duct–dependent circulation.

Signs

Murmur   Ejection systolic
            Upper left intercostal space
            No carotid radiation
            No carotid thrill
            Right ventricular heave

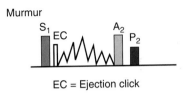

EC = Ejection click

Figure 4.20 Pulmonary stenosis

Heart sounds   Ejection click
               If severe: delayed P2 and soft P2

ECG

RVH

CXR

Post-stenotic dilatation of the pulmonary artery (>age five years)

Management

If the pressure gradient across the pulmonary valve is >50 mmHg, found on Doppler scan (eg. right ventricular pressure 70, pulmonary artery pressure 20) or there is severe pulmonary valve thickening, then transvenous balloon dilatation may be necessary. Surgical valvotomy is performed if balloon dilatation is unsuccessful.

In critical neonatal PS, emergency balloon valvuloplasty or surgical valvotomy is performed.

Aortic stenosis (AS) (Fig. 4.21)

This is usually anatomically a bicuspid aortic valve.

Associations   Aortic incompetence
Coarctation of the aorta
Mitral stenosis

Williams syndrome is *supravalvular* aortic stenosis with hypercalcaemia, elfin facies, mental retardation (see p. 12).

Clinical features

Neonate   Severe heart failure
Duct-dependent circulation
Older child   Asymptomatic murmur
Thrill on the chest
Decreased exercise tolerance
Chest pain, syncope
Endocarditis
Sudden death

Murmur

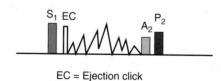

EC = Ejection click

Figure 4.21 Aortic stenosis

Signs

Murmur   Ejection systolic
Aortic area
Radiation to the neck
Carotid thrill
Heart sounds   Paradoxical splitting of second heart sound and soft A2
Apical ejection click (due to opening of deformed aortic valve)
Slow rising plateau pulse

ECG
LVH

CXR
Post-stenotic aortic dilatation

Management

Neonate	Valvotomy (balloon or surgical), then valve replacement later on
Older child	If symptomatic or resting pressure gradient across aortic valve >50–60 mmHg, then valvotomy (balloon or surgical) is required

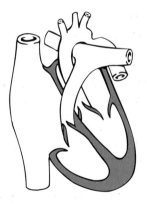

Figure 4.22 Coarctation of the aorta

Coarctation of the aorta (Fig. 4.22)
The descending aorta is constricted at any point between the transverse arch and the iliac bifurcation, but usually just distal to the left subclavian artery. Male: female 2 : 1.

Associations   Bicuspid aortic valve (40%)
Mitral valve anomaly (10%)
VSD
Turner syndrome
Berry aneurysm

Clinical features
This may present early or late.

Early   Circulatory collapse in the first week (duct-dependent circulation)
Late   Murmur discovered
Hypertension (in the upper limbs only)
Heart failure
Subarachnoid haemorrhage (Berry aneurysm or SBE)

Signs

- *Femoral pulses weak or absent (± left radial pulse)*
- *Radiofemoral delay may be observed in older children*
- *Murmur: ejection systolic*
  between the shoulder blades
- *Four-limb blood pressure measurements show BP higher in right arm (± left arm) than legs*

ECG

- *RVH in neonates (because the right ventricle is systemic in the fetus)*
- *LVH in older children*

CXR

- *May be normal*
- *Cardiomegaly with increased pulmonary vascular markings*
- *Rib notching (due to collaterals developing beneath the ribs) > age eight years*

Management

Unstable neonates to be stabilised as for duct-dependent circulation (PGE2, ventilation and inotropes as necessary). Surgical repair with an end-to-end repair or a left subclavian flap procedure. A left thoracotomy is used. The left subclavian flap procedure leaves the child with an absent left radial pulse.

Recoarctation rate approximately 5%. Mortality <2%. Balloon dilatation has been used successfully in older children.

Interrupted aortic arch

This is a form of severe coarctation where there is complete interruption of the aorta.

Associations VSD

Chromosome 22 microdeletion (these can also have truncus arteriosus)

Clinical features

These present as neonates with features of a duct-dependent circulation.

Management

Complete correction is required within days of birth. The operative mortality is around 20%.

Hypoplastic left heart syndrome

This is a condition where there is underdevelopment of the left side of the heart. The features include:

- *small left ventricle*
- *small or atretic mitral valve*
- *aortic valve atresia*
- *small ascending aorta*

Presentation is early in the neonatal period with features of a duct-dependent circulation. The neonate is very sick with collapse, acidosis and impalpable peripheral pulses occurring on closure of the ductus arteriosus.

Associations Coarctation of the aorta, Interrupted aortic arch

Management

The condition may be considered inoperable but surgical treatment is often attempted with a series of palliative operations termed a Norwood procedure (rebuilding the aorta and using the right ventricle as the systolic ventricle) or neonatal cardiac transplant.

CYANOTIC CONGENITAL HEART DISEASE

In cyanotic CHD there is central cyanosis, manifested as a blue-coloured tongue, which occurs when capillary deoxygenated haemoglobin is >3 g per dl (100 ml) of blood. It can be difficult to detect clinically in the presence of anaemia.

Causes of central cyanosis

1. *Lung disease*
2. *Cardiac disease*
3. *Persistent pulmonary hypertension of the newborn (PPHN)*
4. *Methaemoglobinaemia*

Cyanotic congenital heart disease results from:

1. *Right-to-left shunting with decreased pulmonary blood flow, eg. TOF, TA, PA, Ebstein anomaly, or*
2. *Abnormal blood mixing with normal or increased pulmonary blood flow, eg. TGA, TAPVD, double inlet ventricle*

Complications of cyanotic congenital heart disease

1. *Metabolic acidosis (occurs when paO$_2$ <40 mmHg). Treated with sodium bicarbonate*
2. *Increased affinity for oxygen (because the oxyhaemoglobin dissociation curve shifts to the left)*
3. *Polycythaemia, which may lead to thrombosis, embolism, haemorrhage and abscess formation*

The nitrogen washout test

This test is used to distinguish cardiac from respiratory causes of central cyanosis. The baby is given >90% oxygen to breath for 10 minutes.

- *If the paO$_2$ rises to >100 mmHg (14 kPa) the cause is respiratory or a central disorder*
- *If there is no change in the paO$_2$ or a small rise but it remains <100 mmHg (14 kPa) the cause is cardiac or it is PPHN*

Prostaglandin (PGE2)

This is a relatively specific ductal smooth muscle relaxant. It is used as an emergency measure in duct-dependent circulations. It is given as an intravenous infusion.

The common side-effects are: hypotension, fever, apnoea (dose related) and jitteriness.

Methaemoglobinaemia

Iron in haemoglobin is usually in the ferrous form (for both oxygenated and deoxygenated Hb). In methaemoglobin iron is in the ferric form, it is non-functional and brown in colour. Normally methaemoglobin accounts for <2% of total body haemoglobin.

Causes

- *Congenital – autosomal recessive enzyme deficiencies*
- *Nitrites*
- *Nitrobenzine*
- *Aniline dyes*

Clinical features

- *Cyanosis with normal or only slightly reduced oxygen saturations*
- *Cardiac and respiratory distress on exertion*

Investigations

- *Nitrogen washout test (paO_2 rises)*
- *Shaken blood turns brown*
- *Oxygen saturations are 80–100%*
- *Spectrophotometry of blood reveals MetHb*

Management options

1. *Reducing agents (IV) – methylene blue or ascorbic acid*
2. *Exchange transfusion*
3. *Reducing agents (orally) – methylene blue or ascorbic acid*

Tetralogy of Fallot (TOF)

This is the most common congenital cyanotic heart condition. The cyanosis results from right-to-left shunting.

Associations	Down syndrome
	DiGeorge syndrome
	CHARGE syndrome
	VACTERL syndrome
Anatomical features	• Malaligned VSD
	• RV outflow obstruction (valvular + infundibular stenosis)
	• Overriding aorta
	• RV hypertrophy

Clinical presentation

1. *Cyanosis present in the first few days of life (rare)*
2. *Murmur detected at 1–2 months*
3. *Hypercyanotic spells (late infancy):*
   - *occur in the morning and on crying*
   - *cyanosis or pallor*
   - *acidosis*
   - *child assumes squatting position*
   - *murmur becomes inaudible (due to **no** flow through pulmonary valve)*

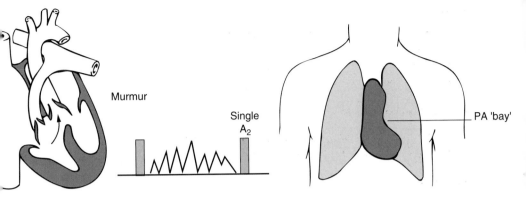

Figure 4.23 Tetralogy of Fallot

Management

- *Put child in knee–chest position holding child over one shoulder with their knees bent and reassure them (increases systemic vascular resistence and therefore pulmonary flow)*
- *IV fluids*
- *Morphine*
- *Propranolol IV (decreases infundibular spasm and peripheral resistance)*
- *Bicarbonate, then as necessary*
- *IPPV (paralysed, therefore decreased oxygen demand)*
- *Noradrenaline (increases systemic vascular resistance and so increases pulmonary flow)*
- *Emergency surgery*

Complications

Cerebral thrombosis, endocarditis, heart failure, myocardial infarction, brain abscess.

Signs

Murmur	Ejection systolic
	Upper left sternal edge (due to flow through pulmonary artery)
Heart sounds	Single second heart sound
Cyanosis	
Clubbing	

ECG

- *RAD*
- *RVH*

CXR

- *Small boot-shaped heart: 'coeur en sabot'*
- *Prominent pulmonary artery bay*
- *Right-sided aortic arch (30%)*
- *Pulmonary oligaemia*

Management

1. *Palliative early surgery in the first few months of life if symptomatic with a Blalock–Taussig shunt:* Classical: *Anastomose subclavian artery to pulmonary artery (child is left with an absent right radial pulse)*
   Modified: *Side-to-side anastomosis of subclavian artery to pulmonary artery.*
2. *Corrective surgery at 4–12 months of age. This involves patch closure of the VSD and relief of the obstruction of the RVOT by removing muscle bundles, pulmonary valvotomy or outflow tract patch. Mortality of total correction is approximately 2%. Long-term problems are those of pulmonary regurgitation.*

Tricuspid atresia

Clinical features

1. *Cyanosis usually present at birth though may become apparent later as is usually progressive*
2. *Systolic murmur at LSE*
3. *Single second heart sound*

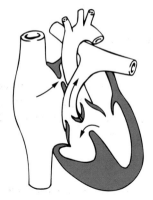

1. *Absence of tricuspid valve*
2. *ASD*
3. *VSD*
4. *Small, non-functional right ventricle*

Figure 4.24 Tricuspid atresia

ECG

- *Superior axis or LAD*
- *Tall P wave in V2*

NB. Severe cyanosis plus superior axis } can only be TA

CXR

Small heart with pulmonary oligaemia

Management
Initial palliation with:

1. *Blalock–Taussig shunt or*
2. *Glenn shunt (SVC to pulmonary artery) if >6 months*

Definitive palliation (usually at 2–5 years) with the Fontan-type procedure (right atrium or SVC and IVC connected to pulmonary artery directly and ASD closed). Long-term problems are due to a single effective ventricle and concern of atrial arrhythmias developing.

Double inlet ventricle
Here both atria empty into a single ventricle. The ventricle may be left, right or indeterminate. Both the aorta and the pulmonary artery arise from this ventricle.

Clinical features
The degree of cyanosis depends on the pulmonary blood flow:

If pulmonary flow is high	Relatively pink with severe heart failure and eventually Eisenmenger reaction
If pulmonary flow is low	Severe cyanosis and no heart failure

CXR
Cardiomegaly with either pulmonary plethora or oligaemia.

Management
Initial palliation with pulmonary artery banding (if no stenosis) or aortopulmonary shunt (if stenosis). Then a bidirectional Glenn shunt (SVC to PA) at 4–12 months. A modified Fontan procedure is performed for later surgical management at 1.5–3 years.

Ebstein anomaly
1. *Abnormal tricuspid valve, leaflets adherent to ventricle wall (anterior cusp most normal)*
2. *Distally displaced TV*
3. *Atrialisation of right ventricle*
4. *ASD*
5. *Functional pulmonary atresia*
6. *WPW syndrome type B*

Clinical features
1. *Cyanosis*
2. *Failure to thrive*
3. *SVT, extrasystoles*
4. *May be asymptomatic, especially if mild anatomical abnormalities*

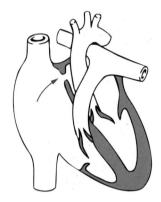

Figure 4.25 Ebstein anomaly

Signs

- *Soft, long systolic murmur (due to tricuspid regurgitation)*
- *Diastolic murmurs, extra heart sounds*

ECG

- *RBBB, RAD*
- *WPW (negative deflection of δ wave)*
- *Tall P waves, long PR interval*

CXR

- *Massive 'box cardiomegaly' and pulmonary oligaemia*
- *May be normal*

Management

Neonate   Consider pulmonary vasodilatation (with O_2, prostacyclin or nitric oxide); if unsuccessful, the duct is opened using PGE2

Older child   Control of SVTs and cardiac failure medically

                Tricuspid repair or replacement with closure of the ASD and ablation of the WPW pathway (this procedure is delayed as long as possible)

Pulmonary atresia

This may be:

1. *complete atresia of the pulmonary valve ± VSD with a PDA or collateral vessels and variable pulmonary arteries*
2. *complete atresia of the pulmonary valve, no VSD, a PDA, unusually small right ventricle and tricuspid valve and good pulmonary arteries. This type is totally duct dependent.*

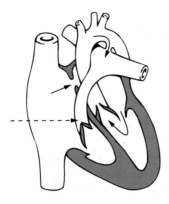

Figure 4.26 Pulmonary atresia

Clinical features and signs

- *Early neonatal cyanosis (duct-dependent circulation)*
- *No murmurs at the front, continuous murmur at the back (from collaterals in those with a VSD)*
- *Single second heart sound*

ECG
RAH + RVH

CXR

- *Prominent right atrium (both types)*
- *Those with a VSD: right-sided aortic arch (30%) and 'coeur en sabot' finding*
- *Pulmonary oligaemia*

Management

- *Emergency neonatal treatment with prostaglandin E2 if duct dependent*
- *Pulmonary valvotomy or outflow patch ± a Blalock–Taussig-type shunt as a neonate*
- *Formation of a systemic-pulmonary connection when older*
- *Unifocalisation (bringing the collaterals together) and shunt formation are often necessary for those with collateral arteries and poor pulmonary arteries*

Total anomalous pulmonary venous drainage (TAPVD) (Fig. 4.27)
All the pulmonary veins drain into the right atrium instead of the left atrium.
There are three types:

1. **supracardiac** – *drainage of pulmonary veins to SVC*
2. **cardiac** – *drainage to right atrium and coronary sinus*
3. **infracardiac** – *drainage below the diaphragm to the IVC, ductus venosus and portal vein. This type is always associated with obstruction to pulmonary venous return.*

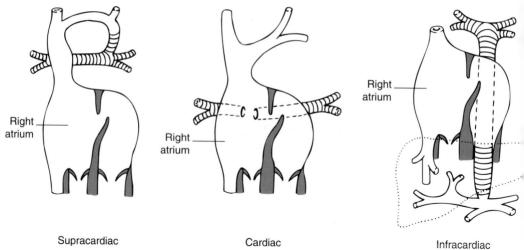

Supracardiac   Cardiac   Infracardiac

Figure 4.27 Total anomalous pulmonary venous drainage

There is mixing of blood between right and left sides at the:

- *patent foramen ovale*
- *ductus arteriosus*
- *ASD*

Clinical features and signs
There are two presentations.

If obstruction present (type 3)	Severe cyanosis as a neonate
	Respiratory distress
	Hepatomegaly
	No murmurs
No obstruction (types 1 and 2)	Mild cyanosis
	Cardiac failure
	Recurrent chest infections
	Pulmonary hypertension

ECG
Normal or RVH

CXR

1. *Infracardiac – small heart and hazy lung fields*
2. *Supracardiac – big supracardiac shadow (classic 'snowman' appearance)*

Management

1. *If obstructive type, emergency prostaglandin infusion in neonates then urgent cardiac surgery*
2. *Elective surgical correction in infancy (pulmonary venous trunk connected to left atrium)*

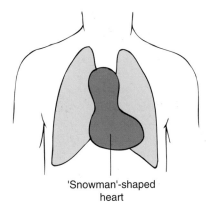

'Snowman'-shaped
heart

Figure 4.28 'Snowman'-shaped heart

Transposition of the great arteries (TGA) (Fig. 4.29)
Association   Maternal diabetes

There are *two parallel* circulations. Survival is due to mixing of blood at the:

- *ductus arteriosus*
- *foramen ovale*
- *ASD*
- *VSD*

Clinical features and signs

1. *Cyanosis within hours (on closure of DA and FO)*
2. *Acidosis*
3. *Mild tachycardia*
4. *No murmur (there may be a systolic murmur from increased pulmonary flow)*
5. *Single second heart sound*

ECG
Normal

CXR

- *'Egg on side' appearance of heart*
- *Increased pulmonary markings*

Management

1. *Emergency neonatal prostaglandin infusion*
2. *Atrial balloon septostomy (Rashkind)*
3. *Corrective surgery with either:*
   - *anatomical correction (switch procedure) – perform within a few weeks of birth*
   - *physiological correction (Mustard/Senning operation of atrial redirection) for later presentation or complicated cases*

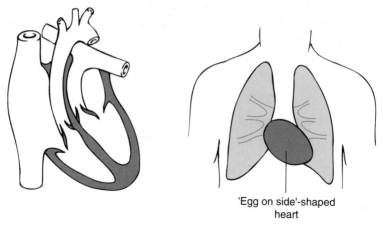

'Egg on side'-shaped
heart

Figure 4.29 Transposition of the great arteries

Duct-dependent circulations

These are circulations that depend on the ductus arteriosus to maintain pulmonary or systemic blood flow and deterioration occurs when the duct closes in the first week.

Causes of collapse in first week	Causes of cyanosis in first week
(duct-dependent systemic blood flow)	(duct-dependent pulmonary blood flow)
1. Coarctation of the aorta	1. Transposition of the great arteries
2. Hypoplastic left heart	2. Pulmonary atresia with a VSD
3. Critical aortic stenosis	3. Critical pulmonary stenosis
4. Interrupted aortic arch	4. Pulmonary atresia with no VSD
	5. Tetralogy of Fallot
	6. Tricuspid atresia
	7. TAPVD with obstruction
	8. Ebstein anomaly

Arrhythmias

SUPRAVENTRICULAR TACHYCARDIA (SVT)

This is the commonest arrhythmia in children. It is a reentry tachycardia causing premature reactivation of the atria. In neonates the rate is >220 bpm; in older children the rate is >180 bpm.

Wolff–Parkinson–White syndrome (WPW) (Fig. 4.30)

A congenital condition caused by an abnormal connection between the atria and the ventricle (an accessory pathway). The features are:

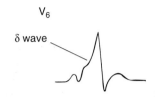

Figure 4.30 Wolff-Parkinson-White syndrome

1. δ *wave*
2. *short PR interval*
3. *wide QRS complexes.*

There are two types:

Type a Activation of the left ventricle via the accessory pathway (most common)

Type b Activation of the right ventricle via the accessory pathway (occurs in Ebstein's anomaly)

The tachycardia may be stopped by IV adenosine, oral digoxin or oral flecanide. Flecanide reduces the recurrence risk of tachycardias.

Clinical presentation of SVT

Older child Palpitations, dizziness, chest pain

Infant Poor cardiac output, pulmonary oedema, cardiac failure

In utero IUD or hydrops fetalis

Investigation

- *ECG (particularly of the tachycardia, recording the response to adenosine if possible)*
- *It is helpful to do an echocardiogram to exclude structural CHD.*

Management

1. *Vagal stimulation*

   - *Diving reflex: babies:*   *Immerse head and face in basin of ice-cold water for five seconds*

       older child: *Place polythene bag full of ice-cold water on face for 15 seconds*

   - *Carotid sinus massage (older children only)*

2. *Adenosine – the treatment of choice, given by rapid IV bolus*
3. *Synchronised DC cardioversion (1–2 J/kg). Anaesthetise or sedate the child (first line if child severely ill, otherwise use if drugs fail). Other drugs that may be used are;*
4. *Verapamil – IV over 20 seconds (contraindicated if <2 years)*

5. *Flecainide – IV over 15 minutes*
6. *Digoxin – oral or IV (slow acting)*

For maintenance therapy to prevent recurrence, the following may be tried:

1. *Flecainide*
2. *Propranolol*
3. *Digoxin*
4. *Amiodarone*

NB. Stop maintenance when over one year of age as 90% will have no further attacks.

Adenosine

Adenosine is an endogenous purine nucleotide. The half-life is very short (3–6 seconds). It acts to block A-V conduction. The side-effects are common and unpleasant.

- *Dyspnoea, flushing, nausea*
- *Chest pain (this is not angina, though feels the same)*
- *Bradycardia (therefore do not use in the presence of sinus node disease)*
- *Heart block*
- *Atrial and ventricular premature beats*
- *If inhaled, bronchoconstriction (therefore do not use in asthmatics)*

The antidote is aminophylline.

VENTRICULAR TACHYCARDIA (VT)

This is the occurrence of three or more ventricular beats in a row, at a rate of at least 120 per minute.

Causes

Long QT syndrome
Metabolic   Calcium, magnesium, potassium imbalances
HOCM
Infantile VT
Postcardiac surgery
    It can be hard to distinguish VT from SVT: see p. 115

Management

1. *Adenosine to make the diagnosis if necessary*
2. *DC cardioversion*
3. *Lignocaine*

NB. If unsure whether it is VT or SVT, always treat as VT.

VT	SVT
Wide complexes	Narrow complexes
Regular complexes	May not be regular
A–V dissociation	A–V association
Intermittent P waves seen	Regular P waves (if seen)
Fusion and capture beats	

Fusion beat – early beat with abnormal QRS
Capture beat – early beat with normal QRS

CONGENITAL COMPLETE HEART BLOCK

This is associated with:

1. *maternal connective tissue disease – SLE and Sjörgren syndrome (maternal anti-Rho antibodies cause atrophy and fibrosis of the AV node)*
2. *structural CHD (in 15% of cases): AVSD*
   congenitally corrected TGA.

Clinical presentation and management

- *Asymptomatic fetal bradycardia*
- *Intrauterine fetal death*
- *Hydrops fetalis*
- *Neonatal heart failure*
- *Syncope (Stokes–Adams attacks)*
- *Investigations include a 24-hour ECG (as it may be intermittent)*
- *Treatment is the placement of a pacemaker and is necessary if symptomatic or if the daytime pulse rate is <60/min in an infant or <50/min in an older child*

PROLONGED QT SYNDROME (*TORSADES DE POINTES*) (Fig. 4.31)

Torsades de pointes is an arrhythmia usually of short duration. The ECG has a prolonged QT between the tachycardias. The arrhythmia usually spontaneously reverts to sinus rhythm; however, it can convert to VF and result in sudden death.

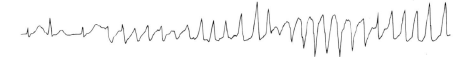

Figure 4.31 Torsades de pointes

Causes of prolonged QT interval

Congenital   1. Jervell–Lang–Neilson

> Autosomal recessive
> Long QT plus congenital deafness. Suffer repeat drop attacks
> Triggering factors: fear, excitement, exercise
> May be misdiagnosed as epilepsy

           2. Romano–Ward

> Autosomal dominant
> Isolated prolonged QT. Prognosis better than Jervell–Lang–Neilson

Acquired   1. Electrolyte disturbances – hypercalcaemia, hypomagnasaemia
           2. Drugs – amiodarone, quinidine, sotalol, MAOIs, tricyclics, erythromycin
           3. Poisoning – organophosphates
           4. Low-protein diets
           5. Anorexia nervosa
           6. Any cause of a bradycardia – myxoedema, complete heart block, head injury

Management

Congenital   β-blockers (mortality reduced from around 80% to 6%)
           Other antiarrhythmic drugs
           Left stellate ganglionectomy
           Implantable defibrillator if future treatment required

Acquired   Isoprenaline IV (this is contraindicated in congenital types)
           Pacing wire if associated heart block

Rheumatic fever

This is an inflammatory disease occurring in response to group A β-haemolytic streptococcal infection. The clinical features involve a pharyngeal infection, followed 2–6 weeks later by a polyarthritis, fever and malaise, the exact symptoms depending on the organs involved. The diagnosis is made on the basis of the Duckett Jones criteria. Two major criteria or one major and two minor criteria are needed to make the diagnosis.

	Major criteria	Minor criteria
1. Carditis:	endo (murmur)	1. Fever
	myo (heart failure)	2. Arthralgia
	peri (pericardial rub,	3. Long PR interval
	pericardial effusions)	4. Raised ESR or CRP
2. Polyarthritis:	medium joints,	5. Leucocytosis
	'flitting'	6. Previous rheumatic fever

	Major criteria	Minor criteria
3. Sydenham chorea:	St Vitus dance lasts 3–6 months	
4. Erythema marginatum:	map-like rash	
5. Subcutaneous nodules:	extensor surfaces hard, painless, pea-like	

Investigations

Evidence of recent streptococcal infection (ASOT raised, throat cultures, serology, recent scarlet fever) is looked for, together with the above signs and symptoms.

Management

- Bed rest (when active fever, carditis or arthritis is present)
- High-dose aspirin
- Steroids
- Treat heart failure
- Benzathine penicillin intramuscularly or oral penicillin course
- Then lifelong penicillin prophylaxis (monthly IM or daily oral penicillin)

Long-term complications

Mitral stenosis ± aortic stenosis.

Infective endocarditis

This is infection of the endocardium, which occurs particularly with congenital heart disease (especially cyanotic) and on previously damaged or prosthetic valves. A high-velocity flow is needed to damage the endocardium. It can be acute (rare) or subacute (SBE).

Infecting organisms

- α-haemolytic streptococcus (viridans) (50% of SBE)
- Staphylococcus aureus (50% of acute endocarditis, occurs with central lines and postcardiac surgery)
- Enterococcus faecalis
- Staphylococcus epidermidis (central lines, postcardiac surgery)
- Candida (central lines, immunosuppressed)
- Aspergillus, brucella, histoplasma, Coxiella burnetii (Q fever) (all rare)

Clinical features

These may be subtle, therefore always think of SBE in a patient with a heart problem who is unwell.

1. Sustained fever, night sweats, malaise
2. Development of new cardiac murmur

3. *Persistence of fever after acute illness (in the acute form)*
4. *Splenomegaly and splenic rub*
5. *Vascular lesions:* splinter haemorrhages
   Roth spots (retinal haemorrhages)
   Janeway lesions (erythematous macules on thenar and hypothenar eminences)
   Osler's nodes (hard, painful embolic swellings on toes, fingers, soles and palms)
6. *Renal lesions – haematuria, focal glomerulosclerosis, renal failure*
7. *Clubbing*
8. *Arthritis of major joints*
9. *Major embolic phenomena – cerebral, coronary, pulmonary and peripheral arterial*

Investigations

Blood tests	Serial blood cultures (at least three sets, more if negative)
	FBC (anaemia)
	ESR and CRP ($\uparrow$), immunoglobulins
	C3 (low due to immune complex formation)
	Serology (chlamydia, candida, coxiella and brucella) if culture negative
Urine	Microscopic haematuria and proteinuria
CXR and ECG	
Echocardiogram	Looking for vegetations

Management

1. *Four to 6 weeks of antibiotic therapy with suitable antibiotic (two weeks IV, then two weeks oral if sensitive)*
2. *Antibiotic prophylaxis in the future for procedures*
3. *Surgery (if extensive valve damage, cardiac failure, vegetations or embolisation)*

NB. 'At Risk' individuals should receive prophylactic antibiotics for certain procedures.

Myocarditis

An inflammation of the heart, with necrosis and fibrosis. May become chronic.

Causes

Infectious	Viral	Most common cause in children
		Coxsackie B, Adenovirus
	Bacterial	Diphtheria, Rikkettsia
	Fungal	
	Parasitic	
Toxic	Pneumonia/sepsis etc.	
Connective tissue disease		
Idiopathic		

Clinical features

Cardiac failure   Tachycardia, weak pulses, respiratory distress

Arrhythmias

Sudden death

Asymptomatic (in adolescents)

Investigations

CXR	Gross cardiomegaly, pulmonary plethora
ECG	Arrhythmias
Bloods	Cardiac enzymes (CK $\uparrow$, LDH $\uparrow$), Viral serology (specific IgM $\uparrow$), PCR
Echocardiography	Poor ventricular function, pericardial effusion

Management

Supportive	Cardiac failure, arrhythmias management, ECMO may be necessary
Cardiac transplant	If refractory heart failure

Cardiomyopathy

DILATED CARDIOMYOPATHY (DCM)

This is a disease involving dysfunction of the cardiomyocytes resulting in dilatation and impaired function of the left $\pm$ right ventricle. Most cases are idiopathic.

Associations

Genetic diseases	Familial, Mitochondrial abnormalities, Friedreich's ataxia, carnitine deficiency, muscular dystrophy, Fabrey's disease, Refsum's disease, Pompe's disease
Infections	Post-viral myocarditis (eg. coxsackie, echovirus), sepsis, diphtheria, rheumatic fever, HIV, trypanosomiasis (Chagas' disease)
Nutrition	Selenium deficiency (eg. TPN, short bowel syndrome, Keshan disease), thiamine, or calcium deficiency, iron overload, severe chronic anaemia
Toxins	eg. Doxorubicin, cyclophosphamide, adriamycin

Clinical features

Heart failure (Tachycardia, cardiomegaly, raised JVP, third and fourth heart sounds present)

Arrhythmias

Embolism

Investigations

CXR	Cardiomegaly and pulmonary plethora
ECG	LVH, nonspecific T wave abnormalities
Echocardiogram	Poorly contracting heart with atrial and ventricular dilatation Reduced ejection fraction, mitral and tricuspid regurgitation

Cardiac biopsy (rarely) Fibrosis, myocardiocyte hypertrophy and white cell infiltration (often unhelpful)

Metabolic screen If necessary for cause

Treatment

1. *Treatment of cardiac failure and anticoagulants (aspirin or warfarin)*
2. *Cardiac transplant if needed*

HYPERTROPHIC CARDIOMYOPATHY

This is characterised by hypertrophy of the interventricular septum and left ventricular wall, in the absence of a cardiac or systemic cause. Left ventricular outflow tract obstruction may be present.

Associations/Causes: Maternal IDDM (transient)
Premature infants receiving steroids for lung disease (transient)
Neurofibromatosis, mucopolysaccharidoses
Autosomal dominant in some cases

In some of the familial cases muations have been found in chromosome 14, cardiac β-myosin heavy chain (β-MCG) defect.

Clinical features

- *Syncope, angina*
- *Arrhythmias (AF and VF)*
- *Sudden death (60–70%)*
- *Family history of sudden death*

Signs

Murmur: ejection systolic (due to left ventricular outflow obstruction)
mid-diastolic ± pan-systolic (mitral regurgitation)
Fourth heart sound (palpable = double apex beat)
Left ventricular failure

Investigations

Echocardiogram
24-hour ECG VT or VF (treat with amiodarone first line)
AF (dangerous as they are dependent on atrial contraction)
ECG Long Q waves (due to thick interventricular septum)
LVH, non-specific T wave changes
Electron microscopy (EM) 'Myocardial dissarray'
CXR Cardiomegaly, prominent left ventricle

Treatment

1. *Amiodarone*
2. *β-blockers*

3. *Cardiac pacing (causes a LBBB)*
4. *Surgical resection of the septum if significant LV outflow obstruction*

Pericarditis

ACUTE PERICARDITIS

This is inflammation of the pericardium.

Causes

- *Coxsackie virus*
- *Staphylococcus, Haemophilus influenze, TB*
- *Rheumatic fever, malignancy (eg. Hodgkin's disease)*

Symptoms

Chest pain: Substernal, sharp, radiating to the neck
Worse on lying flat and respiration
Better on sitting forward

Signs

- *Pericardial friction rub*
- *Fever*

Investigations

- **ECG**

Raised ST segment, concave upwards

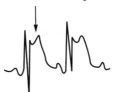

Figure 4.32 ECG in pericarditis

ST elevation, concave upwards
T inversion (Fig 4.32)
- *Cardiac enzymes elevated (if associated myocarditis)*

Treatment

Anti–inflammatory drugs
Drainage if indicated (always in post–viral pericarditis)

PERICARDIAL EFFUSION

All cases of acute pericarditis eventually develop a pericardial effusion.

Clinical features if significant:
Decreased cardiac output, impalpable apex beat
Soft heart sounds, friction rub (quiet)
Pulsus paradoxicus (BP decreases on inspiration)
Kusmaul's sign (neck veins distend on inspiration)
Raised JVP with Friedreich's sign (steep y descent)

Investigations
ECG	Small voltages
CXR	Large, globular heart
Echocardiogram	Diagnostic

Treatment
Pericardiocentesis with pericardial window formation if indicated.

CONSTRICTIVE PERICARDITIS

Causes
TB
Acute pericarditis
Haemopericardium

Clinical features
Cardiac failure – dyspnoea, sweatiness, hepatosplenomegaly
Decreased ventricular filling – pulsus paradoxus, Kusmaul's sign, Friedreich's sign
Atrial fibrillation (30%)
Pericardial knock (loud 3rd heart sound)

Investigations
CXR	Small heart with calcification
ECG	Low voltage QRS complexes and T wave inversion
Echocardiogram	Thick pericardium

Treatment
Surgery (*pericardiectomy* – removal of pericardium)

FURTHER READING

Archer N, Burch M *Paediatric Cardiology – An introduction*, 1st Ed, Chapman & Hall, London 1998

Clinical synopsis of Moss and Adams' *Heart Disease in Infants, Children and Adolescents, including fetus and young adult.* Emmanouilides GC, Allen HD, Reimenschneider TA, Gutgesell HP, Eds. Williams & Wilkins, Baltimore, 1998

Park MD *How to read pediatric ECGs*, Mosby, Philadelphia, 1992

Freedom RM, Benson LN *Congenital Heart Disease: Textbook of Angiocardiography*, Futura Publishing Company inc, 1997

5

Respiratory

- *Physiology*
- *ENT conditions*
- *Upper respiratory tract*

- *Lower respiratory tract*
- *Parenchymal lung disease*

Physiology

LUNG FUNCTION TESTS

Peak respiratory flow rate (PEFR)
The PEFR is a useful and very simple lung function test. It varies with height, sex, age and ethnic group. It also varies during the day, being lowest in the early morning, and with exercise, being low shortly after moderate exercise. It is used to assess asthma severity by comparing a child's PEFR to normal corrected PEFR and to the individual child's normal PEFR.

Spirometry
Spirometry provides timed measurements of expired volumes from the lung. It enables one to distinguish between obstructive and restrictive lung conditions.

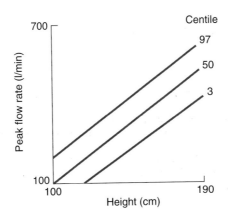

Figure 5.1 Peak flow readings

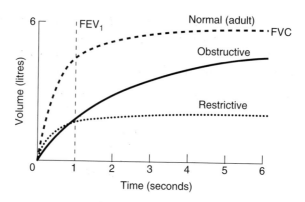

Figure 5.2 Spirometry

Obstructive lesions	Restrictive lesions
Low FEV$_1$: FVC ratio, RV↑, FVC↓, TLC↑	FVC↓, TLC↓, FEV$_1$: FVC ratio↑ or N
Asthma	Cystic fibrosis (both)
Bronchiolitis/bronchitis	Sarcoidosis
Emphysema (α1–antitrypsin)	Myaesthenia gravis
Cystic fibrosis (both)	Fibrosing alveolitis
	Scoliosis

Lung volumes

Methods of measuring the lung volumes:

1. *Helium dilution*
2. *Nitrogen washout*
3. *Whole-body plethysmography*

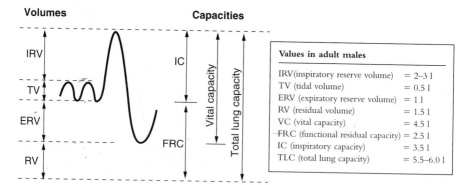

Values in adult males	
IRV (inspiratory reserve volume)	= 2–3 l
TV (tidal volume)	= 0.5 l
ERV (expiratory reserve volume)	= 1 l
RV (residual volume)	= 1.5 l
VC (vital capacity)	= 4.5 l
FRC (functional residual capacity)	= 2.5 l
IC (inspiratory capacity)	= 3.5 l
TLC (total lung capacity)	= 5.5–6.0 l

Figure 5.3 Lung volumes and capacities

Transfer factor

This measures the rate at which a gas will transfer from the alveoli into the blood. It is a function of both the membrane-diffusing capacity and pulmonary vascular components, which together reflect the alveolar-capillary unit function. Carbon monoxide is used to measure this. Normal diffusing capacity (Dco) is 25–30 ml/min/mmHg.

Decreased Dco	Increased Dco
Anaemia	Polycythaemia
Cystic Fibrosis	Pulmonary haemorrhage
Interstitial lung disease:	Heart failure
pneumonia	Left-to-right shunt
pulmonary fibrosis	Hyperkinetic states
Pulmonary vascular disease:	Exercise
pulmonary emboli	Asthma
pulmonary hypertension	

Flow–volume curves

These are constructed from spirometric data and are used to locate the site of an airway obstruction.

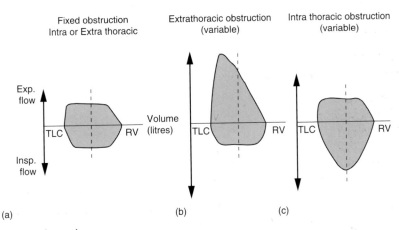

Figure 5.4 Flow–volume curves

PLEURAL EFFUSIONS

Pleural effusions are the accumulation of an excessive amount of fluid in the pleural space. They are divided into transudates and exudates, depending on the protein content of the effusion.

Transudate (protein <30 gm/l)	Exudate (protein >30 gm/l)
Heart failure	Pneumonia
Hypoproteinaemic states	TB
Hypothyroidism	Pulmonary infarct
Constrictive pericarditis	Connective tissue disease
	Pancreatitis
	—Familial Mediterranean fever
	Yellow-nail syndrome

HEARING TESTS

Hearing impairment is detected using different methods at various ages (see p. 364).

Tuning fork hearing tests
These tests are used on older children to distinguish sensorineural hearing loss from conductive hearing loss.

Rinne test Tuning fork held in front of the ear (air conduction) and then on the mastoid process (bone conduction):
Rinne positive (+) = heard louder in front of the ear
Rinne negative (−) = heard louder on the mastoid process
Weber test Tuning fork held on the forehead in the midline. A conductive loss in one ear results in the sound being referred to that ear and heard as a louder sound

Possible test results

Interpretation	Right ear	Left ear
Normal or mild bilateral sensorineural loss	Rinne +	Rinne +
	Weber central	
Left conductive or mixed loss	Rinne +	Rinne −
	Weber referred to the left	
Left severe sensorineural loss	Rinne +	Rinne −
	Weber referred to the right	
Bilateral conductive or mixed loss	Rinne −	Rinne −
	Weber central	

ENT Conditions

EARS

Acute Otitis media
This is infection of the middle ear.

Causes
Bacterial Pneumococcus, *Haemophilus influenzae*, *Moxarella catarrhalis* group A β-haemolytic streptococcus and *Streptococcus pyogenes*

Viral RSV

Clinical features

- *Severe earache*
- *Fevers*
- *URTI*

Signs
Injected tympanic membrane (TM), bulging drum, loss of light reflex, perforated drum, discharge.

Management

1. *Analgesia for 24 hours; if no improvement, commence oral antibiotics*
2. *Ear toilet*
3. *Oral antibiotics, IV antibiotics if oral therapy fails*
4. *Myringotomy and drainage rarely required*

Glue ear (Otitis media with effusion)
Glue ear occurs after acute otitis media when fluid persists for >8 weeks without signs of inflammation. Incidence and prevalence are high but the majority of effusions resolve spontaneously. The initial infection may not be noticed.

Associations Down syndrome, cleft palate and other craniofacial abnormalities
IgG subclass deficiency, food allergies

Clinical features

- *Conductive hearing loss*
- *Speech and learning difficulties*

Signs

- *Retracted drum, loss of light reflex, bubbles and fluid levels on the TM*
- *There may be a normal-looking drum*
- *Rinne test negative (if >5 years)*
- *Tympanometry shows a flat (type B) response*
- *Pure tone audiometry shows a conductive hearing loss*

Management

- *Initial observation for spontaneous resolution 'watchful waiting' for three months*
- *Trial of antibiotics may benefit some children (eg. one month of augmentin)*
- *Grommet insertion*
- *Adenoidectomy may be combined with grommets (leads to higher resolution rates)*

Chronic suppurative otitis media

This consists of a chronic discharge from the ear and a perforation in the tympanic membrane. There are two forms.

Tubotympanic disease

Central tympanic membrane perforation, so-called *'safe'* perforation, with no cholesteatoma. May be active, with discharge either intermittently or continuously, or quiescent when the only sign is the perforation. There is conductive deafness of variable degree and in long-standing cases there is often a coexistent sensory loss. Surgical repair of the drum may be performed if indicated.

Atticoantral disease

Marginal tympanic perforation or severe retraction with squamous epithelia and granulation tissue in the middle ear cleft. This is cholesteatoma disease arising from a failure of epithelial migration which goes on to destroy neighbouring structures. This is an *'unsafe'* perforation. Management is surgical.

Complications of cholesteatoma:

Extracranial	VII nerve palsy, suppurative labyrinthitis, perimastoid abscess
Intracranial	Extradural, subdural and intracerebral abscess, meningitis, sigmoid sinus thrombosis and hydrocephalus

Otitis externa

This is relatively uncommon in children. It comprises an infected, oedematous external auditory canal and usually presents as a discharging ear which then becomes painful (unlike otitis media which is initially painful and then may discharge). Treatment is with aural toilet and topical antibiotics given as eardrops or impregnated onto a wick.

Mastoiditis

Clinical features

This is a serious condition, which presents with symptoms of acute otitis media, plus swelling and tenderness in the postauricular region.

Investigations

CT Scan	Opacification of the mastoid air cell system with breakdown of bony septa.
Blood tests	FBC (neutrophilia), blood cultures

Treatment

Admit immediately for IV antibiotics and analgesia. Surgical exploration and mastoidectomy are performed as soon as possible.

Complications

The concern with this condition is the development of *brain abscess, meningitis* or *venous sinus thrombosis*.

NOSE

Rhinitis

This is divided into allergic rhinitis (where known allergens trigger the symptoms) and non–allergic rhinitis. The symptoms are very similar.

Clinical features

- *Persistently runny nose, clear discharge, occasionally becoming purulent.*
- *Sneezing and itchy nose*
- *Nasal obstruction*
- *Mouth breather, hyponasal speech*
- *Family history of atopy*

Signs and investigations

- *Nasal mucosa pale and purple (normally pink)*
- *Serum IgE (↑) and RAST tests may be done (allergic rhinitis)*
- *Postnasal space X-ray if concern about enlarged adenoids*

Management

- *Avoidance of allergens*
- *Topical steroids (nasal drops)*
- *Decongestants for short-term (<1 week) usage for acute exacerbations eg. ephedrine, xylomethyzoline*
- *Antihistamines (nasal or systemic)*
- *Mast cell stabilisers eg. disodium chromoglycate*
- *Check for nasal foreign body (if unilateral discharge)*

Sinusitis

Infection of the sinuses in children usually involves the maxillary sinuses as the frontal sinuses are not fully developed. The serious complication of *orbital cellulitis* or *abscess* may be the presentation.

Clinical features

- *Purulent nasal discharge, fever, local tenderness and pain*
- *Postnasal drip and chronic cough in chronic sinusitis*

Investigations

Sinus X-ray Opaque maxillary sinuses ($\pm$ MRI)
Blood tests FBC and blood cultures (if acutely unwell)

Management

- *Broad-spectrum antibiotics (IV if acutely unwell)*
- *Steam inhalations*

If orbital cellulitis is present, an ophthalmologist must be involved to assess and help make the differentiation between pre- and postseptal cellulitis, and an ENT surgeon should also be involved. A CT of the sinuses will show sinus involvement as well as intraorbital complications necessitating surgical intervention.

Progression of orbital cellulitis:
- Pre-septal
- Post-septal
- Subperiosteal abscess
- Orbital abscess
- Cavernous sinus thrombosis

Danger signs indicating need for surgery:

Decreased acuity
Impaired globe mobility
Decreased colour vision
Proptosis

Epistaxis

This is a common problem in childhood, usually involving bleeding from Little's area of the nasal mucosa. Immediate management involves applying pressure to the soft part of the nose; vasoconstrictors such as otrivine or cocaine will usually arrest bleeding if this fails. A nasal pack can be inserted (with admission) if this fails. If recurrent nose bleeds are occurring, underlying defects of coagulation, hypertension and neoplasms should be excluded. Cauterisation of Little's area can be carried out if necessary.

THROAT

Pharyngitis

This is a common infection usually caused by a virus (adenovirus or para-influenza virus) or, more rarely, a bacteria.

Clinical features

- *Sore throat, nasal congestion, fever*
- *Oropharyngeal inflammation*

Treatment

Symptomatic treatment with antipyretics and plenty of fluids, unless bacterial infection is suspected.

Differential diagnoses

- *Infectious mononucleosis, measles, scarlet fever, diphtheria, chronic adenoiditis, HIV*
- *Presentation of actue leukaemia or lymphoma*

Acute tonsillitis

Clinical features

- *Sore throat, fever, malaise*
- *Red tonsils ± pus*
- *Cervical lymphadenopathy*

Investigations

- *Throat swab*
- *FBC and Monospot test*

Management

- *Analgesics, antipyretics and plenty of fluids*
- *Antibiotics may be required (penicillin V as first-line management – usually streptococcal if bacterial)*

Complications

1. Quinsy *(peritonsillar abscess) – surgical drainage required.*
2. Post-streptococcal complications
3. Chronic tonsillitis *presents with a persistent sore throat, poor general health, bad breath, cervical lymphadenopathy and erythematous anterior faucal pillars. A three-week course of appropriate antibiotics may help. Tonsillectomy may have a place.*

Tonsillectomy indications

1. *At least six attacks of tonsillitis per year for two years.*
2. *Three attacks per year over a number of years for the older child.*
3. *Obstructive sleep apnoea is a strong indication.*

Upper respiratory tract

CAUSES OF STRIDOR

Stridor is a harsh sound caused by upper airway obstruction. Inspiratory stridor is caused by extrathoracic obstruction and expiratory stridor is caused by intrathoracic obstruction. Stridor arising from the subglottis and cervical trachea is often biphasic. Associated hoarse voice or cry, barking cough, tracheal tug or sternal recession may be seen.

Causes of stridor

Intraluminal

- *Foreign body*
- *Tumour*
- *Papilloma*

Intramural

- *Laryngomalacia*
- *Subglottic stenosis*
- *Laryngeal web*
- *Haemangioma*
- *Tracheomalacia*
- *Infection (croup, epiglottitis, diptheria, bacterial croup)*
- *Vocal cord paralysis or prolapse*
- *Angioneurotic oedema*
- *Hypocalcaemia*

Extramural

- *Goitre*
- *Cystic hygroma*
- *Haemangioma*
- *Mediastinal tumour*

CROUP (acute laryngo tracheobronchitis)

This is the commonest cause of acute stridor in children. It is a viral condition caused by parainfluenza virus, respiratory syncytial virus (RSV) or rhinovirus. The child's already small airway is narrowed by secretions and oedema.

Clinical presentation

- *Usual age 1–2 years*
- *Stridor, mild fever, hoarse voice, barking cough and little constitutional disturbance. Sometimes viral croup can deteriorate into a much more severe condition.*

Management

- *Calm atmosphere with avoidance of unnecessary blood tests, direct airway vision and neck X-rays which may frighten the child, making the condition worse*
- *Mist therapy (unproven benefit)*
- *Oxygen as necessary (keep oxygen saturations >92%)*
- *Steroid nebulisers (budesonide 1 mg 12 hourly)*
- *Adrenaline nebuliser 1 ml 1/1000 if necessary (NB. Rebound increased stridor common 30–45 minutes later)*
- *Systemic steroids (oral or IV)*
- *Intubation and IPPV are needed in approximately 1% of children and tracheostomy very rarely*

Indications for IPPV

- *Drowsiness due to hypoxia*
- *Tiring*
- *Rapid deterioration*

BACTERIAL TRACHEITIS (PSEUDOMEMBRANOUS CROUP)

An uncommon condition usually caused by *Staphylococcus aureus*. The child is unwell for 2–3 days and is usually severely unwell on presentation. Intubation with IPPV for several days is usually required together with antibiotic therapy.

ACUTE EPIGLOTITIS

This is an infection caused by *Haemophilus influenzae* type b. It presents between one and seven years (peak 2–3 years). It has become much less common since the introduction of the Hib vaccine.

Clinical presentation

- *Toxic child*
- *Drooling, no cough, stridor, high fever and a short history (usually <6 hours)*
- *Muffled voice, pain in throat*

Management

- *Intensive care or high-dependency setting with immediate involvement of ENT surgeon and anaesthetist*
- *Intubation with IPPV for 24 hours electively or in response to hypoxia*
- *Antibiotic therapy – 3rd generation cephalosporin eg. cefuroxime, IV for five days.*
- *Steroids – oral or IV*
- *Rifampicin prophylaxis for contacts*

Lower respiratory tract

CONGENITAL MALFORMATIONS

1. *Laryngomalacia*
2. *Tracheooesophageal fistula* } *See Chapter 16*
3. *Congenital lobar emphysema*
4. *Bronchogenic cyst*
   These are usually asymptomatic at birth and present when secondarily infected or they enlarge in size and compromise an adjacent airway. There is an air–fluid level on CXR and treatment is with surgical excision.
5. *Cystic adenomatoid malformation (CAM lung). This is the second most common congenital lung malformation after congenital lobar emphysema. A single lobe of one lung is enlarged and cystic and usually causes mediastinal shift with compression of the other lung. It presents with neonatal respiratory distress, a pneumothorax or recurrent respiratory infections. It may be seen on CXR and CT scan of the thorax. Management is surgical.*

CAUSES OF WHEEZE

Infection:
  bronchiolitis
  viral-induced wheeze (<1 year of age)
  whooping cough
  pneumonia
Reflux with aspiration
Asthma (>1 year of age)
Cystic fibrosis
Immunodeficiency

Vascular ring
Congenital lobar emphysema
Mediastinal mass (glands, tumours, cysts)
Foreign body aspiration
Heart failure
Fibrosing alveolitis
Tumour

BRONCHIOLITIS

This is a common condition usually presenting between one and nine months. It is due to the respiratory syncytial virus (RSV) in 80% of cases and is otherwise due to adenovirus types 3, 7 and 21.

Clinical features

- Coryza, cough, dyspnoea, wheeze
- Feeding difficulties
- Apnoea in small babies

Signs

- Tachypnoea, tachycardia, intercostal, subcostal and suprasternal recession
- Cyanosis, crackles, wheeze and fever

Investigations

CXR   Hyperinflation (horizontal ribs and flattened diaphragm)
Nasopharyngeal aspirate   Immunofluorescence test for RSV antibodies
Blood tests   Paired antibody titres (for RSV)
               Viral culture

Treatment

- Moist oxygen via a head box
- NG feeding or IV fluids as necessary
- Ribavirin via SPAG machine for high-risk infants only (eg. BPD, CHD, CF, immunodeficiency or <6 weeks old)
- Antibiotic therapy if secondary bacterial pneumonia suspected
- CPAP or intubation with IPPV if exhaustion, deterioration in level of conciousness or persistent apnoeas
- ECMO if above management is failing

Complications

1. **Bronchiolitis obliterans** – *severe persistent airways damage (usually with adenovirus)*
2. **Macleod syndrome** – *persistent overdistension of one lung*

INHALATION OF FOREIGN BODY

Clinical features

- *Acute coughing episode followed by stridor or wheeze*
- *Positive history of small object inhaled (commonly a peanut)*
- *Recurrent lobar pneumonias involving the same lobe*
- *Persistent wheeze*

Investigations
CXR with inspiratory film (both sides equal) and expiratory film (foreign body (FB) side lung hyperinflated). NB. Peanuts are radiolucent.

Management
Removal of FB using **rigid bronchoscopy** under general anaesthesia.

ASTHMA

This is an endemic condition. It is a chronic inflammatory disease of the airways characterised by:

1. *bronchoconstriction*
2. *mucosal oedema*
3. *excessive mucus production.*

Associations: Atopic conditions 33% have eczema, 50% have allergic rhinitis ± conjunctivitis.

Asthma presents as recurrent wheeze, breathlessness, and cough ± nocturnal cough. In long-standing disease there may be chest hyperinflation, pectus carinatum (Pigeon chest) and Harrison sulci (a permanent groove in the chest wall at the insertion of the diaphragm).

Clinical features of an exacerbation

- *Dyspnoea*
- *Wheeze, crackles in younger children*
- *Respiratory distress (tachypnoea, recession, tachycardia, cyanosis)*

Features of a life-threatening attack

- *Unable to speak or feed*
- *Central cyanosis*
- *Exhaustion/confusion/level of consciousness decreasing*

- *Silent chest (due to minimal air entry)*
- *Peak flow <30% of predicted*
- *Pulsus paradoxus (fall of inspiratory systolic BP >10 mmHg from expiratory systolic BP)*

Management

Acute attack

- *Oxygen*
- *Nebulised β-agonist as frequently as necessary*
- *Ipatropium bromide nebulised six hourly*
- *Systemic steroids (oral prednisolone 2 mg/kg (max. dose 40 mg) or IV hydrocortisone)*
- *Steroids nebulised (in babies)*

NB. A short course of steroids is usually required to treat an acute exacerbation. Then, if necessary, progress to:

- *IV aminophylline (or IV salbutamol) NB. Caution with aminophylline if on oral theophylline*
- *Intubation and ventilation if deterioration in general condition, peak flow, blood gases or drowsiness.*

Long-term therapy

This is outlined in the British Guidelines on Asthma Management summarised in the box below. For full guidelines see British Guidelines on Asthma Management. Thorax 1997: 52 (supp 1): 1–21. The lowest step to control the asthma should be used. Management should be reviewed every 3–6 months and a step down in treatment is possible if control is sustained for >3 months.

Children under five years			
Step 1	**Step 2**	**Step 3**	**Step 4**
• Occ.β_2–agonist Inh. or oral	• β_2-agonist inh. +	• β_2-agonist inh. +	• β_2-agonist inh. +
If > 1/day go to step 2	a) cromoglycate or	• inh. steroids higher dose	• inh. steroids high dose
	b) inh. steroids low dose	± long-acting β-agonist or slow-release xanthine	± long-acting β-agonist (spacer or neb) or slow-release xantheine
Low-dose steroids	1. *Beclomethasone or budesonide <400 μg daily* 2. *Fluticasone <200 μg daily*		
Higher dose steroids	1. *Beclomethasone or budesonide 800 μg daily* 2. *Fluticasone 500 μg daily*		
High-dose steroids	*Beclomethasone or budesonide up to 2 mg/day*		

Adults and school children

Step1	Step 2	Step 3	Step 4	Step 5
● Occ. β_2-agonist Inh.	● β_2-agonist inh. +	● β_2-agonist inh. +	● β_2-agonist inh. +	● β_2-agonist inh. +
If > 1/day go to step 2	a) inh.steroids low dose or	a) inh.steroids high dose or	● inh. steroids high dose +	● inh.steroids high dose +
	b) cromoglycate	b) inh. steroids low dose and salmeterol	● trial regular one or more of : 1. salmeterol 2. theophylline SR 3. ipatropium bromide 4. salmeterol oral 5. inh. bronchodilator 6. cromoglycate	● Long acting bronchodilator + Regular oral steroids

Low-dose steroids   1. *Beclomethasone or budesonide 100–400 µg BD*
                  2. *Fluticasone 50–200 µg BD*
High-dose steroids 1. *Beclomethasone or budesonide 800–2000 µg daily*
                  2. *Fluticasone 400–1000 µg daily*

Available medications

Quick-relief medications

1. *β-2-agonists, bronchodilator*

Generic name	**Device**
Salbutamol	MDI, tabs, syrup, injection, resp sol, accuhaler, rotacaps, diskhaler
Terbutaline	MDI, turbohaler, tabs, syrup, resp sol, injection
Salmeterol	MDI, accuhaler, diskhaler
Rimiterol	MDI
Reproterol	MDI
Fenoterol	MDI

2. *Anticholinergics*

Ipatropium bromide	MDI, resp sol, autohaler, aerocaps
Oxitropium	MDI

Long-term preventive medications

1. *Inhaled steroids*

Beclomethasone	MDI, autohaler, rotacaps, diskhaler
Budesonide	MDI, turbohaler, resp sol
Fluticasone	MDI, diskhaler, accuhaler

2. *Anti-inflammatory agents*

Sodium cromoglycate	MDI, spinhaler, resp sol
Necrodomil	MDI

3. *Methyl xanthines*

Aminophylline	Tabs
Theophylline	Tabs, caps, syrup

Spacer devices

There are two spacer devices, which connect with different medications.
1. *Nebuhaler – terbutaline, budesonide, ipatropium bromide*
2. *Volumatic – salbutamol, beclomethasone, fluticasone*

Age-related medications

<3 years	MDI + spacer + mask, or nebuliser
3-5 years	MDI + spacer (may require a mask as well), or nebuliser
5-12 years	MDI + spacer, or dry powder device (turbohaler, diskhaler, accuhaler, spinhaler, rotocaps), or nebuliser
>12 years	MDI alone, or dry powder device, or nebuliser

NB. Only 10–15% of the medication reaches the lungs in MDI or nebuliser therapy.

Important questions in Asthma History and Management

History

1. *What triggers the asthma (pets, exercise, cold, dust mite, pollen, respiratory infections, smoking, aerosols)?*
2. *Does the asthma affect their daily living (eg. school, sport)?*

Management

1. *Can they measure peak flow properly to monitor asthma?*
2. *Can they use their device properly?*
3. *Do they recognise a deterioration and have a good management plan?*
4. *Do they recognise a severe attack and know to seek medical attention?*
5. *Do they understand the difference between quick-relief and preventive medications?*

CAUSES OF CHRONIC COUGH

- *Asthma*
- *Aspiration*
- *Prolonged infection, eg. pertussis, mycoplasma, RSV, TB*
- *Foreign body*
- *Habit cough. NB. These will not cough during sleep*

- *Lung disease, eg. cystic fibrosis, bronchiectasis, congenital cysts, primary ciliary dyskinesia*
- *Immunodeficiency, eg. HIV, cancer therapy*

PERTUSSIS (WHOOPING COUGH)

This is an infection caused by the Gram-negative coccobacillus, *Borditella pertussis*.

Clinical features
Usually occurs <5 years of age
Incubation period 7–14 days

Catarrhal stage	Mucoid rhinorrhoea, conjunctivitis, malaise, highly infectious
Paroxysmal stage	This begins 3–7 days later. Paroxysms of coughing with inspiratory whoop and vomiting. Conjunctival petechiae and epistaxis occur. Severe in young babies. May last 10–12 weeks (usually 2 weeks).

Investigations
A clinical diagnosis, confirmed by:

Per nasal swab	Microscopy and culture. Fluorescent antibody testing for rapid diagnosis.
FBC	Lymphocytosis

Management
- *Isolate child*
- *Erythromycin early in disease and for contacts*
- *Prevention by immunisation*

Complications
- *Rectal prolapse, inguinal hernia, lobar pneumonia, atelectasis*
- *Cerebral anoxia with convulsions in young children, apnoea and death*
- *Bronchiectasis (late sequelae)*

CYSTIC FIBROSIS

This is a congenital autosomal recessive disorder of salt and water transport resulting in viscid secretions in the lungs and from exocrine glands. Highest prevalence in Northern Europeans: carrier rate one in 25, one in 2500 affected.

Chromosome 7 is involved, with loss of phenylalanine at position 508 (DF 508) in 78% of CF cases. The defect is of CFTR (cystic fibrosis transmembrane regulator), which is a cAMP chloride channel blocker.

Clinical features

Respiratory	Recurrent infections classically in the following order: *Staphyloccocus aureus, Haemophilus influenzae*, pseudomonas, cepacia
	Lobar collapse, pneumothorax, haemoptysis, allergic aspergillosis, bronchiectasis, abscesses and nasal polyps
	Restrictive lung disorder, with obstructive component in one-third

Pancreas	Decreased enzymes (lipase, amylase, proteases), causing steatorrhoea IDDM (10% of teenagers)
Liver	Involved in 15%. Cirrhosis, pericholangitis, portal hypertension, cholesterol gall stones
Gut	Meconium ileus (15% present with this), meconium ileus equivalent, constipation, intussusception, rectal prolapse, fibrosing colonopathy (side-effect of some high strength pancreatic enzymes)
Reproductive	Males infertile (vas deferens secretions too thick), females reduced fertility

Examination findings

General	Poor growth and nutritional state
	Finger clubbing, finger prick marks (from monitoring IDDM)
Respiratory	Hyperinflation, scoliosis. (NB. Auscultation may be normal if post physiotherapy)
Cardiovascular	Right heart failure
Abdominal	Palpable liver and/or spleen, faecal masses, pubertal delay, jaundice Surgical scars, eg. from meconium ileus, liver transplant, gastrostomy, Portacath
ENT	Nasal polyps
Joints	Swelling (cystic fibrosis-related arthropathy)

Diagnosis

This is usually suspected on the basis of:

- *failure to thrive*
- *malabsorption*
- *recurrent chest infections*

Investigations

Immune-reactive trypsin (IRT)	Immune-reactive trypsin, increased. Used <3 months of age. May be performed on Guthrie test
Sweat test	The *gold standard*. Two tests needed, with >100 mg sweat, pilocarpine used
	In CF, high sodium–Na > 60mmol/l, diagnostic. Chloride also high (>50)
Gene analysis	PCR technique looking for common mutations. This is possible on the Guthrie test
Stool	Elastase low, fat content high, chymotrypsin absent
Electrolytes	The pattern seen in CF is *hypokalaemic alkalosis* secondary to sodium and potassium loss in the sweat. It is known as *Pseudo-Bartters syndrome*
CXR	Bronchial wall thickening
	Hyperinflation with flattened diaphragms
	Rings
	Mottling

Management

Aims of management are to ensure optimal physical and emotional growth, delay the progress of the pulmonary disease and normalise the lifestyle of the child and family as much as possible.

Lung disease	Physiotherapy twice daily (more as necessary)
	Antibiotics for infections (may be long term or pulsed as prophylaxis)
	Nebulised antibiotics (eg. colistin and gentamicin) as prophylaxis
	Bronchodilators (useful in 30%)
	Oxygen at night if necessary
Gastrointestinal disease	Pancreatic enzymes, eg. creon®, pancrease®, nutrizym®
	Nutrition: High-calorie, high-protein diet.
	Vitamins if poor intake or ill health
	Salt required in hot weather and for babies
	Bile acids (ursodeoxycholic acid)
Others	DNase therapy (Pulmozyme)
	Gene therapy (in development)
	Fully immunise including influenza vaccine
	Heart-lung transplantation if necessary (complications of bronchiectasis obliterans, infection and rejection)

Regular review

Looking at growth, chest infections, PEFR, school, and later fertility and genetic counselling.

Causes of a false-positive sweat test

Addison's disease	Muccopolysaccharidoses
Ectodermal dysplasia	Flucloxacillin therapy
Hypothyroidism	Congenital adrenal hyperplasia
Nephrogenic diabetes insipidus	HIV
Glycogen storage disease type 1	Eczema
Hypoproteinaemia (severe)	Fuscidiosis

BRONCHIECTASIS

This is a condition of dilatation of the bronchi. There are inflamed bronchial walls, decreased mucociliary transport and recurrent bacterial infections.

Causes

- *Inhaled foreign body*
- *Cystic fibrosis*
- *Post-whooping cough and measles*
- *Tuberculosis (classically right middle lobe)*

- *IgA deficiency IgG subclass deficiency*
- *Primary ciliary dyskinesia*

Clinical features

- *Productive cough*
- *Dyspnoea*
- *Haemoptysis*
- *Clubbing*

Investigations

CXR   Hyperinflation and peribronchial thickening of affected area
CT scan thorax   Dilated bronchi seen

Management

- *Postural drainage*
- *Antibiotics (for acute infections or prophylaxis)*
- *Bronchodilators*
- *Surgical resection of affected lobe if necessary and possible*

PRIMARY CILIARY DYSKINESIA

This is an inherited condition caused by an absence of dynein arms (ATPase) on the cilia, which results in defective cilia action. First described as *Kartagener syndrome* (situs inversus, chronic sinusitis and airway disease). Also known as *immotile cilia syndrome*.

Autosomal recessive condition, affecting one in 20 000 caucasians; 50% also have situs inversus (see p. 90).

Clinical features

- *Neonatal respiratory distress*
- *Chronic sinusitis*
- *Otitis media (conductive hearing loss)*
- *Chronic productive cough ± wheeze*
- *Males infertile (sperm motility poor)*

Diagnosis

1. *Ultrastructural changes of dynein arms on the cilia (gold standard)*
2. *Nasal mucosal scrapings – motility decreased*
3. *Mucociliary clearance – time to taste saccharine placed on inferior nasal turbinates (prolonged)*
4. *Liver function tests – obstructive picture*
5. *CXR and CT scan as for bronchiectasis*

Management

As for bronchiectasis with ENT involvement.

α1-ANTITRYPSIN DEFICIENCY

See p. 199. The lung disease in α1-antitrypsin deficiency generally presents as emphysema at 30–50 years of age, though younger presentation occurs. Hyperinflation is seen on CXR. Management is with aggressive treatment of infections, vaccination for pneumococcus and influenza, bronchodilators if necessary and advice against smoking.

Parenchymal lung disease

PNEUMONIA

A common disease of childhood caused by many pathogens.

Clinical features

- *Respiratory distress symptoms and signs*
- *Fever and malaise*
- *Abdominal pain (children)*

Causes

Newborn	Group B β-haemolytic streptococcus, *Escherichia coli*, *Listeria monocytogenes*, chlamydia, TB
Infants	*Streptococcus pneumoniae*, *E. coli*, *Staphylococcus aureus*, *Haemophilus influenzae*, chlamydia, TB, RSV
Children	Mycoplasma, *Streptococcus pneumoniae*, TB
Immunocompromised	PCP, atypical TB

Investigations

CXR   Lobar pneumonia (dense) or bronchopneumonia (patchy)
Blood tests   FBC, blood cultures, viral immunofluorescence, blood gas if unwell

Sputum or oropharyngeal suction specimen for M, C and S.

Management

1. *Humidified oxygen as needed to keep saturation >92%. Use head box, nasal cannulae, or face mask*
2. *Physiotherapy*
3. *Oropharyngeal suctioning (infants)*
4. *Therapy with appropriate antibiotic*

Complications

- *Pneumococcal pneumonia – meningitis, pleural effusion*
- *Staphylococcal pneumonia – empyema, lung abscess, pneumothorax*

TUBERCULOSIS

This is a disease caused by infection with mycobacteria (usually *M. tuberculosis*), an acid- and alcohol-fast bacillus.

In children tuberculosis is usually a *primary* lung infection (or rarely in disseminated form), whereas in adults it is usually a *reactivation* of pulmonary infection. Children with primary pulmonary TB are not infectious, unlike adults with the disease.

Types of TB in children

TB infection	Asymptomatic, normal CXR, *only* a positive Mantoux
	Subclinical TB or TB contact is infection without disease
TB disease (tuberculosis)	Positive Mantoux + either symptoms, signs of pulmonary or extrapulmonary TB or abnormal CXR
	In children this is usually 'complicated' or 'progressive' primary TB. A disseminated illness may occur (eg. miliary TB)

Pathogenesis

TB infection

Children generally become infected from an adult with pulmonary TB. The immune response mounted by the child is primarily responsible for the lung manifestations. A primary lung focus develops consisting of a small parenchymal component and regional lymph node involvement. This is asymptomatic and not visible on CXR. This usually evolves into a small area of fibrosis, which can calcify over 1–2 years and become visible on CXR. This primary healed complex may reactivate later and cause 'open' pulmonary TB, which is highly infectious.

Complicated primary TB

Sometimes the primary complex develops and a *complicated primary TB* occurs, which is symptomatic and visible on CXR. There are few organisms present and release of organisms with rupture causes a marked hypersensitivity reaction, as delayed hypersensitivity to TB has developed by this time. The complications include:

- *Obstruction of a bronchus – Cough, localised wheeze*
- *Rupture into a bronchus – Bronchitis, bronchopneumonia,*
- *Rupture into the pleural cavity – pleural effusion*

Disseminated tuberculosis

This occurs if the organisms enter the bloodstream. This is more likely to occur in children <4 years. It can result in miliary TB, TB meningitis or other (eg. bone, kidney or joint) infection.

Clinical features

TB infection is usually asymptomatic. Complicated primary pulmonary TB may present with wheeze, fever, cough and dyspnoea. Disseminated TB may include:

Miliary TB	Acutely unwell, fever, weight loss, 'miliary' picture on CXR, hepato-splenomegaly, choroidal tubercles in retinal blood vessels
TB meningitis	Slow, insidious onset
	Weight loss, night sweats, malaise
	Symptoms of meningeal irritation occur later
	CSF shows mainly a lymphocytic response, protein ↑, glucose ↓
	Mycobacteria TB seen on microscopy (in 33%) and on culture (in 50–90%)
	CXR abnormalities in 50%
TB pericarditis	Constrictive pericarditis
GI tract	Presentation similar to Crohn's disease
Lymph nodes	Tender lump in anterior triangle of the neck or the groin
Skin features	Erythema nodosum

NB. Atypical mycobacterial infection commonly presents with unilateral cervical lymphadenopathy in children.

Diagnosis

Mantoux test
Intradermal test of delayed hypersensitivity to tuberculin. 0.1 ml of 1:1000 (or 1:10 000 initially if high risk) purified protein derivative (PPD) injected intradermally. The induration is measured 48–72 hours later. Interpretation is variable depending on the population:

- *if child at high risk >5 mm considered positive*
- *If child at medium risk >10 mm considered positive.*

NB. The Heaf test is not recommended because the exact dose injected is variable and there is poor repeatability.

Other tests to look for TB:

1. *CXR*
2. *Sputum* ⎱ *ZN (Ziehl–Neilsen) stain for AAFB*
3. *Gastric washings* ⎰ *Culture 4–8 weeks plus four weeks sensitivities*
4. *Bronchoscopy washings* ⎱ *(on Lowenstein–Jensen medium)*
5. *Early morning urine*
6. *Biopsies* *Of lymph nodes, pleura, gut, tuberculoma as appropriate*

Treatment

1. *Chemoprophylaxis* For TB infection Isoniazid 6–9 months
   (Give to all children with a positive Mantoux test)

2. *Chemotherapy*
   Pulmonary disease 1. Isoniazid + rifampicin 6–9 months *or*
   2. Isoniazid + rifampicin 6 months with ethambutol and pyrazinamide also for the first 2 months (only use this option if >7 years)
   3. Isoniazid + rifampicin 6 months with pyrazinamide also for the first 2 months.

Disseminated disease   At least 12 months therapy. Use options 2 or 3 above (isoniazid + rifampicin 12 months with pyrazinamide ± ethamb-
utol also for the first 2 months)

Antituberculous drugs	
Drug	**Features and side-effects**
Isoniazid	Increased effects in slow acetylators
	Skin rashes and hepatoxicity (rare in children)
	Psychosis rarely occurs (due to pyridoxine deficiency)
Rifampicin	A liver enzyme inducer
	Pink/orange secretions <4–8 hours
	Skin rashes, gastrointestinal upset and hepatotoxicity (rare)
Pyrazinamide	Skin rashes, gastrointestinal upset and hepatotoxicity
Ethambutol	Ocular effects (colour-blindness, blurred vision, scotoma)
	Ophthalmological opinion with visual acuity assessment must be done prior to commencing. Not recommended <7–8 years as children not capable of reporting visual disturbances

Prevention
Vaccination with the BCG (Bacille Calmette-Guerin, 1954, live bovine attenuated strain) gives approximately 50% protection. This is given at birth to high-risk groups (Asian, African, certain areas of London) and at 10–14 years to tuberculin test-negative children.

EXTRINSIC ALLERGIC ALVEOLITIS

This is a diffuse inflammatory reaction of the small airways and alveoli.

Causes
Inhalation of allergens:

- *Farmer's lung – mouldy hay (aspergillus)*
- *Bird fancier's lung – pigeons, budgerigars (proteins in excreta)*
- *Maltworker's lung – barley (aspergillus)*
- *Humidifier fever – air conditioning (bacteria)*

Clinical features

- *Fever, malaise, weight loss*
- *Dyspnoea and cough (worse immediately postexposure)*
- *Tachypnoea, wheezes, coarse end-expiratory crackles, cyanosis, progression to fibrosing alveolitis*

Investigations
CXR   Fluffy nodules and streaks in upper zones
Serum   For precipitating antibodies
         Neutrophilia
PFT   Restrictive lung function defect

Management

1. *Remove source*
2. *Steroids*

PULMONARY FIBROSIS

This is a rare condition resulting in 'honeycomb' lung seen on CXR. Progression to respiratory failure is inevitable.

Causes

Localised	Widespread
TB	Cryptogenic fibrosing alveolitis
Sarcoid (on CXR)	Langerhans cell histiocytosis
Systemic sclerosis	Neurofibromatosis
Post-pneumonia	Tuberose sclerosis
Asbestosis	Rheumatoid lung
	Drugs – busulphan, bleomycin, cyclophosphamide

Management
Supportive, with steroids to alleviate symptoms.

SARCOIDOSIS

A multisystem granulomatous disease, uncommon in children, most usually seen in young adults.

Clinical features
Very variable depending on the organs involved and the severity. Organs involved include:

Lungs	Parenchymal infiltrates, miliary nodules, _restrictive_ lung changes
	Hilar and paratracheal lymphadenopathy
Eyes	Uveitis, iritis
Joints	Arthritis
Other	Skin rashes, peripheral lymphadenopathy, liver involvement
	Hypercalcaemia may lead to renal damage

Clinical presentation

Young child	Cough, fatigue, weight loss, anaemia, bone and joint pain
Older child	Maculopapular erythematous rash, uveitis, arthritis and minimal lung involvement

Investigations

Biopsy	Of involved area (non-caseating, granulomatous lesions)
Serum	ESR ↑
	Ca ↑
	ACE (Angiotensin-converting enzyme) ↑, a measure of disease activity
Urine	Hypercalciuria
Lung function tests	Restrictive defect
CXR/CT scan	Perihilar lymphadenopathy, parenchymal infiltrates.

Management

- *Regular assessment for lung, renal, eye and other involvement*
- *Supportive and symptomatic treatment. Steroids may be used*
- *Prognosis is very variable*

FURTHER READING

Kendig's disorders of the respiratory tract in children. Chernick and Boat, 6th Ed, Saunders, Philadelphia, 1997

British Thoracic Society. The British Guidelines on Asthma Management, *Thorax* 1997 Vol 52: Suppl 1, 1–21

6

Gastrointestinal disorders

- *Physiology*
- *Upper gastrointestinal conditions*
- *Malabsorption*
- *Gastroenteritis*
- *Diarrhoea*
- *Chronic abdominal pain*
- *Peptic ulcer*
- *Inflammatory bowel disease*

- *Constipation*
- *Pancreatitis*
- *Gastrointestinal tract bleeding*
- *Gastrointestinal tract tumours*
- *Failure to thrive*
- *Nutritional disorders*
- *Eating disorders*

Physiology

OESOPHAGUS

The oesophagus propels food along with normal peristaltic waves, which are disturbed in motility disorders. It has two sphincters:

Upper oesophageal sphincter (UOS)   Normally closed by the cricopharyngeus muscle
Lower oesophageal sphincter (LOS)   A high resting tone to prevent reflux of gastric contents
Composed of oesophageal smooth muscle, under vagal and hormonal control.
The intra-abdominal oesophagus also acts as a flap valve

STOMACH

Function   Food reservoir, mixes food, produces acid, emulsifies fats, intrinsic factor secretion and minimal absorption

Gastrin (hormone)

Released with: Antral distension
Amino acids in antrum
Vagal nerve stimulation
pH > 1.5

Actions: Release of gastric acid, pepsin, IF
Gastric emptying
Pancreatic bicarbonate release

Stimulation of gastric acid secretion	Inhibition of gastric acid secretion
Vagal stimulation Hormonal stimulation (gastrin) Histamine release (H2 receptors on oxyntic cells) Pepsin	Low gastric pH Higher centres, eg. fear (sympathetic NS) Intestinal peptides – CCK-PZ, GIP, secretin

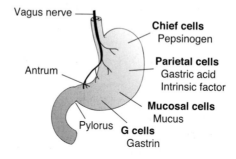

Figure 6.1 The stomach

PANCREAS

Exocrine function (98%)	Endocrine function	
These enzymes are produced in the acinar cells.	In islets of Langerhans:	
Enzymes Maltase, lipases, amylase, nucleases	1. β-cells	Insulin
Proenzymes Trypsinogen, chymotrysinogens,	2. α-cells	Glucagon
proaminopeptidase, procarboxypeptidases,	3. D-cells	Somatostatin
co-lipase	4. pp-cells	Pancreatic polypeptide

DUODENUM AND JEJUNUM

Function   Digestion, absorption, hormone production and defence organ
Produces 2 litres of fluid per day, made from:

- *Brunner's glands – bicarbonate juice*
- *Panneth cells – watery juice*
- *Enterocytes – digestive enzymes and absorption*

Principal gastrointestinal polypeptide hormones

Secretin	Pancreatic bicarbonate release↑
	Delays gastric emptying, inhibits gastric acid and pepsin secretion
Cholecystokinin-pancreozymin (CCK-PZ)	Pancreatic enzyme and bicarbonate release↑, gall bladder contraction, inhibits gastric emptying
Gastric inhibitory peptide (GIP)	Insulin secretion↑, inhibits gastric acid secretion
Motilin	Increases bowel motility
Gastrin	Action as above (p. 150)
Pancreatic polypeptide (PP)	Inhibits pancreatic secretion
	Gall bladder relaxation
Somatostatin	Inhibits secretion and action of many hormones
Vasoactive intestinal peptide (VIP)	Intestinal and pancreatic secretion↑, inhibits gastric acid and pepsin secretion
Substance P	Increases small bowel motility

Digestive enzymes

Amylase, lactase, sucrase, maltase, isomaltase, lipases and enterokinase

Absorption

- *Passive – water, salts, folic acid, vitamins B and C*
- *Active – amino acids and monosaccharides*
- *Released from micelles then passive – fatty acids, cholesterol, monoglycerides, vitamins A, D, E, K*

ILEUM

Function is absorption (though this occurs mainly in the jejunum and duodenum), with bile salts and vitamin B_{12} absorbed in the terminal ileum.

Bile Acids

Function	Digestion of fats
Bile contains	Bile acids, cholesterol, phospholipids, bile pigments (bilirubin and biliverdin) and protein
Primary bile acids	Cholic acid
	Chenodeoxycholic acid

Secondary bile acids Deoxycholic acid ⎫
 Lithocholic acid ⎬ from breakdown of primary acids

ENTEROHEPATIC CIRCULATION (EHP)

This occurs 6–8 times a day. It is increased by parasympathetic stimulation, gastrin and secretin and decreased by sympathetic stimulation and cholestyramine.

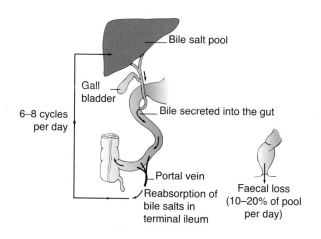

Figure 6.2 The enterohepatic circulation

COLON

Function Absorption of water, sodium and chloride (passive and active)
 Secretion of potassium, bicarbonate and mucous

Stool is 70% water.

Upper gastrointestinal conditions

CAUSES OF VOMITING

Gut pathology
Medical
Possetting (not pathological)
Overfeeding
GO reflux
Gastroenteritis
Food intolerance
Cyclical vomiting
Coeliac disease

Surgical
Obstruction:
  Atresias/stenoses
  Intussusception
  Malrotation
  Achalasia
  Foreign body
Acute abdomen any other cause
Other – peptic ulcer

Other pathology
Acute infection
Metabolic disorder, eg. IDDM
CNS disease, eg. migraine, ICP↑
Psychogenic, eg. anorexia nervose, bulimia
Severe illness
Poisoning

GASTRO-OESOPHAGEAL REFLUX

This is the passage of gastric contents involuntarily into the oesophagus. It is the result of an incompetent lower oesophageal sphincter secondary to immaturity.

Clinical features

- *Vomiting at end of feeds (± altered blood)*
- *Crying, food refusal, poor sleeping, irritability*
- *Usually resolves spontaneously by 1–2 years of age*

Complications

1. *Failure to thrive*
2. *Oesophagitis ± oesophageal stricture*
3. *Apnoea, SIDS*
4. *Aspiration, wheezing, recurrent chest infections*
5. *Iron deficiency anaemia*

Associations

Cerebral palsy, hiatus hernia, thoracic stomach, Coeliac disease, raised intracranial pressure, UTIs, Munchhausen by proxy

Investigations

These are necessary only if there is failure to resolve with simple measures or the reflux is complicated. The investigations are complementary to each other.

1. *Oesophageal pH measurement:*
   percentage of time pH < 4.0 in 24 hours: *>10% = abnormal if <1 year old*
                                                    >6% = abnormal if >1 year old
2. *Barium swallow and meal:*
   looking for malrotation, hiatus hernia, oesophageal stricture
3. *Endoscopy:*
   looking for oesophagitis, stricture, enteropathy

Other investigations

- *CXR*
- *Urine M, C and S*
- *Hb and iron studies*
- *Faecal occult bloods*
- *Remember raised intracranial pressure*

Management

Position	Nurse on side (left lateral)
Thicken feeds	Add thickeners (eg. Carobel, Nestargal) or use prethickened feeds (eg. Enfamil AR)
Change feeds	Consider changing feeds to casein-hydrosylated (eg. Nutramigen, Pregestamil, Peptijunior)
Drugs	Antacid, eg. Gaviscon
	Prokinetic, eg. cisapride, domperidone
	H$_2$ blocker, eg. ranitidine, cimetidine
	Proton pump inhibitor, eg. omeprazole
Surgery	If medical management fails over a three-month period, consider a Nissen fundoplication.

NB. *Cisapride* – Prolonged QTc and arrhythmias may occur if given with certain antibiotics (eg. erythromycin) or azole antifungals.

POSSETTING

This is small-volume vomits that occur during or between feeds. The infant will be thriving and there is no cause for concern. Management is with reassurance.

HIATUS HERNIA

This is herniation of the stomach through the oesophageal hiatus and may be of the sliding type (gastro-oesophageal junction slides into the thorax) or para-oesophageal (a portion of the stomach herniates beside the gastro-oesophageal junction).

Sliding hiatus hernia	Paraoesophageal hiatus hernia
Common type Associated with GO reflux	No reflux occurs Complication of fundoplication (Nissen) Upper abdominal pain common symptom

Management

- *Antireflux medication*
- *Surgery if necessary (rarely so)*

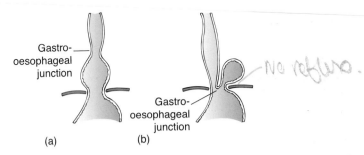

Figure 6.3 Types of hiatus hernia. (a) Sliding hiatus hernia. (b) Para-oesophageal hiatus hernia.

Malabsorption

Malabsorption may be *generalised* or *specific* where individual transport mechanisms or enzymes are defective. Generalised malabsorption presents with failure to thrive, growth retardation and steatorrhoea. Specific malabsorption may present with different features.

CAUSES OF MALABSORPTION

Generalised

Gut	Short gut syndrome, blind loop syndrome, chronic infection (giardiasis, immunodeficiency), coeliac disease, food intolerance (eg. cow's milk protein, soya) Diffuse mucosal lesions (eg. congenital microvillous atrophy)
Pancreas	Cystic fibrosis, chronic pancreatitis, Schwachman–Diamond syndrome
Liver	Cholestasis of any cause, eg. biliary atresia

Specific

Protein	Amino acid transport defects (eg. Hartnup disease, cysteinuria)
Carbohydrate	Disaccharidase deficiencies (eg. lactase, sucrase-isomaltase)
	Glucose-galactose malabsorption
Fat	Abetalipoproteinaemia
Elements	Chloride diarrhoea, acrodermatitis enteropathica (zinc)
Vitamins	Juvenile pernicious anaemia

INVESTIGATIONS

The list is exhaustive and therefore investigations must be symptom led. Some investigations to consider are:

Bloods	FBC, iron studies, bicarbonate, U&Es, creatinine, plasma lipids
	Coeliac screen, CF genotype
Stool	Electrolytes, fats, reducing substances
	Microscopy and culture (cysts, parasites)
	Faecal elastase ($\downarrow$) and α1-antitrypsin ($\uparrow$ in pancreatic insufficiency)
Sweat test	Looking for cystic fibrosis
Radiology	AXR, CXR, barium studies
Endoscopy	With biopsies and duodenal juice culture
Breath tests	Lactose, sucrose and lactulose breath tests (for bacterial overgrowth)

FOOD INTOLERANCES

Dietary protein intolerance

This is most commonly due to cow's milk protein (CMP) intolerance. Other protein intolerances occur to soya, fish, wheat and eggs.

Associations   Atopy, IgA deficiency

Clinical features

- *Diarrhoea, vomiting, failure to thrive*
- *Recurrent mouth ulcers, pancolitis*
- *History of contact allergy or anaphylaxis (rare) to cow's milk, family history of reaction to foods*
- *Atopic history (eczema, asthma)*

Investigations

Diagnosis may be established by:

1. *trial of cow's milk protein elimination diet without biopsy or*
2. *small intestinal biopsy – patchy, partial villous atrophy, eosinophils in lamina propria.*

Other investigations:

- *IgE $\uparrow$*
- *Eosinophilia*

Management

Elimination diet using casein-hydrosylate based formula. Breastfeeding mothers need to avoid cow's milk.

NB. 35–40% of children with CMP sensitivity also have soya sensitivity and need CMP and soya-free diet, eg. Nutramigen, Pregestamil, Peptijunior. 50% of children recover by one year and most of the rest by two years of age.

Postgastroenteritis intolerance

This is a transient condition, occurring after acute gastroenteritis and resulting in persistent diarrhoea (>14 days). Patients have usually developed a temporary intolerance to lactose secondary to cow's milk protein sensitisation. Diagnosis is on the history and presence of reducing substances in the stool (positive Clinitest). Test for glucose in the stool (Clinistix) is negative. The condition usually resolves after 2–3 days on a lactose-free diet. Other transient intolerances can develop (eg. to monosaccharides).

Lactose intolerance

Lactase, the enzyme necessary for digesting lactose (the sugar in milk), appears late in fetal life and falls after age three. 40% of Orientals have late-onset lactose intolerance.

Causes

1. *Transient postgastroenteritis*
2. *Primary lactase deficiency (very rare)*
3. *Late-onset lactase deficiency (common)*

Clinical features

After ingestion of lactose: explosive watery diarrhoea, abdominal distension, flatulence, loud borborygmi.

Investigations

1. *Stool chromatography positive for lactose (ie. > 1% present)*
2. *Lactose hydrogen breath test*

Management

- *Lactose-free formula feed for infants*
- *Milk-free diet with calcium supplements for older children*

SUCRASE-ISOMALTASE DEFICIENCY

Autosomal recessive. This is a congenital enzyme deficiency of the disaccharidases sucrase and isomaltase and is worth considering as a differential diagnosis in toddler's diarrhoea.

Symptoms are of diarrhoea and bloating. Sucrose may be seen in stool chromatography. This is not a reducing sugar. Enzyme assays show the specific deficiencies and hydrogen breath test is positive after sucrose ingestion. Management is with dietary sucrose restriction.

GLUCOSE-GALACTOSE MALABSORPTION

Autosomal recessive. This is due to a congenital deficiency of the glucose-galactose transport sites. The condition presents with severe diarrhoea, bloating and dehydration. Management is with glucose and galactose-free diet, using fructose-containing formula.

COELIAC DISEASE

A dietary *gliadin* intolerance resulting in small bowel mucosal damage. Gliadin, a fraction of the protein gluten, is in wheat, barley, oats and rye.

Associations   HLA-B8, DR3, DR7, DQW2

Presentation is usually with the introduction of dietary gluten at around 4–6 months.

Clinical features

- *Failure to thrive, anorexia, vomiting, diarrhoea*
- *Irritable, unhappy*
- *Abdominal pain, rectal prolapse, smelly stools*
- *Signs of pallor, abdominal distension, clubbing and malabsorption*

Investigations

IgA antiendomysial abs with total IgA level	Very sensitive and specific
	Antibodies not seen in IgA-deficient individuals
Jejunal biopsy	Gold standard
	Total or subtotal villous atrophy seen
Gluten challenge	Now only necessary in children diagnosed under two years, as they may be normal when > 2 years
Other findings include	Anaemia (dimorphic blood film from iron and folate deficiency)
	Hypoalbuminaemia
	Antibodies to gliadin, casein, reticulin (non-specific)

Associations

1. *Intestinal lymphoma*
2. *Oesophageal carcinoma*
3. *Malabsorption*
4. **Dermatitis herpetiformis** – *very itchy vesicles on extensor surfaces improve on a gluten-free diet. IgA abs in normal and perilesional skin but* not *active lesions. Treatment is with dapsone until diet effective. All children with dermatitis herpetiformis have coeliac disease.*
5. *IDDM*
6. *Selective IgA deficiency*

Management

Lifetime gluten-free diet (this reduces intestinal lymphoma risk).

Causes of villous atrophy on jejunal biopsy

Subtotal	Partial
Coeliac disease	Cow's milk protein intolerance
Giardia lamblia	Soya intolerance
Tropical sprue	Postgastroenteritis
Enteropathy	Immunodeficiency, eg. SCIDS, chemotherapy

INTESTINAL LYMPHANGIECTASIA

This is a group of disorders involving dilatation of the intestinal lymphatic vessels with leakage of lymph into the intestine and peritoneal cavity.

Associations   Noonan and Turner syndrome, Klippel–Trenauney–Weber syndrome

Causes
Congenital
Acquired   Lymphatic obstruction from abdominal or thoracic surgery, malrotation, right heart failure or constrictive pericarditis

Clinical features

- *Fat malabsorption with steatorrhoea*
- *Protein-losing enteropathy*
- *Lymphocyte depletion*
- *Anaemia*
- *Oedema*
- *Chylous ascites*
- *Hypoalbuminaemia and hypogammaglobulinaemia*
- *Features of vitamin E deficiency*

Diagnostic investigations

1. *Small bowel biopsy – distorted villi with dilated lacteals*
2. *Faecal α1-antitrypsin ↑ due to protein-losing enteropathy*
3. *Laparotomy (in some cases)*
4. *Lymphangiogram (generally unhelpful)*

Management

1. *High-protein, high medium chain triglyceride (MCT) diet*
2. *Fat-soluble vitamin supplements*

ABETALIPOPROTEINAEMIA

Autosomal recessive. Severe fat malabsorption with neuropathy secondary to vitamin E deficiency. Underlying deficiency of microsomal triglyceride transfer protein in the small bowel.

Clinical features

Gastrointestinal   Failure to thrive, steatorrhoea, abdominal distension
Neurological   (After age 10 years)
Ataxia (spinocerebellar degeneration), loss of proprioception and vibration sense, peripheral neuropathy and retinitis pigmentosa
Mental retardation and regression

Investigations

- Acanthocytes *in the blood (spiky red cells)*
- *Decreased cholesterol and triglycerides*
- *No vitamin E in serum*
- *Jejunal biopsy (fat accumulation in intestinal cells)*

Management

- *Supplements of fat-soluble vitamins (A, D, E and K)*
- *Special diet with increased MCTs*

SCHWACHMAN-DIAMOND SYNDROME

An inherited autosomal recessive condition, 1: 20 000 births, male: female = 1 : 2. The syndrome involves:

1. *pancreatic insufficiency (with subsequent malabsorption)*
2. *neutropenia – often cyclic, progression to myeloid arrest can occur*
3. *neutrophil chemotactic defects*
4. *metaphyseal dysostosis*
5. *thrombocytopenia (70%), anaemia (50%)*
6. *short stature and failure to thrive*
7. *high HbF*

Management is with pancreatic enzyme replacement therapy and steroids or androgens. Average survival time is 35 years. BMT and GCSF have been used.

Gastroenteritis

Causes

Viral   Rotavirus (winter epidemics, cause in 60% <2 years old in winter)
Norwalk virus, adenovirus (40 and 41), astrovirus
Bacterial   Staphylococcus (exotoxin)
Watery diarrhoea   *Enterotoxigenic E. coli* (ETEC, traveller's diarrhoea)
Vibrio cholerae

Bloody diarrhoea   *Enteroinvasive E. coli* (EIEC)
                    Enterohaemorrhagic E. coli (EHEC)
                    Shigella, *Campylobacter jejuni*,
                    Salmonella enteritidis, yersinia
Protozoal   Giardia, cryptosporidium, amoebiasis

Clinical features

- *Acute-onset vomiting and diarrhoea*
- *Abdominal pain and distension*
- *Mild pyrexia*
- *Invasive bacterial infection – unwell, high fever, blood and mucoid stool*

Differential diagnosis

Acute infection   Septicaemia, meningitis, UTI, respiratory infection
Surgical   Intussusception, appendicitis
Metabolic   Diabetic ketoacidosis
Other   Reye syndrome, coeliac disease

Examination findings

1. *Assess child for dehydration, which is difficult to do accurately. Below 5% dehydration there are not usually obvious clinical findings. The dehydration is usually hyponatraemic or isotonic.*
2. *Other possible findings:*   *Acidosis*   *- Hyperpnoea*
                                Potassium depletion   *- Hypotonia, weakness*
                                Hypocalcaemia   *- Neuromuscular irritability*
                                Hypoglycaemia   *- Lethargy, coma, convulsions*

DEHYDRATION ASSESSMENT

	Moderate 5–10%	Severe >10%
Condition	Restless/lethargic	Drowsy
Eyes	Sunken	Very sunken
Fontanelle	Sunken	Very sunken
Tears	Reduced	Absent
Mucous membranes	Dry	Very dry
Tissue elasticity	Reduced	Absent
Cap refill time	2–4 seconds	>4 seconds
Pulse	Tachycardia	Thready, very tachycardic
BP	Normal	Normal or low
Urine output	Reduced	Reduced/absent

Hypernatraemic dehydration

- *Unusual and potentially serious*
- *Irritable with doughy skin and relatively good circulation*

- *Water shifts from intracellular to extracellular and therefore the* signs of extracellular fluid loss are reduced
- *Rehydration should be slow (over 48 hours) to avoid rapid brain rehydration and subsequent raised intracranial pressure*

Investigations
These depend on the clinical state of the child.

Stool   Virology, M, C and S, 'hot stool' for cysts and ova
Bloods   FBC, haemtocrit, U and Es, creatinine, glucose, capillary blood gas
Plasma and urine osmolality, as necessary.

Management

Mild <5%   Oral rehydration therapy (ORT) for 24 hours or until diarrhoea settles, then milk and light diet. ORT fluid contains glucose and sodium because they are absorbed across even a damaged mucosa by a joint mechanism and water absorption follows by osmosis. NB. Breastfeeding can continue with initial ORT.

Moderate/severe >5%   Admit. If the CRT >3 seconds or acidotic breathing is apparent, intravenous rehydration is necessary.
If in shock: IV volume expansion with 20–30 ml/kg normal saline.
Then rehydrate over 24 hours.
Rehydration fluid: 1. Deficit = % dehydration $\times$ wt (kg)
                            2. Maintenance
                            3. Continuing loss
             Use N.saline with dextrose 5–10%
If severe acidosis (pH <7.0) treat with bicarbonate (half the deficit).

Maintenance fluid calculation

Weight	Fluid requirements
0–10 kg	100–120 ml/kg/24 h (4mls/kg/hr)
10–20 kg	1000 ml + 50 ml/kg/24 h (2mls/kg/hr) for each kg >10
>20 kg	1500 ml + 20 ml/kg/24 h (1ml/kg/hr) for each kg >20

Bicarbonate calculation
Half deficit (mmol) = wt (kg) $\times$ 5 $\times$ 0.3 $\times$ (24 − plasma bicarbonate)

Complications

1. *Renal*

- *Oliguria (<200 ml/m2/day or <0.5 ml/kg/h)*
  NB. If prerenal renal failure: Urine osmolality >500
  Urine Na <10 mmol/l
  Urine urea >250 mmol/l
  Urine: plasma osmolality ratio >1.3
- *Renal vein thrombosis (haematuria + renal mass)*
- *Haemolytic uraemic syndrome (haematuria + thrombocytopenia + fragmented red cells)*

Management of oliguria
Urgent intravenous volume re-expansion. If no recovery of renal function, then give minimal maintenance fluid plus losses only, with no potassium. Dialysis is necessary if the fluid, electrolyte or acid-base status does not correct. Recovery is seen with the polyuric phase of acute tubular necrosis.

2. *Pulmonary oedema, from fluid overload*
3. *Convulsions:*

- *Several possible causes: hypernatraemia, cerebral haemorrhage, hypoglycaemia, febrile convulsions, other electrolyte disturbance, cavernous sinus thrombosis*
- *Check blood glucose, U and Es, Mg, Ca and cranial USS and treat accordingly*

4. *Prolonged diarrhoea >14 days (see postgastroenteritis diarrhoea, p. 157)*

Diarrhoea

The pathogenesis of most episodes of diarrhoea can be explained by osmotic, secretory or motility disorders or a combination of these. In *osmotic diarrhoea* the underlying mechanism is a high osmotic load of intraluminal content and in *secretory diarrhoea* the mechanism is active chloride secretion.

Osmotic diarrhoea	Secretory diarrhoea
Common	Rare
Stops when feeding discontinued	Does not stop when feeding discontinued
Reducing substances in stool	Very watery, severe diarrhoea
Stool electrolytes ↓ (Na < 50 mEq/l)	Stool electrolytes ↑ (Na > 90 mEq/l)
Examples	*Examples*
Lactase deficiency	Cholera, toxigenic *E. coli*
Disaccharidase enzyme deficiencies	Congenital chloride diarrhoea
Drugs, eg. lactulose	Neural crest tumours, eg. carcinoid, VIP
Maldigestion, eg. Crohn's, CF	Bile salt/fatty acid malabsorption
Transport mechanism disorder	
eg. Glucose-galactose malabsorption	

Motility disorders

Increased motility   A decreased transit time results in diarrhoea
                        Causes include IBS, postvagotomy and dumping syndrome
Decreased motility   Bacterial overgrowth results in diarrhoea
                        Causes include intestinal pseudo-obstruction

Combined mechanisms

1. This occurs with *mucosal invasion*, resulting in inflammation, decreased colonic reabsorption and increased motility. This is seen in dysentery from bacterial infection (eg. salmonella) and amoebic infection.
2. A *decreased surface area* results in both osmotic and motility disorders, as seen in short bowel syndrome.

CAUSES OF DIARRHOEA

Chronic	Acute
Toddler diarrhoea	Gastroenteritis
Overflow constipation	Systemic infection
Anxiety	Toxic ingestion
Irritable bowel syndrome	
Postinfection	
Chronic infection (eg. giardia, cryptosporidium)	
Coeliac disease	
Food intolerance	
Pancreatic dysfunction	
Inflammatory bowel disease	
Hirschsprung disease	
Immunodeficiency	
Inborn error of metabolism, eg. congenital chloride diarrhoea	
Carbohydrate malabsorption, eg. sucrase-isomaltase deficiency	
Congenital lactase deficiency	
Protein-losing enteropathy, eg. intestinal lymphangiectasia	
Hyperthyroidism	

TODDLER'S DIARRHOEA

A chronic diarrhoea in infants, with loose stools at a frequency of 3–6 per day and normal growth and nothing abnormal on examination. The cause is not clearly understood and may be due to decreased gut transit time leading to colonic bacterial degradation of partially digested foods and subsequent release of secretagogues.

Management is with reassurance and dietary changes ($\uparrow$ fat, $\downarrow$ fibre, $\downarrow$ juice) to increase gut transit time. The condition usually resolves by three years spontaneously.

CHRONIC DIARRHOEA

Prolonged diarrhoea may be due to any of the above causes and the child will quickly become malnourished.

Investigations

Stool	M, C and S, reducing substances, fats and electrolytes
	Faecal elastase (pancreatic insufficiency)
Bloods	FBC (immunodeficiency?), electrolytes, ESR, CRP
	Coeliac screen (Antiendomysial IgA and total IgA)
AXR and CXR	Obstruction? bronchiectasis?
Sweat test	Cystic fibrosis?
Trial off oral feeds	(Secretory or osmotic diarrhoea)
Endoscopy	With small biopsy and duodenal juice culture (enteropathy, infection)

Management

Nutritional support while the diagnosis is being arrived at. A hypoallergenic modular feed with supplementation (eg. Neocate) can be tried at first. If enteral feeds fail then a period of TPN will be necessary.

A trial of metronidazole for five to seven days may be considered (as giardia is only usually detected in 20% of stool specimens).

Chronic abdominal pain

CAUSES

Psychiatric	Psychogenic recurrent abdominal pain
Abdominal	Constipation, food intolerance (including lactose intolerance), IBD, coeliac disease, Meckel's diverticulum, abdominal TB, peptic ulcer irritable bowel syndrome
Pancreas/liver	Chronic pancreatitis, cystic fibrosis, cholecystitis, chronic hepatitis
Renal	UTI, pyelonephritis, renal calculi
Metabolic	IDDM, porphyria, lead poisoning
CNS	Migraine
Other	Referred testicular pain, ovarian pain, sickle cell crisis

PSYCHOGENIC RECURRENT ABDOMINAL PAIN

This is a very common condition. In order to arrive at this diagnosis, a thorough history and examination must be done. It is defined as >3 episodes of life-altering pain per week for 3 months (Apley's criteria). Typical findings are:

- *pain periumbilical*
- *association with family history of migraine and irritable bowel syndrome*
- *no other findings of ill health*

NB. UTI must be excluded by checking urine sample. Any other investigations depend on the history.

Management involves giving a good explanation to parents and child and not dismissing the symptoms but explaining them (eg. as an increased sensitivity to bowel movements).

Rapid recovery is seen in 50%, slow recovery in 25%, and continuation of symptoms in 25%.

Peptic ulcer

Duodenal ulcers are seen in children with gastric ulcers being very rare.

Zollinger Ellison syndrome	Multiple ulcers due to a gastrin-secreting tumour (see p.273)
Association	*Helicobacter pylori* infection (this can be asymptomatic or cause chronic gastritis or peptic ulceration)

Clinical features

- *Intermittent abdominal pain, worse at night*
- *Nausea, vomiting*
- *Iron deficiency anaemia, gastrointestinal bleeding*

Investigations

1. *Endoscopy with biopsies*
2. *CLO test on biopsy specimen to detect H. pylori; H. pylori makes urease, which changes the colour in the agar.*

Management

- *H$_2$ antagonists or proton pump inhibitor (eg. omeprazole)*
- *Helicobacter pylori eradication therapy: omeprazole and a combination of two of amoxycillin, clarythromicin and metronidazole for 1–2 weeks*

Inflammatory bowel disease

CROHN'S DISEASE

A disease of chronic inflammation of the bowel, involving any part from the mouth to the anus, classically the terminal ileum, and the rectum is often spared. Incidence increasing, male = female.

Differential diagnosis

1. *Gastrointestinal TB*
2. *Infectious enteropathies, esp. Yersinia ileitis*
3. *Small bowel lymphoma*

Clinical features

Gastrointestinal	Abdominal pain, diarrhoea, anorexia, aphthous ulcers
	Abdominal mass, perianal lesions (tags, abscess, fistulae), stricture and fistulae common
Systemic features	Fever, malaise, weight loss, anaemia, nutritional deficiencies, growth retardation, amenorrhoea
Extraabdominal features	See box p.169

Investigations

Bloods	FBC, iron studies, folate, B_{12}, ESR, CRP, LFTs, serum proteins ($\downarrow$)
	Yersinia serology
Stool microscopy and culture	Enterocolitides (salmonella, shigella, campylobacter, *entamoeba histolytica*)
Plain AXR	Partial small bowel obstruction, *thumb-printing* colon wall
Barium meal and follow-through	*Cobblestone appearance* (linear ulcers), deep fissures
	Strictures and fistulae common, discontinuous disease with normal "*skip*" lesions
Upper endoscopy and ileocolonoscopy with biopsies	
Histology of lesions	Non-caseating granulomas, transmural inflammation, patchy involvement

Management options

Polymeric elemental diets	Effective as initial therapy instead of steroids. Give elemental feed (eg. Modulin IBD, AL110) for eight weeks orally or via NG tube, as tolerated.
Steroids	Oral or IV. High dose for 3–4 weeks, then alternate days and reduce as able
Aminosalicylates	Sulphasalazine or olsalazine for colon disease
	Delayed-release 5-ASA (Asacol) for terminal small bowel disease
Azathioprine	If steroid dependent or not responding
Metronidazole or ciprofloxacin	If fistulae or peranal disease
Steroid creams	For perianal disease
TPN	May be necessary temporarily
Surgery	Reserved for special indications as recurrence risk high
	Resection of disease unresponsive to medical therapy (right hemicolectomy or sub-total colectomy)
	Abscess, perforation, obstruction, bleeding

ULCERATIVE COLITIS

This is a chronic inflammatory disease of the colon with ulceration, classically involving large bowel from the rectum upwards. Small bowel may be involved. Incidence: male = female.

Differential diagnosis
Crohn's colitis, amoebic colitis, bacillary dysentery.

Clinical features
Gastrointestinal	Diarrhoea with blood and mucus
General	Anaemia (iron loss from bleeding), growth retardation (malabsorption rare)
Extra-abdominal features	See box below (p. 169)

Investigations
Blood tests	FBC (Hb$\downarrow$, leucocytosis), iron studies, B$_{12}$, LFTs, ESR, CRP, albumin ($\downarrow$)
AXR	Decreased haustrations
	Dilated colon, NB. *Toxic megacolon* = colon width >2.5 vertebrae
Double contrast barium (air) enema	Continous pathology, '*Collar button ulcers*', '*lead pipe*' (smooth) colon, *backwash ileitis*, double contour
Colonoscopy with biopsies	
Histology of lesions	Mucosal involvement only, gland destruction, crypt abscesses, decreased goblet cells, pseudopolyps, friability, ulceration

Management options
Aminosalicylates	Oral, eg. sulphasalazine. For mild colitis and prevention of relapses
Enemas	Aminosalicylate or steroid for left sided disease distal to splenic flexure
Steroids	Oral or intravenous at 1–2 mg/kg/day, prednisolone equivalent (maximum dose 40 mg), for cases unresponsive to aminosalicylates
Other drugs	Azathioprine, 6-MP, cyclosporin, tacrolimus, metronidazole may be used in steroid-dependent or uncontrolled disease
TPN	In preparation for surgery
Surgery	Colectomy is performed for fulminant disease unresponsive to medical therapy or pancolitis of >10 years' duration

Complications

- *Toxic megacolon*
- *Fulminating colitis*
- *Colon cancer (longterm), therefore regular colonoscopy after >10 years active disease*

Extraabdominal features of Crohn's disease and ulcerative colitis

There are many extraabdominal features associated with inflammatory bowel disease. Some are more common in Crohn's disease and others in ulcerative colitis.

Crohn's (most commonly)	Both equally	Ulcerative colitis (most commonly)
Erythema nodosum	Uveitis	Pyoderma gangrenosum
Peripheral arthritis	Conjunctivitis	Ankylosing spondylitis
Aphthous ulcers	Fatty liver	Sclerosing cholangitis
Clubbing	Cholangiocarcinoma	Chronic active hepatitis
Episcleritis		Cirrhosis
Renal stones (oxalate, uric acid)		Pericholangitis
Gall stones		

Constipation

This is a difficulty in defaecation. When prolonged, there is overflow diarrhoea due to liquid faeces escaping around a hard lump of faeces in the rectum.

NB. Important differential diagnosis is Hirschsprung disease.

Causes

Non-organic

Organic	Intake	Low-residue diet, dehydration
	Gut	Hirschsprung disease, stricture
	Metabolic	Hypothyroidism, cystic fibrosis, hypercalcaemia
	Neuromuscular	Cerebral palsy, spinal cord lesions, myotonic dystrophy, absent abdominal wall muscles
	Drugs	Narcotics, antidepressants

Complications

1. *Short-term constipation. This quickly resolves with fluids and stool softeners, usually with no sequelae.*
2. *Long-term constipation:*

   - *acquired megacolon (decreased sensation of a full rectum)*
   - *anal fissures*
   - *overflow incontinence*
   - *behavioural problems (fear of defaecation, embarrassment of overflow)*

Clinical findings

Hard faeces on abdominal examination

PR Not always necessary
Faecal mass, soiled anal region, sacral tuft (spina bifida occulta)
Sphincter tone ($\downarrow$ in simple constipation, $\uparrow$ in Hirschsprung disease)
AXR Loaded with faeces

Management

1. *Positive reinforcement*
2. *Increase fluids and fibre intake*
3. *Oral medications:*

   - *softener, eg. lactulose, paraffin oil*
   - *stimulant, eg. Senekot, sodium picosulphate*
   - *bulking agent, eg. Fibogel*

4. *Enema if necessary for disimpaction, eg. phosphate enema*
5. *Anal fissure treatment with local topical anaesthetic cream*

HIRSCHSPRUNG DISEASE

Incidence: 1 in 5000. Polygenic inheritance, 3–5% recurrence.

Associations Down syndrome
Lawrence–Moon–Beidel syndrome
Waardenburg syndrome

This disease is due to the absence of parasympathetic ganglions in Auerbach's and Meissner's plexi. The unopposed sympathetic activity results in hypertonus of the affected segment of bowel. The disease occurs from the rectum upwards.
There are two types:

1. *Short aganglionic segment – common, male > female*
2. *Long aganglionic segment – rare, male = female, familial*

Presentation

Neonatal (>80%) Acute obstruction
Older child Chronic constipation, history of delayed passage of meconium (>48 hours), failure to thrive

Investigations

AXR	Constipation
Barium enema	Narrow aganglionic segment, dilated proximal segment
Rectal biopsy	1. Rectal suction biopsy (mucosa + submucosa)
	2. Full thickness biopsy
Anorectal manometry	Failure of internal sphincter pressure to drop with rectal distension
Histology of affected bowel	Acetycholinesterase staining shows *increased* number of hypertrophied nerve bundles that stain positively for acetylcholinesterase

Management

This is surgical, with an immediate definitive repair or a temporary neonatal colostomy with definitive repair at 3–6 months of age. Definitive repair is with direct resection and anastomosis or an endorectal pull-through.

Ultrashort segment disease can be treated with anal dilatation and partial sphincterotomy.

ENCOPRESIS

This is the passage of faeces into inappropriate places. It is a complex psychological condition, requiring the input of a child psychiatrist.

Pancreatitis

ACUTE PANCREATITIS

This involves inflammation of the pancreas with autodigestion, localised necrosis and haemorrhage. Complications can be severe.

Causes

Biliary sludging	
Congenital abnormalities	
Blunt abdominal trauma	
Viral infections	Mumps, varicella, measles, EBV, coxsackie virus
Drugs	Azathioprine, steroids, total parenteral nutrition
Diseases associated	HUS, Kawasaki disease, bone marrow transplant, brain tumour

Clinical features

- *Abdominal pain (epigastric, radiating straight through to the back), nausea, vomiting, fever*
- *Tender abdomen, guarding, absent or obstructed bowel sounds, abdominal mass*
- Acute haemorrhagic pancreatitis:
  - *Very unwell, shocked, jaundiced*
  - Cullen sign *(bluish periumbilical region)*
  - Grey Turner sign *(bluish flanks)*
  - *50% mortality with DIC, renal failure, RDS*
  - *Sepsis, gastrointestinal bleeding*

Investigations

Serum amylase	> 500 iu/l seen in first 72 hours
Other bloods	FBC (leucocytosis), glucose ($\uparrow$), Ca ($\downarrow$), Clotting screen (prolonged clotting), LFTs (raised)
CXR	Left pleural effusion, atelectasis

AXR	Ileus, ascites, pseudocyst, pancreatic calcification (in recurrent disease)
USS and/or CT abdo	Oedematous pancreas, abscess, pseudocyst

Management

1. *Analgesia*
2. *Keep NBM with intravenous fluids and nasogastric suctioning until amylase normal. Treat shock if necessary*
3. *Fluid and electrolyte balance with careful monitoring*
4. *Surgical drainage if abscess or pseudocyst*

CHRONIC PANCREATITIS

Causes

Hereditary	Autosomal dominant. Progressively more severe attacks
Congenital pancreatic or biliary ductal anomalies	
Predisposing disorders	Hyperlipidaemia, cystic fibrosis, ascariasis, Wilson disease Cystinuria, hyperparathyroidism, cystinosis, α1-antitrypsin disease, drugs

Complications

Pancreatic pseudocysts, calcifications and pancreatic insufficiency.

Investigations

As for acute pancreatitis.
Also check: Sweat test
Stools for ascaris
ERCP (necessary prior to any surgery)

Management

Endoscopic treatment with sphincterotomy, pancreatic or biliary endoprostheses and stone extraction is possible as necessary.

Gastrointestinal tract bleeding

This has many causes, the frequency of which depends on the age of the child.

Clinical presentations

- *Haematemesis – fresh blood or 'coffee grounds'* (altered by gastric juices)
- *Melaena (altered blood per rectum) – tarry smelly stool*

- *Fresh rectal bleeding*
- *Massive bleeding with collapse*
- *Small bleeds with iron deficiency anaemia*

Causes

Infant	Child	Adolescent
Swallowed maternal blood	Colonic polyps (painless)	Bacterial infections
Haemorrhagic disease of	Anal fissure	IBD
the newborn	Bacterial infections	Anal fissure
NEC	Intussusception	Colonic polyps
Cow's milk protein allergy	Mallory–Weiss tear	Peptic ulcer/gastritis
Anal fissure	HUS	Mallory–Weiss tear
Intussusception	Henoch–Schönlein Purpura	Oesophageal varices
Volvulus	Oesophageal varices	Telangiectasia
Meckel's diverticulum	Meckel's diverticulum	
	Oesophagitis	
	Peptic ulcer/gastritis	
	IBD	
	AV malformation, haemangioma	
	Telangiectasia	
	Sexual abuse	

Investigations and management

1. *Assess circulation and resuscitate if necessary*
2. *Bloods – FBC, clotting studies, iron studies*
3. *Faecal occult bloods*
4. *Endoscopy – this is the emergency management also. For varices oesophageal banding, sclerotherapy and insertion of a Sengstaken–Blakemore tube may be employed*
5. *Laparotomy if necessary*

Swallowed maternal blood

This is a common event with small babies. Maternal blood is identified with the APT test.

APT test: Bloody vomit or stool is mixed with water, centrifuged and the supernatant mixed with 1% sodium hydroxide.
If it remains pink = infant blood
If it turns brown = maternal blood

Gastrointestinal tract tumours

JUVENILE COLONIC POLYPS

These occur in 3–4% population in the colon only. Symptoms usually occur between 2 and 10 years. Uncommon >15 years. They are usually benign hamartomas (unless they have an adenomatous element).

Presentation

Bright red rectal bleeding, autolysis, prolapse of a polyp, anaemia, abdominal pain (unusual).

Diagnosis

Rectal examination, colonoscopy with polyp removal, barium enema.

FAMILIAL POLYPOSIS SYNDROMES

Familial adenomatous polyposis coli (FAP)

Autosomal dominant, incidence 1 in 8000, premalignant condition. The APC (adenomatous polyposis coli) gene has been identified on the long arm of chromosome 5; many different mutations may occur within this gene, resulting in FAP. Multiple adenomas occur on the distal bowel (100–1000), onset <10 years.

Annual colonoscopy needed after age 10 and pancolectomy after 10 years of disease.

Congenital hypertrophy of the retinal pigment epithelium (CHRPE)
Seen in association with APC gene mutations (55–75%). When present CHRPE lesions are an early clinical marker for familial polyposis coli and may be used in risk assessment.

Turcot syndrome
APC gene defects
Primary medulloblastoma
Multiple colorectal polyposis

Gardner syndrome
APC gene defect
Multiple colorectal polyps
Soft tissue and bone tumours (especially the mandible)
Extracolonic cancers

Peutz–Jegers syndrome

Autosomal dominant, 50% new mutations.
Syndrome of:

- *mucosal pigmentation (freckles) of lips and gums*
- *stomach and small bowel hamartomas*
- *malignant tumours (not of the GI tract) develop in 50% of patients*

ENDOCRINE TUMOURS

1. *APUDomas – these hormone-secreting tumours arise from APUD cells (neural crest cell derivatives of the gastroenteropancreatic endocrine system). They are:*
   - *carcinoid*
   - *VIPomas, gastrinoma (see p. 273)*
   - *mastocytoma, medullary carcinoma thyroid, somatostatinoma*
2. *Neurogenic tumours:*
   - *ganglioneuroma*
   - *phaeochromocytoma (see p. 258)*

NB. **APUD** = **a**mine **p**recursor **u**ptake and **d**ecarboxylation

Carcinoid tumours

These tumours of the intestine usually arise in the appendix in children. They are benign or low-grade malignancy and when symptomatic present as appendicitis. Tumours elsewhere in the GI tract are likely to metastasise. They produce the *carcinoid syndrome*, the result of serotonin (5-HT) and other hormone production, when *metastatic.*

Carcinoid syndrome

- *All have liver metastases*
- *Intestinal hypermobility, with watery diarrhoea and abdominal pain*
- *Bluish-red facial flushing with telangiectasia*
- *Bronchoconstriction*
- *Tricuspid incompetence or pulmonary stenosis*
- *Diagnosis:*
  urine 5HIAA ↑ *(serotonin metabolite)*
  Plasma serotonin ↑
  Bradykinin, histamine, tachykinins and/or prostaglandins ↑

Management

- *Resection of primary tumour if possible*
- *Octeotride (somatostatin analogue) inhibits release of gut hormones*

Failure to thrive

This is the failure to gain adequate weight or achieve adequate growth during infancy. The child falls across two major centiles.

CAUSES

Organic	Non-organic
1. *Inadequate food intake*	1. *Undernutrition*
Breastfeeding poorly	Poor parental understanding
Bottle feeds too dilute	Low income
Exclusion diets	Poor social support
Cleft palate	2. *Child abuse*
Vomiting/reflux	Deliberate starvation
2. *Malabsorption*	Parental psychiatric illness
Pancreatic disease	
Short gut syndrome	
Enteropathy, eg. coeliac, giardia,	
Cow's milk protein intolerance	
3. *Increased loss of nutrients*	
Protein-losing enteropathy	
Protein intolerance	
4. *Chronic illness*	
Cardiac, renal, respiratory, GIT	
5. *Increased energy requirements*	
Tumour, catabolic state	
6. *Metabolic*	
Hypothyroidism	
Congenital adrenal hyperplasia	

Nutritional disorders

MALNUTRITION

Malnutrition has traditionally been classified into marasmus, kwashiorkor and marasmic–kwashiorkor. A new classification based on wasting (weight for height ratios) and stunting (height for age and sex ratios) using standard scores has been devised.

Marasmus
This is a mixed deficiency of both protein and calories, resulting in non-oedematous malnutrition. Decreased weight for age and sex ratios (<60% of the mean average).

Features

- *Hungry, emaciated child*
- *Loose, wrinkled skin, 'old man' appearance, decreased skin turgor*
- *Muscle atrophy and little subcutaneous fat*
- *Thin sparse hair, hair colour changes unusual*

- *Hypothermia, bradycardia, hypotension (basal metabolic rate ↓)*
- *Listlessness*

Kwashiorkor *oedema*

This malnutrition results in oedema which is due to unknown causes, though it has historically been attributed to a disproportionately low protein intake compared with calorie intake. There is a near normal weight for age ratio (weight for age and sex ratio <80%) and oedema.

Features

- *Lethargy, miserable, no appetite*
- Oedema – *hypoalbuminaemic, overall 'fatness' appearance, moon face*
- *Hepatomegaly (fatty infiltration)*
- *Skin lesions (flaking paint rash, ulcers, fissures, pellagra-type rash)*
- *Thin, red hair and darkened skin*
- *Cardiomegaly*
- *Infections, secondary immunodeficiency*

Marasmic kwashiorkor (mixed type)

A combined type exists where there are features of both marasmus and kwashiorkor, with a weight for age and sex ratio of <60% with oedema.

Management

1. *Initial rehydration*
2. *Dilute milk for five days, increasing volume gradually to 150 ml/kg/day*
3. *High-energy feeds as strength builds up*

NB. If feeds are too strong too early, hepatomegaly and a slower recovery result.

ACRODERMATITIS ENTEROPATHICA (ZINC DEFICIENCY)

Autosomal recessive. This is an inability to absorb sufficient zinc.

Clinical features

Skin   Eczematous, vesicobullous, scaly or psoriaform rash. Symmetrical distribution involving cheeks, elbows, knees, perioral region and perineum Dystrophic nails, glossitis and stomatitis

Hair   Red with areas of alopecia

Eyes   Photophobia, conjunctivitis, blepharitis, corneal dystrophy

Growth   Retardation

Others   Irritability, delayed wound healing, chronic diarrhoea, recurrent bacterial and candida infections

Diagnosis is made on clinical suspicion with confirmation with low plasma zinc level.

Management is with oral zinc supplementation with monitoring of plasma levels. Any other cause of zinc deficiency results in the same clinical features.

SCURVY (VITAMIN C – ASCORBIC ACID – DEFICIENCY)

Ascorbic acid is a reducing agent involved in collagen synthesis. It is found in fruit and vegetables, oxidised by heat and leaks into water.

Deficiency features

1. *Perifollicular haemorrhages, follicular hyperkeratosis and 'corkscrew' hair on back, arms and legs*
2. *Spontaneous bruising and bleeding with subperiosteal haemorrhages of long bones*
3. *Swollen, spongy gums*
4. *Delayed wound healing*
5. *Irritability*
6. *Muscle pain and weakness, pseudoparalysis of the legs*
7. *Anaemia*

Diagnosis is made by checking plasma ascorbic acid levels or giving a trial of vitamin C. Management is with oral vitamin C 1 g/day.

PELLAGRA (NIACIN DEFICIENCY)

A lack of niacin (nicotinamide) results in this condition. Niacin forms part of the enzymes NAD (nicotinamide adenine dinucleotidase) and NADP (nicotinamide adenine dinucleotide phosphatase). It is found in fish and meat and in small amount in cereals. Niacin can be made from tryptophan (found in milk and eggs).

Features of deficiency

Dermatitis Erythema on sun-exposed areas ('Casals' necklace' on the neck), hyperkeratosis, ulcers, progressing to atrophy. Red tongue and angular stomatitis

Dementia Tremor, depression, encephalopathy, psychosis

Diarrhoea Also constipation

Management is with oral nicotinamide or vitamin B complex therapy. Other causes include:

- *isoniazid (causes B$_6$ deficiency, needed for nicotinamide manufacture)*
- *generalised malabsorption, low-protein diets*
- *Hartnup disease (tryptophan not absorbed)*
- *Phaeochromocytoma, carcinoid (metabolism of niacin altered)*

VITAMIN A DEFICIENCY

Vitamin A (retinol) is found in milk, eggs, liver and green vegetables. Deficiency occurs with dietary deficiency (rare), fat malabsorption, liver disease.

Clinical features

Eyes	Night blindness, xerophthalmia, photophobia, keratomalacia and blindness
Developmental delay	
Growth retardation	
Skin	Follicular hyperkeratosis, dry and scaly

Diagnosis can be confirmed with low vitamin A levels. Management is with oral vitamin A.

BERIBERI (THIAMINE DEFICIENCY)

Thiamine (vitamin B_1) is a cofactor for many enzyme reactions. It is found in most foods, especially legumes. Deficiency occurs with dietary deficiency (eg. polished rice only diet, alcoholics) and babies breastfed by a deficient mother. Clinical features involve cardiac and neurological problems.

Cardiac features	Dilated heart with cardiac failure and oedema
(wet beriberi)	Tachycardia, tachypnoea, hepatomegaly, QT prolongation
Neurological features	Slow onset
(dry beriberi)	Symmetrical polyneuropathy, commencing with lower limbs (absent lower limb tendon reflexes, paraesthesias, loss of vibration sense)
	CNS involvement (Wernicke–Korsakoff syndrome):

1. *Occular*   *Nystagmus, papilloedema, lateral rectus palsies Conjugate gaze palsies, fixed pupils, ptosis, optic atrophy*
2. *Ataxia*   *Cerebellar signs*
3. *Confusion* *Irritability, amnesia, apathy and coma*

Diagnosis is based on a rapid clinical response to therapy. Management is with IV or IM thiamine if in cardiac failure. Otherwise oral thiamine is given to the mother and child.

Eating disorders

ANOREXIA NERVOSA

This is seen mostly in teenagers and in Western countries. Females > males, 10: 1. Complex family dynamics involved. The 1994 DSM-IV criteria are:

- *a fear of becoming obese*
- *a disturbance of perception of body size, shape and weight*
- *refusal to maintain body weight over the age/height minimum*
- *amenorrhoea*

The typical psychological profile includes: overachiever, poor self-esteem, distorted body image, strong-willed, distrustful, irritable, uncommunicative, obsessive thoughts of food and body shape.

Physical features

Body weight	Below expected for age/height
Skin	Dry skin, fine *lanugo* hair on face
Cardiac	Bradycardia, BP ↓ with pronounced postural drop, long QT interval, arrhythmias (may cause sudden death)
Hormones	GH↑, T3↓, rT3↑, hypothalamic–pituitary–ovarian disorders (amenorrhoea)
	Loss of diurnal variation in cortisol
Electrolyte	Disturbances (eg. K ↓ and hypochloraemic alkalosis due to vomiting)
Other	Hypothermia, constipation

Management

This is with a combination of expert psychotherapy and nutritional rehabilitation.

BULIMIA

More common than anorexia nervosa. This is characterised by high-calorie binge eating followed by purging, laxative abuse and/or episodes of fasting. The individual is usually of normal weight or mildly overweight. Diagnosis is made by history. Electrolyte and cardiac abnormalities as for anorexia nervosa may occur. Teeth enamel erosion, salivary gland enlargement and cheilosis may be seen from recurrent vomiting.

OBESITY

Infants/children	Body mass index (BMI) >85th percentile. This is commonly due to overfed infants and children and lack of exercise.
Other causes	Prader–Willi syndrome (gene probe available), Laurence–Moon–Beidel syndrome, Cushing's syndrome.
Problems	Advanced bone age, increased height (early), early puberty
	Psychological effects (poor self-image, depression)
	Sleep apnoea (severe obesity)
	Obesity throughout life increased
	Long-term effects: hypertension, diabetes, cardiovascular disease

FURTHER READING

Walker WA, Durie PR, Hamilton JR, Walker-Smith JA, Watkins JBBC Eds. *Pediatric Gastrointestinal disease*, 3rd Ed, Mosby, Philadelphia, 2000

7

Liver

- *Physiology and anatomy*
- *Clinical manifestations of liver disease*
- *Jaundice*
- *Metabolic disorders*
- *Congenital hepatic fibrosis*

- *Hepatitis*
- *Portal hypertension*
- *Gall bladder disease*
- *Liver transplantation*

Physiology and anatomy

FUNCTIONS

Protein

Metabolism Principal site of synthesis of all circulating proteins (except γ globulins), eg. albumin, coagulation factors (except factor VIII), complement system components, carrier proteins (transferrin, caeruloplasmin), α-fetoprotein, and α1-antitrypsin. Factors II, VII, IX and X are vitamin K dependent.

Degradation Amino acids are deaminated. The amino groups and ammonia are converted to urea

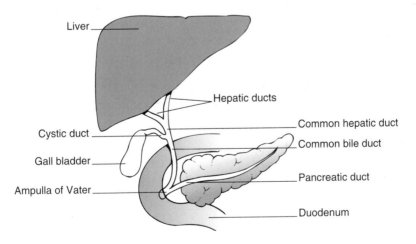

Figure 7.1 Anatomy of the liver and ducts

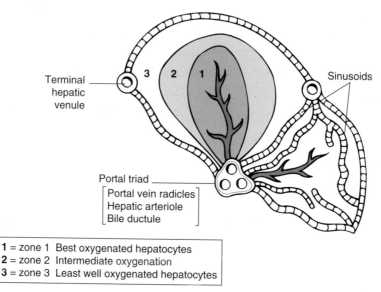

Figure 7.2 A functional liver acinus

Carbohydrate metabolism

Postprandially, glucose converted to glycogen and stored, and to fatty acids and transported to adipose tissue. In starvation, glucose released from glyogen (**glycogenolysis**) and glucose synthesised from amino acids, lactate and glycerol (**gluconeogenesis**). Preterm infants have inefficient regulation of this.

Lipid metabolism

Synthesis of lipoproteins VLDL and HDL, fatty acid oxidation and cholesterol excretion. Young infants have reduced capacity for hepatic ketogenesis.

Bile

Bile acids	Synthesis from cholesterol
Bilirubin metabolism	See Figure 7.3
Bile secretion	Containing bile acids, water, bilirubin, electrolytes, cholesterol and phospholipids. Neonates have inefficient ileal reabsorption and hepatic clearance of bile acids from portal blood and therefore raised serum levels of bile acids

Hormone and drug metabolism

Many hormones inactivated in the liver or targeted to the liver. Drugs metabolised by enzymes including the P450 system (eg. alcohol). Newborn infant has decreased capacity to metabolise certain drugs.

Immunological function

Involving the reticuloendothelial system of the liver. Kupffer cell (macrophages on endothelium) functions include:

- *phagocytosis*
- *secretion of interleukins, TNF, collagenase and lysosomal hydrolases*

IMPORTANT INVESTIGATIVE LIVER BLOOD TESTS

Laboratory tests examine the functions of the liver and include markers of liver cell damage. As the liver has a very large functional reserve, functional tests alter later in disease.

Albumin
Synthetic function marker.

Prothrombin time (PT)
Synthetic function marker. Very sensitive (as short half-life). NB. Must exclude vitamin K deficiency as cause of prolonged PT.

Bilirubin
Raised bilirubin level may be:

- *conjugated = 'direct' reading*
- *or unconjugated = 'indirect' reading*

Aminotransferases (transaminases)
Enzymes in hepatocytes which leak into blood with liver cell damage (also raised in increased red cell degradation). Sensitive markers.

1. *Aspartate aminotransferase (AST) – mitochondrial enzyme, also in heart, muscle, kidney, brain*
2. *Alanine aminotransferase (ALT) – cytosol enzyme, more specific to liver than AST*

Alkaline phosphatase (AP)
In canalicular and sinusoidal membranes. Also in bone, intestine and placenta. Isoenzymes used to determine specific origin. Raised in cholestasis, cirrhosis and liver metastases.

γ-Glutamyl transpeptidase (γGT)
Microsomal enzyme which increases in cholestasis and is induced by some drugs (eg. phenytoin, alcohol).

Serum proteins

- *Albumin (hypoalbuminaemia as above)*
- *Globulins (hyperglobulinaemia due to decreased phagocytosis of antigens by Kupffer cells)*
- *Immunoglobulins (raised in chronic disease)*

α-Fetoprotein
Normally produced by the foetal liver. Seen in teratomas, hepatocellular carcinoma, hepatitis, chronic liver disease and in pregnancy with foetal neural tube defects.

Immunological tests

- *Antimitochondrial antibody (AMA) in primary biliary cirrhosis and autoimmune hepatitis*
- *Antinuclear (ANA), antismooth muscle (ASM) and liver/kidney microsomal (LKMA) antibodies seen in autoimmune hepatitis*

Other biochemical alterations

Hypoglycaemia, electrolyte imbalance, hyperammonaemia.

Clinical manifestations of liver disease

Liver disease may be acute or chronic and may manifest with the following.

ACUTE LIVER DISEASE

- *Asymptomatic*
- *General malaise (fever, anorexia)*
- *Hypoglycaemia*
- *Hepatomegaly*
- *Jaundice*
- *Pruritis*
- *Spider naevi and liver palms (rare in acute)*
- *Encephalopathy, bleeding disorders and renal impairment may occur*

CHRONIC LIVER DISEASE

Asymptomatic	
Anorexia	
Liver size	Increased (hepatomegaly), decreased or no change
Jaundice	
Pruritis	Seen in cholestasis, due to conjugated hyperbilirubinaemia
Other skin changes	Palmar erythema, spider naevi (telangiectasia in the distribution of the superior vena cava), xanthomata, purpura, clubbing
Portal hypertension	An increase in portal venous pressure to >10–12 mmHg Caput medusae, varices, splenomegaly
Ascites	Due to hydrostatic pressure from sinusoidal blockade and hypoalbuminaemia
Encephalopathy	Portosystemic encephalopathy (PSE), a chronic syndrome involving neuropsychiatric disturbance, drowsiness, foetor hepaticus and liver flap. Due to metabolic abnormalities
Endocrine abnormalities	Testicular atrophy, gynaecomastia, parotid enlargement
Renal abnormalities	Secondary impairment of renal function. Hepatorenal syndrome (renal failure of no other demonstrable cause in a patient with cirrhosis)
Gastrointestinal bleeding	Due to coagulation dysfunction and portal hypertension

FULMINANT HEPATIC FAILURE (FHF)

This is an acute clinical syndrome resulting from massive impairment or necrosis of hepatocytes in a patient without pre-existing chronic liver disease. The prognosis is poor with a mortality without transplant of around 70%.

Causes

Viral hepatitis	Combined B and D especially
Drugs	eg. paracetamol, sodium valproate
Hypoxic liver damage	
Metabolic disorders	eg. Wilson disease, galactosaemia, neonatal haemochromatosis, mitochondrial cytopathy, tyrosinaemia

Clinical manifestations

- *Progressive jaundice, foetor hepaticus, fever, vomiting, abdominal pain*
- *Rapid decrease in liver size with no clinical improvement (ominous sign)*
- *Defective coagulation*
- *Hypoglycaemia*
- *Sepsis*
- *Fluid overload*
- *Occult gastrointestinal or intracranial bleeding*
- *Pancreatitis*
- *Hepatic encephalopathy with cerebral oedema (lethargy, sleep rhythm disturbance, confusion, progressing to coma)*

Poor prognostic features

- *Onset of liver failure <7 days*
- *<10 years*
- *Shrinking liver size*
- *Renal failure*
- *Paracetamol overdose*
- *Hypersensitivity reactions of unknown aetiology*

Investigations

1. *PT↑*
2. *Transaminases (raised initially, then may decrease with no clinical improvement, indicating little or no functioning liver remaining)*
3. *Ammonia↑*
4. *Glucose↓*
5. *Hyperbilirubinaemia (conjugated and unconjugated)*
6. *Metabolic acidosis, K↓, Na↓*
7. *EEG (monitor of cerebral activity, occult seizures may be present)*

Management

The aims of management include close monitoring to prevent complications, maintenance of blood glucose >4 mmol/l, support of the cardiovascular, renal and respiratory systems and close monitoring of CNS function. Liver transplant should be considered early if recovery is considered unlikely.

Specific management includes the following:

- *Fluid restriction to 50–75% maintenance (to avoid ICP↑)*
- *Use colloid to maintain intravascular volume*
- *Sodium and potassium additives depending on electrolytes*
- *Maintain blood glucose with IV hypertonic glucose as needed*
- *Monitor with CVP, MAP, urine output, ICP, blood gases, serum electrolyte and glucose status*

Cerebral complications	Avoid sedation as this masks encephalopathy
	Monitor for ↑ICP and maintain normal ICP with mannitol, hyperventilation, thiopentone and haemofiltration as necessary
	Convulsions may be occult and EEG or cerebral function monitoring should be performed if concern exists. Any convulsions are treated (eg. phenytoin IV, paraldehyde in oil PR, phenobarbitone IV or thiopentone IV may be required)
Renal	Nephrotoxic drugs and arterial hypotension should be avoided. Hepatorenal syndrome may occur
	Established renal failure treated with haemofiltration
Sepsis	Daily culturing for infection and empirical use of broad-spectrum antibiotics with antifungals. Acyclovir if herpetic origin suspected
Bleeding	Vitamin K IV given daily. Avoid invasive procedures if possible
Respiratory	ARDS equivalent may occur
Cardiovascular	Inotropic support as required. Prostacyclin or N-acetyl cysteine may improve microcirculation
Gastrointestinal	Prophylaxis for stress ulceration with IV ranitidine or omeprazole. GI haemorrhage managed with blood products and emergency endoscopy as necessary

CIRRHOSIS

This is a histological diagnosis identified by **fibrosis and nodule formation** with **abnormal liver architecture** and results from necrosis of liver cells. It may be macronodular (nodules up to 5 cm), micronodular (nodules <3 mm) or mixed. Progressive scarring in cirrhosis leads to restricted blood flow with further impairment of liver function and portal hypertension.

Causes

- *Acute viral hepatitis*
- *Autoimmune CAH, primary biliary cirrhosis*
- *Metabolic liver disease eg. Wilson disease, tyrosinaemia*

- *Veno-occlusive disease (especially post BMT)*
- *Alcohol (adults)*
- *Idiopathic*

The prognosis is variable and the five-year survival rate is around 50%, depending on the aetiology.

CAUSES OF HEPATOMEGALY

Inflammation
Hepatitis viral, bacterial, toxic
Autoimmune chronic hepatitis, SLE, sarcoidosis, sclerosing cholangitis

Tumour
Primary neoplasm hepatoblastoma, hepatocellular carcinoma, haemangioma
Secondary deposits Leukaemia, lymphoma, neuroblastoma, histiocytosis

Posthepatic portal hypertension
Hepatic vein obstruction
Cardiac failure, pericardial tamponade (constrictive pericarditis)

Biliary obstruction
Extrahepatic obstruction

Haematological
Sickle cell disease, thalassaemia, spherocytosis

Metabolic disease
Fatty liver   Reye syndrome, TPN, CF, IDDM
Lipid storage disease   Gaucher, Neimann-Pick, Wolman syndrome
Glycogen storage disease GSD 1, GSD 3, GSD 6
Other   Wilson disease, haemochromatosis, α1-antitrypsin disease

Cysts
Polycystic, hydatid

Apparent
Chest hyperexpansion due to lung disease, Reidel's lobe.

Jaundice (Icterus)

Serum bilirubin >35 μmol/l is clinically detectable. Jaundice is traditionally classified as prehepatic, hepatocellular and obstructive (cholestatic) but this is inaccurate, as cholestasis occurs in hepatocellular as well as obstructive jaundice. It may help to consider jaundice as:

1. *haemolytic*   *(prehepatic)*
2. *congenital hyperbilirubinaemias*   *(hepatocellular)*
3. *cholestatic – intrahepatic*   *(hepatocellular and/or obstructive)*
        – extrahepatic   *(obstructive)*.

BILIRUBIN METABOLISM

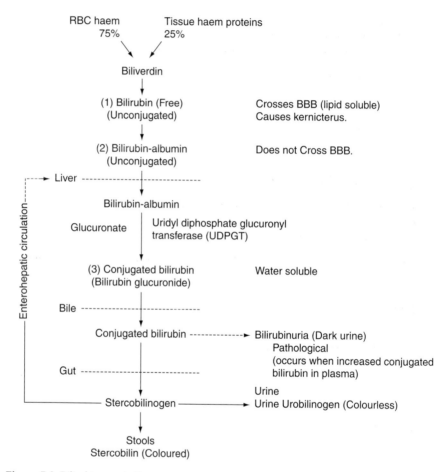

Figure 7.3 Bilirubin metabolism

HAEMOLYTIC JAUNDICE

Unconjugated bilirubin ↑ (not water soluble, therefore not in urine) = acholuric jaundice (ie. *no bilirubinuria*). Therefore urine and stools normal colour.

Urine urobilinogen ↑
Transaminases
Alkaline phosphatase } Normal
Albumin
Haemolytic features:

- *Plasma haptoglobins* ↓
- *Lactate dehydrogenase (LDH)* ↑
- *Reticulocytes* ↑
- *Bone marrow erythroid hyperplasia*
- *Spherocytes, red cell fragments, sickle cells may be present*

In intravascular haemolysis:

- *Haemosiderinuria, haemoglobinuria*
- *Methaemalbumin*
- *FDPs* ↑, *haptoglobins* ↓

CHOLESTATIC JAUNDICE

- *Conjugated bilirubin* ↑ *(>20% total bilirubin)*
- *Pale stools*
- *Dark urine (bilirubinuria)*

Altered synthetic function and transaminases may sometimes accompany the picture as outlined below.

1. Intrahepatic
This may be due to:

- *parenchymal disease (hepatocellular)*
- *bile canalicular excretion problem*

Additional features may include:

- *AST, ALT*   ↑↑
- *Alk.phos*   (↑)
- *PT*   ↑
- *Albumin*   ↓
- *γGT*   ↑

2. Extrahepatic (large duct obstruction)
Additional features may include:

- *Alk.phos*   ↑↑
- *AST, ALT*   (↑)
- *PT*   ↑
- *Albumin*   ↓
- *γGT*   ↑

NEONATAL JAUNDICE

Over 60% of neonates become jaundiced. The cause may be due to unconjugated or conjugated hyperbilirubinaemia.

Management depends on the bilirubin level and rate of increase, the gestational and chronological age, the clinical condition of the infant and the cause (and type) of jaundice.

When levels of unconjugated bilirubin are high, they exceed the albumin-binding capacity of the blood and exist as *free unconjugated bilirubin* which is harmful. Premature infants, sick neonates, neonates with a severe metabolic acidosis and those with low albumin levels tolerate lower levels of bilirubin. Guidelines with bilirubin levels at which phototherapy and exchange transfusion are necessary exist for different gestations and weights and for well and ill babies.

Kernicterus

Unconjugated bilirubin when *free* (not bound to albumin) is fat soluble and therefore crosses the blood–brain barrier (BBB), where it causes bilirubin neurotoxicity (kernicterus).

- *Immediate effects*   *Lethargy, irritability, increased tone and opisthotonus*
- *Long-term effects*   *Choreoathetoid cerebral palsy, sensorineural deafness and learning difficulties*

Management

NB. Regular monitoring of serum bilirubin (SBR) to monitor progress is advised throughout these treatments. Phototherapy or exchange transfusion as indicated.

Phototherapy

Converts unconjugated bilirubin to conjugated bilirubin (does not cross BBB).

Method	Eyes covered to prevent damage
	Extra fluid 30 ml/kg/day given to avoid dehydration
	'High strength' may be used if necessary
Side-effects	Loose stools, overheating, dehydration, 'bronze baby syndrome'

Exchange transfusion (partial or total)

Removes bilirubin from the bloodstream. Repeat transfusions may be necessary.

Blood	Fresh whole CMV-negative blood
Group	O Rh negative (or infant's ABO type if mother is the same group), compatible with infant and maternal blood
Method	Via peripheral arterial and venous lines (umbilical vein catheter may be used if necessary), alternate aspirations of 10 ml infant blood and infusions of 10 ml donor blood are performed over a set time period

Complications   Hypoglycaemia, acidosis, hypoxia, bradycardias and apnoeas, thrombosis, NEC.

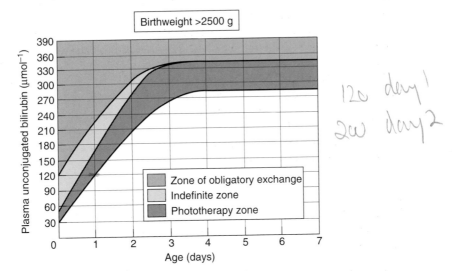

Figure 7.4 Phototherapy treatment chart (Redrawn from Cockington, 1979).

Neonatal unconjugated (UC) hyperbilirubinaemia

Causes
Physiological
Breast milk jaundice
Haemolytic   Blood group incompatibility

        1. *Rhesus incompatibility*
        2. *ABO incompatibility*

Red cell shape abnormality, eg. spherocytosis, elliptocytosis
Red cell membrane instability, eg. G6PD deficiency, pyruvate kinase deficiency

Sepsis   (UC and C)
Hypothyroidism   (UC and C)
Congenital hyperbilirubinaemias   (UC and C), eg. Crigler–Najjar types I and II, Gilbert disease
Metabolic disease   (UC and C), eg. galactosaemia, fructosaemia
High intestinal obstruction
Drugs
Excessive bruising
Infant of diabetic mother

Physiological jaundice
This occurs in 65% of term babies and 80% of preterm babies. It commences after 24 hours and usually lasts 5–7 days.

Causes

1. *Immature foetal liver with inefficient bilirubin metabolism*
2. *Red cell lifespan short in infants (70 days: adult 120 days)*
3. *Haemolysis occurs after birth with rapid fall in Hb*

Investigations

1. *SBR only*
2. *If SBR raised to near treatment levels, then check:*
   - *blood group, Coombs' test, FBC*
   - *bilirubin conjugated and unconjugated fractions*
   - *urine (MC and S)*

Management

- *Keep well hydrated*
- *Phototherapy only if SBR above treatment level (> 350 μmol/l on day 3)*
- *Check regular SBRs*

Breast milk jaundice

A diagnosis of exclusion, which is poorly understood. It lasts for several weeks. No treatment is necessary and breast feeding should not be discontinued.

Haemolytic jaundice due to rhesus or ABO incompatability

1. *A rapid rise in SBR is seen on the first day*
2. *Haemolytic anaemia (hydrops fetalis most severe scenario)*

Causes

1. *Rhesus incompatibility*
   - *Maternal antibodies to rhesus C, D or E antigen (usually anti-D)*
   - *Mother – group Rhesus negative; baby – group Rhesus positive*
2. *ABO incompatibility*
   - *Maternal antibodies to A or B antigen*
   - *Mother – group O; baby – group A or B, usually*

NB.ABO incompatability is a more common cause of severe jaundice than Rhesus disease.

Investigations

Cord blood for Hb, PCV (anaemia, low PCV)

Blood group (incompatible, as above)

Coombs' test (positive in Rhesus, may be negative in ABO)

Bilirubin level (rapid rise)

Maternal antibodies (anti-D, anti-A, anti-B)

Management

1. *Phototherapy*
2. *Regular six-hourly SBR, Hb or PCV and blood glucose (hyperinsulinaemia may occur)*
3. *Exchange transfusion if necessary (ie. bilirubin level > exchange line, rapid bilirubin rise or cord Hb <10 gm/dl)*

Neonatal conjugated hyperbilirubinaemia

Causes

1. *Extrahepatic bile duct obstruction*
   - *Biliary atresia*
   - *Choledochal cyst*
2. *Intrahepatic disease*
   - *Intrahepatic bile duct obstruction*
     Intrahepatic biliary hypoplasia, eg. Alagille syndrome
     Intrahepatic biliary dilatation (Caroli's disease)
     Progressive familial intrahepatic cholestasis (PFIC)
   - *Hepatocyte injury*
     Infections: Hepatitis eg. HSV, CMV, enteroviruses, hepatitis B and C
                Systemic eg. listeria, toxoplasmosis, UTI
     Metabolic disease
       Galactosaemia, fructosaemia, tyrosinaemia,
       α1-antitrypsin deficiency
       Glycogen storage disease
       Cystic fibrosis
       Peroxisomal disease
       Inborn error of bile acid biosynthesis
     Other:
       Idiopathic neonatal hepatitis
       Hypothyroidism
       TPN therapy
       Chromosomal
       Hypoxic ischaemic damage

NB. 'Neonatal hepatitis syndrome' refers to intrahepatic cholestasis of many causes (idiopathic, infectious hepatitis or intrahepatic bile duct paucity).

Examination and investigations

Examination	Liver and spleen size
	Cystic mass below the liver (choledochal cyst)
	Skin lesions, purpura, choroidoretinitis (congenital infection)
	Cataracts (galactosaemia, hypoparathryroidism)
	Cutaneous haemangioma (hepatic haemangioma)
	Situs inversus (extrahepatic biliary atresia)
	Abnormal facies, embryotoxon, systolic murmur (bile duct hypoplasia)
	Dysmorphic features (trisomy 13, 18 or 21)
	Micropenis, optic nerve hypoplasia (septo–optic dysplasia)
Biochemistry	Fractionated bilirubin (conjugated >20% of total is pathological)
	LFTs
	Blood glucose, U&E, creatinine

Galactose-l-phosphate uridyl transferase
α1-antitrypsin phenotype
Metabolic screen (urine and serum amino acids, urine-reducing substances)
IRT, ΔF508
Thyroid function tests
Cholesterol profile

Haematology   FBC, prothrombin time, blood group

Infection screen   Culture of urine, blood and CSF
Serology for congenital infection and hepatitis B and C (ie. HBSAg, VDRL, HIV, other specific viral serology)

Urine   Succinylacetone (↑ in tyrosinaemia – suspect if parents consangiuneous)

Sweat test   Cystic fibrosis screening

Imaging   USS liver and gall bladder (?choledochal cyst ?biliary tract dilatation)
TEBIDA or DISIDA scan following 3–5 days of phenobarbitone which will help distinguish neonatal hepatitis (some excretion) from biliary atresia (no excretion). A HIDA scan was done in the past
Direct cholangiography at operation
Other systems eg. skeletal X-rays, echocardiography

Liver biopsy   Biliary tract and hepatocellular differentiation (NB. Coagulation correction prior to and during biopsy if abnormal)

Biliary atresia

Incidence 1: 10–15 000. A condition of ***progressive*** obliteration of part or all of the extrahepatic biliary ducts (an obliterative cholangiopathy). This leads to chronic liver failure and death. It should be suspected if there is prolonged jaundice beyond 14 days.

Clinical manifestations

- *Normal at birth*
- *Jaundice persisting from day 2*
- *Pale stools and dark urine*
- *Hepatosplenomegaly with progressive liver disease*

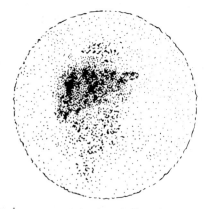

Figure 7.5 TEBIDA scan shows no excretion into the bowel

Investigations

LFTs	Often normal enzymes, with conjugated hyperbilirubinaemia
USS	May be normal, gall bladder may be absent
Fasting TEBIDA radioisotope scan	Isotope uptake into liver unimpaired, excretion into the intestine absent
Liver biopsy	Perilobular oedema and fibrosis, proliferation of bile ductules, bile plugs, basic hepatic architecture intact
Laparotomy with operative cholangiography	

NB. It can be difficult to differentiate **biliary atresia** from **neonatal hepatitis**.

Management

1. *The Kasai procedure (hepatoportoenterostomy)*
   Success rate 80%
   Later complications: cholangitis, fat malabsorption, cirrhosis, portal hypertension
   NB. Surgery must be performed <60 days of life to increase chances of success
2. *Liver transplantation usually necessary at a later date*

Alagille syndrome (arteriohepatic dysplasia)

Autosomal dominant with variable penetrance, incidence 1 : 100 000 births. Gene mapping is now possible.

Liver	Progressive intrahepatic bile duct paucity, pruritis
Facial dysmorphism	Broad forehead, hypertelorism, deep-set eyes, long nose, small mandible
Eyes	Posterior embryotoxon
CVS	Peripheral pulmonary stenosis, tetralogy of Fallot
Skeletal	'Butterfly vertebrae' (vertebral arch defects)
Renal	Tubulointerstitial nephropathy
Other	Cholesterol ↑, tuberous xanthomas

Zellweger syndrome (cerebrohepatorenal syndrome)

Autosomal recessive. Incidence 1 : 100 000 births. A peroxisomal disorder.

Liver	Progressive degeneration, hepatomegaly. Absence of **peroxisomes** in hepatocytes
Kidneys	Progressive degeneration, renal cortical cysts
Neurological	Neurological impairment, severe hypotonia, psychomotor retardation
Dysmorphism	Abnormal-shaped head, distinctive facies (similar to Down syndrome)
Skeletal	Stippled calcification of patellae and greater trochanter (chondrodysplasia punctata)
Eyes	Congenital cataracts, hypoplastic, pale optic disc, retinal pigmentary changes

Caroli's disease

Autosomal recessive. A congenital cystic dilatation of the intrahepatic bile ducts.

Symptoms are of recurring episodes of acute cholangitis, biliary lithiasis and there is increased risk of cholangiocarcinoma.

- Caroli's disease   *Isolated ductal dilatations*
- Caroli's syndrome   *Ductal dilatations with congenital hepatic fibrosis and autosomal recessive polycystic kidneys*

Neonatal jaundice related to time		
<24 hours of birth	Haemolytic disease	
	Congenital infection	
24 hours to 2 weeks	Physiological jaundice	Breast milk jaundice
	Prematurity	Sepsis
	Hypothyroidism	Galactosaemia
	Haemolysis	Bruising
	Congenital hyperbilirubinaemias	
>2 weeks	Breast milk jaundice	Neonatal hepatitis
	Sepsis	Biliary atresia
	Haemolysis	Choledochal cyst

CONGENITAL HYPERBILIRUBINAEMIAS

Unconjugated	Conjugated
Gilbert's syndrome	**Dubin–Johnson syndrome**
2–5% population	Aut. recessive
Aut. dominant	Hepatocyte secretion of biliruin glucuronide ↓
↓ Hepatic UDPGT activity	Bilirubin excretion defective
(+ other biochemical defects)	Mild conjugated hyperbilirubinaemia
Asymptomatic	LFTs normal
Bilirubin levels 50–60	Usually asymptomatic
(↑ during illness and fasting)	Pigment in the liver → black liver
Crigler–Najjar syndrome	**Rotor syndrome**
Type I (Aut. recessive)	Aut. recessive
No glucuronyl transferase	Deficiency in uptake and storage of bilirubin
Severe or fatal kernicterus	
Treatment: neonatal exchange transfusion	
phototherapy into childhood	
liver transplant	
Type II (aut. dominant)	
Decreased glucuronyl transferase	
Neonatal unconjugated hyperbilirubinaemia	
Survive to adults, usually asymptomatic	
Treatment: phenobarbitone	
liver transplant	

Metabolic disorders

WILSON DISEASE (HEPATOLENTICULAR DEGENERATION)

Autosomal recessive. Incidence 1 : 100 000 births. Gene mapped (ATP7B) to chromosome 13 q14–21.

The underlying problem is a copper transport defect. A defect in the hepatocytes prevents entry of copper into the caeruloplasmin compartment. Copper therefore accumulates in the liver and then escapes to the circulation and other organs such as the brain, kidneys and eyes.

Copper metabolism

Ingested copper is absorbed in the stomach and small intestine and transported bound to albumin to the liver. In the liver it is incorporated into caeruloplasmin for transport to the rest of the body. It is excreted into the biliary system or incorporated into copper storage proteins.

Clinical manifestations

Liver	Manifest >5 years. Subacute or chronic hepatitis, hepatomegaly ± splenomegaly, fulminant hepatic failure, cirrhosis, portal hypertension, manifestations of chronic liver disease
Brain	Manifest >10 years. Copper deposition in the basal ganglia. Intention tremor, severe 'wing-beat' tremor later, dysarthria, choreoathetosis, dystonia, behavioural change (bizarre or psychotic), school performance deterioration. Occasionally behavioural changes may be the only manifestation
Kidney	Proximal renal tubular acidosis (Fanconi syndrome), renal failure
Blood	Haemolysis, may be initial presentation, severe
Cornea	Kayser-Fleischer ring is **pathognomonic** (golden brown ring at periphery of cornea due to deposition in Descemet membrane)
Others	Arthritis, endocrinopathies (eg. hypoparathyroidism)

Diagnostic Investigations

Urine	24-hr copper excretion ↑
	24-hr copper excretion after penicillamine given ↑↑

Serum caeruloplasmin ↓

Liver biopsy	Characteristic histology and periportal copper deposition present
Serum copper	Raised early in disease, may be normal

Management

Symptoms and signs improved with therapy, presymptomatic disease treated in relatives.

Copper chelation agents	Penicillamine orally. (NB. This is an antimetabolite to vitamin B_6, therefore this is also given.)
	TETA (triethylene tetramine dihydrochloride) if penicillamine not tolerated
Copper intake	Reduce to <1 mg/kg/day
	Foods high in copper: liver, nuts, chocolate, shellfish

| *Liver transplant* | If fulminant liver disease |

Screening

All family members are screened for presymptomatic disease:

1. *caeruloplasmin* ($\downarrow$)
2. *urine copper* ($\uparrow$)
3. *liver biopsy if diagnosis suspected.*

Antenatal diagnosis is possible.

HAEMOCHROMATOSIS

Autosomal recessive 1 in 300 heterozygotes.
Associations: HLA A3 (72%), HLA B7 (Australia), HLA B14 (France).
Gene (C282Y) on chromosome 6p.

A disease of excess iron deposition and absorption. The underlying defect is unknown.

Clinical manifestations

Liver	Fibrosis, cirrhosis, of which 30% will develop primary hepatocellular carcinoma
Skin	Slate-grey discolouration
Pancreas	IDDM, 'bronzed diabetes'
Heart	Cardiomyopathy, arrhythmias
Endocrine glands	Pituitary (failure), growth failure, hypothyroidism, hypoparathyroidism
Gonads	Testicular atrophy
Joints	Chondrocalcinosis (calcium pyrophosphate deposition), asymmetrical, all joints

Investigations

Serum	Ferritin $\uparrow$
	Iron $\uparrow$
	TIBC (saturated)
Bone marrow	Biopsy (Perls' stain)
Liver biopsy	Fibrosis and iron deposition
Liver CT/MRI	
Desferrioxamine test	Iron excretion increases with chelation

Investigations to assess individual organ damage:
- *Liver* — LFTs, CT/MRI, biopsy
- *Cardiac* — CXR, ECG, echocardiogram
- *Endocrine* — Pituitary function tests, TFTs, GH, parathyroid, adrenal and gonadal function

Management

1. *Venesection regularly*
2. *Iron chelation therapy with desferrioxamine subcutaneously five nights a week*

Neonatal haemochromatosis

An acquired condition secondary to severe prenatal liver disease. Severe liver dysfunction, with liver transplantation usually required. Aggressive chelation and antioxidant regime can, rarely, avoid the need for liver transplantation. Diagnosis most accurate by estimation of extrahepatic iron deposition, eg. lip biopsy.

Transfusion-induced haemochromatosis

This occurs with multiple chronic transfusions and results in a similar pathology due to the excess iron deposition. Therefore chelation therapy must be given.

α1-ANTITRYPSIN DEFICIENCY

Autosomal dominant. Incidence 1 : 2000–5000 live births. Common in Northern Europeans (one in 10 carries a deficiency gene). Gene located on chromosome 14q31–32.3.

This disease is the result of a deficiency of α1-antitrypsin in varying degrees of severity. α1-antitrypsin is a protease inhibitor (Pi) made by hepatocytes; it is a glycoprotein and accounts for >80% of the circulating α1-globulin.

The disease results in

1. *liver disease – childhood onset*
2. *lung disease – 20–40 year onset*

Proteases are inherited as a series of codominant alleles (over 20 phenotypes exist). The genetic variants are characterised by their electrophoretic mobilities as medium (M), slow (S) and very slow (Z). Example genotypes are:

PiMM   = normal phenotype
PiSS   = α1-AT 60% activity
PiZZ   = α1-AT 15% activity. 1 : 3400 births. Most clinical disease. 20% have
              neonatal cholestasis
Pinullnull = not associated with liver disease. 0% α1-AT activity

Clinical manifestations

Liver   Very variable. Neonatal cholestasis, transient jaundice in first few months of life, hepatomegaly ± splenomegaly, childhood cirrhosis
Respiratory Emphysema (see p. 143)
Skin   Persistent cutaneous vasculitis, cold-contact urticaria, acquired angio-oedema, red, tender nodules on trunk and proximal extremities

Investigations

1. *Serum α1-antitrypsin* ↓
2. *Liver biopsy (globules of α1-antitrypsin in the periportal cells)*
3. *Pi phenotype*
4. *Parental genotype*

Antenatal diagnosis is possible.

Management

- Liver transplant if severe liver disease.
- Lung disease – give danazol (increases α1-antitrypsin), enzyme replacement therapy available.
- Genetic counselling required for future pregnancies

REYE SYNDROME

A syndrome of acute encephalopathy and fatty degeneration of the liver. The incidence has markedly declined over recent years, due to decreased aspirin use in children and greater recognition of the differential diagnoses.

- Associations: aspirin therapy, viral infections (influenza B, varicella), mitochondrial cytopathy
- Usual age 4–12 years, mortality 40%

Clinical manifestations

- Prodromal URTI or chicken pox
- 4–7 days later: vomiting +++
  encephalopathy
  moderate hepatomegaly, no jaundice, not icteric
  ± hypoglycaemia

Clinical staging of Reye syndrome

Grade	Signs
I	Lethargic, vomiting
II	Confusion, delirium
III	Light coma, decorticate rigidity, seizures
IV	Deeper coma, decerebrate rigidity, seizures
V	Isoelectric (flat) EEG, respiratory arrest

Investigations

Blood	Ammonia ↑ (>125 μg/dl)
	AST, ALT, LDH, CK (↑)
	Glucose (↓, in small children especially)
	Clotting deranged (PT↑)
CSF	Normal analysis, raised ICP
Liver biopsy	Fatty infiltration, specific mitochondrial morphology on EM

Management

This is supportive, with correction of hypoglycaemia and coagulation defects and IPPV intensive care as necessary. It is important to:

1. control raised ICP
2. make sure the diagnosis is correct

Differential diagnoses

- *Metabolic disease, eg. fatty acid oxidation defects, organic acidurias, urea cycle defects*
- *CNS infections*
- *Drug ingestion*
- *Haemorrhagic shock with encephalopathy*

Congenital hepatic fibrosis (see p. 239).

Autosomal recessive. This is a congenital disease involving:

1. *liver disease*   *diffuse fibrosis $\pm$ abnormal bile ducts*
                          hepatosplenomegaly, portal hypertension
2. *renal disease (75%)*   *renal tubule ectasia, ARPKD, nephronopthisis.*

Clinical features

- *Hepatosplenomegaly, bleeding from varices*
- *Cholangitis (when bile duct abnormal)*

Investigations

LFTs   Alkaline phosphatase $\uparrow$
                Other LFTs (AST, ALT, bilirubin, albumin and PT) usually normal
Liver biopsy   Needed for the diagnosis

Management

Treatment of varices.

Hepatitis

VIRAL HEPATITIS

This may be caused by the hepatitis viruses, CMV, EBV, HSV, varicella, HIV, rubella, adenovirus, enteroviruses and arboviruses.

Hepatitis A (HAV)

RNA picornavirus, the commonest cause of viral hepatitis. Transmission is faecal–oral (especially water, seafood, poor sanitation).

Clinical features

Incubation (2 weeks)   Infective until just after jaundice appears (while faecal HAV excreted)
Prodrome (2 weeks)   Malaise, nausea, vomiting, diarrhoea, headaches (mild in young children)
Jaundice (2–4 weeks)   Cholestatic jaundice, mild hepatosplenomegaly, symptoms improving
Rare complications   Fulminant hepatic failure, vasculitis, arthritis, myocarditis, renal failure

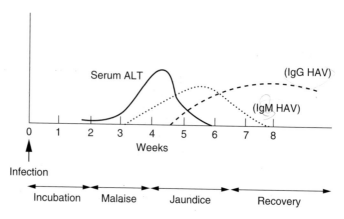

Figure 7.6 HAV serology. (NB. IgG indicates past infection).

Investigations

Prodrome	Jaundice
Serum bilirubin (N)	Bilirubin (↑)
Urine bilirubin and urobilinogen (↑)	AST (↑) for up to six months
AST (↑↑)	Alk. phos (↑)
FBC (WCC ↓ with relative lymphocytosis, aplastic anaemia,	Anti-HAV IgM
Coombs +ve haemolytic anaemia)	
ESR ↑, PT (↑ indicates liver injury)	
Stool EM positive for HAV	

Management
Supportive only. No carrier state.

Prevention

1. *Passive immunisation – standard immunoglobulin, three months protection*
2. *Active immunisation – vaccine available*

Hepatitis B (HBV)
DNA hepadnavirus. Transmission by intravenous, close contact or vertical

Clinical features
These are as for hepatitis A but more prolonged and severe.

Investigations

As for hepatitis A.

Specific markers for hepatitis B:

Antigen	Antibody
HBsAg	Anti-HBsAg
HBcAg	Anti-HBcAg
	IgM anti-HBcAg
HBeAg	Anti-HBeAg

PCR for HBV DNA also available (indicates continued viral replication)

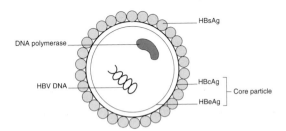

Figure 7.7 HBV particle

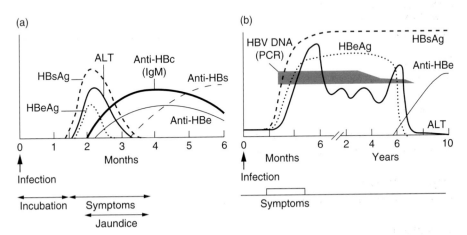

Figure 7.8 HBV serology: (a) acute infection (b) chronic carrier

Clinical Course

Most make a full recovery.

- *1% Fulminant hepatitis*
- *10% Chronic infection:*   *HBsAg (normal carrier state)*
  HBeAg (very infectious)
  70–90% asymptomatic carrier → chronic hepatitis,
  cirrhosis, hepatocellular carcinoma (few)
  10–30% chronic hepatitis → cirrhosis → hepatocellular
  carcinoma
  common among infants infected <1 yr

Carriers may be treated with interferon-α which may seroconvert them (though <40% effective). Other antiviral drugs such as lamivudine are receiving attention.

Infants of hepatitis B carrier mothers		
These are at risk of contracting hepatitis B.		
If mother is:	HBsAg positive	Vaccine within 12 hours of birth, 0.5 ml
	Anti-HBeAb positive	(10 μg) IM thigh
		Repeat doses of vaccine at one and six months
If mother is:	HBsAg positive	Vaccine within 12 hours of birth, 0.5 ml
	HBeAg positive	IM thigh
		Hepatitis B immune globulin (HBIG) <1 hour, 200 IU, IM, opposite thigh
		Repeat doses of vaccine at one and six months

Hepatitis C (HCV)

RNA virus with 6 subtypes. Types I, II and III common in Europe, Type IV is common in the Far East.

Transmission   Intravenous, close contact.
Vertical (uncommon)

This causes a mild flu-like illness.
Rare complications are aplastic anaemia, arthritis, agranulocytosis, neurological problems.
Diagnosis is with Anti-HCV antibody detection (these are negative until 1–3 months after clinical onset of illness).
Chronic liver disease occurs in 50% --> Cirrhosis (25%) --> Hepatocellular carcinoma (15%).
No prophylaxis for maternal transmission.
Interferon-α can be given to chronic carriers but there is a high relapse rate when it is stopped. Ribavirin is also receiving attention.

Hepatitis D (HDV)

Hepatitis D virus (delta virus) is an incomplete RNA particle enclosed in the HBsAg. It can only replicate in the presence of hepatitis B infection. Common in drug addicts. Two patterns of infection are seen: **superinfection** in a person already infected with HBV and **coinfection** with HBV. Features are similar but more severe with more fulminant hepatitis occurring than in other viral hepatitis.

Transmission   Percutaneous, close contact, vertical

Coinfection	Superinfection
Acute hepatitis common	Chronic hepatitis common
Similar to HBV but more severe	Fulminant hepatitis more common
Biphasic AST rise	IgM anti-HDV and IgG anti-HBcAg
IgM anti-HDV and IgM anti-HBcAg	

- *Diagnosis is by detecting IgM antibody to HDV*
- *Chronic infection is very serious as 70% get cirrhosis*
- *α-interferon therapy causes a remission only*

Hepatitis E (HEV)

RNA virus.

Transmission   Enteral route

Clinical illness is similar to hepatitis A though often more severe. NB. Pregnant women have high rate of fulminant hepatic failure (20% v. 2% in others infected) and fatality.

- *Diagnosis is by HEV RNA detection in serum or stools*
- *No effective prophylaxis*
- *No carrier state exists*

CHRONIC HEPATITIS

This is the presence of hepatic inflammation (manifest by elevated transaminases) for longer than six months. There are two subdivisions of chronic hepatitis, distinguished histologically:

1. *chronic persistent hepatitis – benign, self-limiting usually*
2. *chronic active hepatitis – progressive disease with eventual cirrhosis*

The clinical manifestations are variable:

1. *asymptomatic*
2. *chronic liver disease*
3. *hepatic failure*

Causes
Persistent viral infection

Autoimmune

Drugs   eg. isoniazid, nitrofurantoin, sulphonamides, dantrolene

Metabolic   eg. Wilson's disease, haemochromatosis, α1-antitrypsin disease, cystic fibrosis

Chronic persistent hepatitis (CPH)

Usual cause   Hepatitis B or C

Histology   Inflammation limited to portal triads, no fibrosis or cirrhosis

Clinical manifestations   Usually asymptomatic, may have non-specific malaise and mild hepatomegaly. Sometimes chronic liver disease occurs

Investigations   Transaminases ↑, bilirubin ↑

                             Alkaline phosphatase, albumin, PT all normal

                             Autoantibodies negative

                             Liver biopsy essential

Management   Interferon-α may help in hepatitis B or C disease

Chronic active hepatitis (CAH)

Usual cause   Hepatitis B or C, autoimmune disease

Histology   Inflammatory infiltrates beyond portal areas, 'piecemeal' necrosis of hepatocytes, fibrosis and necrosis between neighbouring triads, cirrhosis

Clinical manifestations   Very variable, ranging from asymptomatic to cirrhosis or hepatic failure

Associations   Arthritis, rash, nephritis, vasculitis, haemolytic anaemia in autoimmune disease

Investigations   Transaminases ↑, bilirubin ↑, γ-globulins ↑, PT ↑

                             Anaemia, thrombocytopenia, leucopenia

                             ANA ↑, ASM ↑, AMA ↑, LKM (liver-kidney microsomal antibodies) ↑ and IgG↑ in autoimmune disease

                             Liver biopsy essential

Management   Steroids and azathioprine in autoimmune disease

                             Course of interferon-α injections in hepatitis B or C

                             Liver transplant in endstage liver disease

Portal hypertension

This occurs when the portal pressure is elevated >10–12 mmHg (normal = 7 mmHg). Increased portal venous pressure results in collaterals (varices) developing (portosystemic shunting) and a hyperdynamic circulation. These together can cause varices to rupture and result in GI bleeds. Important sites of collaterals (varices):

1. *oesophagus*
2. *anorectal*
3. *periumbilical (caput medusae. NB. These flow away from the umbilicus)*
4. *retroperitoneal*
5. *perivertebral/perispinal*

Causes

It is caused by obstruction to the portal flow anywhere along the portal system.

Prehepatic	Hepatic	Posthepatic
Small liver, big spleen	Liver small/large/normal Big spleen	Big liver, big spleen
Portal/splenic vein thrombosis:	Hepatocellular:	Hepatic vein thrombosis
Neonatal sepsis	Cong. hepatic fibrosis	(Budd–Chiari syndrome):
Dehydration	Viral hepatitis	Cong. venous web
Hypercoagulable state	Metabolic cirrhosis	Polycythaemia
Increased portal flow:	Hepatotoxicity	Leukaemia
AV fistula	(TPN)	Coagulopathy
	(Methotrexate)	Sickle cell disease
	Biliary tract disease:	Oral contraceptive pill
	Sclerosing cholangitis	GVHD
	Choledochal cyst	Right heart failure
	Biliary atresia	Constrictive pericarditis
	Intrahepatic bile	Veno-occlusive disease
	duct paucity	(seen with DXT in BMT)

Clinical features

- Bleeding oesophageal varices
- Cutaneous collaterals (periumbilical, away from umbilicus)
- Splenomegaly (depending on the site of the obstruction)
- Liver size may be normal, enlarged or small and there may be signs of underlying liver disease
- Haemorrhagic encephalopathy secondary to massive GI bleed

Investigations

USS	Outlining portal vein pathology, direction of flow of the portal system, presence of oesophageal varices
CT/MRI scan	Findings as for USS
Arteriography	Can be done from the coeliac axis, superior mesenteric artery or splenic vein
Endoscopy	Outlining oesophageal and gastric varices

Management

Emergency	Resuscitation (clear fluids and blood)
	Treatment of coagulopathy (FFP, vitamin K, platelets)
	NG tube
	H_2 antagonist intravenously
	Other drugs if necessary (vasopressin, GTN)
	Endoscopy – sclerosis, elastic band ligation of varices or insertion of Sengstaken–Blakemore tube (gastric balloon only) or Linton tube

Elective	Endoscopic operations (as above)
	Portosystemic shunts, eg. TIPSS (transjugular intrahepatic portosystemic shunt), Complication of encephalopathy
	Liver transplantation (for intrahepatic disease or hepatic vein obstruction)

Gall bladder disease

Gall stones are relatively rare in children. They are of the pigment type in 70% of children and cholesterol stones in 20%. Conditions associated with gall stone formation include:

- *chronic haemolysis (sickle cell disease, spherocytosis). Pigment stones*
- *Crohn's disease*
- *ileal resection*
- *cystic fibrosis*
- *TPN*
- *obesity*
- *sick premature infants*

Clinical features
Intolerance of fatty foods
Recurrent colicky, right upper quadrant (RUQ) abdominal pain
Acute cholecystitis: RUQ pain, tenderness and guarding, fever, jaundice, nausea, vomiting

Investigations
USS   Liver and gall bladder
Blood   LFTs, blood cultures (in acute cholecystitis)

Management
Cholecystectomy (open or laparoscopic, once acute infection subsided)

Liver transplantation

Orthotopic liver transplant is available for chronic liver disease or acute/subacute liver failure.

Transplant should be considered before irreversible nutritional deficit and growth and developmental delay. Biliary atresia and metabolic liver disease are common indications in children.

Combined small bowel and liver transplantation is now an effective treatment for short-gut or intestinal failure. However, isolated small bowel transplant is recommended unless endstage liver dysfunction accompanies bowel disease.

Indications and contraindications for urgent liver transplantation:

Indications	Contraindications
Deteriorating liver synthetic function	Irreversible cerebral damage
INR >4	Multisystem disease not correctable by
↓ transaminases reflecting ↓ hepatic mass	transplant (eg. mitochondrial cytopathies)
Blood glucose and albumin ↓ if unsupported	

Chronic indications also include poor quality of life, severe pruritis (eg. Alagille's syndrome), persistent encephalopathy, recurrent hepatic complications, persistent hyperbilirubinaemia > 120 μmol/l.

Complications
Early Renal impairment, hypertension, GI haemorrhage, graft dysfunction, acute rejection, hepatic artery thrombosis
Late Infection (especially bacterial, CMV and PCP), organ rejection, lympho-proliferative disease (with excessive immunosuppression)

Prognosis
80–90% five-year survival rate for elective transplantation

FURTHER READING

Kelly D *Diseases of the liver and biliary tract in children*, Churchill Livingstone, London, 1999
Shah N, Thompson M *The liver in intensive care in: a manual of paediatric intensive care.* Ed: Henderson J, Fleming P Edward Arnold, London, UK 1999

8

Renal

- *Physiology*
- *Urinary tract infection*
- *Vesicoureteric reflux*
- *Congenital urinary tract obstruction*
- *Nocturnal enuresis*
- *Renal calculi*
- *Nephrotic syndrome*
- *Glomerulonephritis*

- *Haemolytic uraemic syndrome*
- *Renal venous thrombosis*
- *Disorders of tubular function*
- *Congenital structural malformations*
- *Urate metabolism*
- *Renal failure*
- *Hypertension*

Physiology

FUNCTIONS OF THE KIDNEY

1. *Excretion of waste products*
2. *Regulation of body fluid volume and composition (salt and water balance)*
3. *Endocrine and metabolic (renin, prostaglandins, erythropoietin, vitamin D metabolism)*

GLOMERULAR FILTRATION

Glomerular filtration rate (GFR) = the total volume of plasma per minute filtered through the glomerulus

$$GFR = \frac{\text{Urine flow} \times [\text{urine}]}{[\text{plasma}]} \qquad [\ ] = \text{concentration of substance}$$

The GFR is very low at birth and rises to reach adult levels at around two years of age.

Normal value = 80–130 ml/min/1.73 m^2 (55–75 ml/min/m^2)   (Adult)

$$\text{Approximation} = \frac{\text{Height (cm)} \times 40}{\text{Plasma-creatinine} (\mu mol/l)} \qquad \text{(Child)}$$

Renal clearance = the volume of plasma from which all of a given substance is removed per minute by the kidneys

$$\text{Cr clearance} = \frac{(\text{Urine Cr} \times \text{urine (vol/min)})}{\text{Plasma Cr}} \qquad (\text{Cr} = \text{creatinine})$$

GFR can be estimated using endogenous substances or by injecting a substance and comparing the rate of urinary excretion with the plasma concentration. The ideal substance for this estimation is:

1. *not metabolised*
2. *freely filtered (ie. not protein bound)*
3. *neither secreted nor reabsorbed*
4. *the concentration in the plasma remains in a steady state during the collection of urine (ie. the rate of production = the rate of clearance).*

If all these criteria are met then the *renal clearance* = GFR. Substances that may be used for measurement:

Creatinine	Commonly used (endogenous), some tubular secretion
Inulin	The gold standard, used for research purposes
Cr EDTA	Used for accurate GFR calculation.

RENAL BLOOD FLOW (RBF)

This is dependent on the BP and the renal vascular resistance. RBF is low at birth and gradually increases to adult levels (25% of the cardiac output). The RBF remains constant throughout a BP range of 80–180 mmHg in adults.

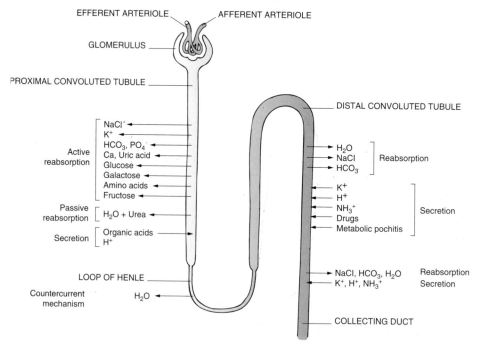

Figure 8.1 Schematic diagram of sites of electrolyte absorption and excretion

The *countercurrent mechanism* ensures a concentrated environment surrounding the distal collecting duct and thus water is reabsorbed at this point (the amount dependent on ADH status), resulting in more concentrated urine.

THE RENIN-ANGIOTENSIN-ALDOSTERONE SYSTEM

This system is involved in the control of BP. The juxtaglomerular apparatus (JGA) is made up of specialised arteriolar smooth muscle cells which secrete renin in response to various stimuli (see Figure 8.2). Renin cleaves angiotensin I from angiotensinogen, which is then converted to active angiotensin II. This results directly in vasoconstriction and also in sodium retention via aldosterone release. These changes mediate an increase in BP and salt and water retention.

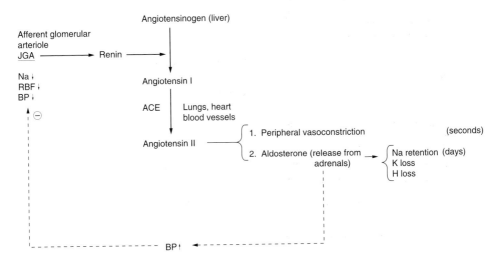

Figure 8.2 Renin-angiotensin-aldosterone system

ATRIAL NATRIURETIC PEPTIDES (ANP)

These are peptides secreted from the cardiac atria in response to increased stretch, increased pressure and increased osmolality and are involved in cardiovascular and fluid homeostasis. ANP has the following actions.

1. GFR $\uparrow$
2. Na excretion $\uparrow$
3. H_2O excretion $\uparrow$
4. BP $\downarrow$
5. Renin $\downarrow$, aldosterone $\downarrow$

ACID-BASE HOMEOSTASIS

Normal arterial blood gases:

pH	7.35–7.45	
pO_2	10.0–13.3 kPa	(75–100 mmHg)
pCO_2	4.8–6.1 kPa	(36–46 mmHg)
HCO_3	23–30 mmol/l	
BE	±2.3 mmol/l	

The anion gap

This is used to evaluate acid-base disturbances. It is the apparent disparity between the total cation (+) and the total anion (−) concentration in the blood. It occurs because some anions are not routinely measured.

$$\text{Anion gap} = [Na] - [Cl + HCO_3]$$
$$= 10\text{–}12 \text{ mmol/l (normally)}$$

The anion gap in metabolic acidosis is dependent on chloride concentration and may be normal or increased, depending on the cause of the acidosis:

Acidosis with Normal anion gap (chloride ↑)

Bicarbonate loss ↑   GIT losses

Renal losses (eg. proximal RTA, interstitial nephritis, hypoadrenalism)

H^+ excretion ↓   eg. distal RTA, chronic renal failure

Acidosis with Increased anion gap (chloride normal)

Acid increased   Lactic acidosis

Ketoacidosis

Chronic renal failure

Inborn errors of metabolism

DIURETICS

Drug	Mechanism	Side-effects
Loop diuretics eg. frusemide	Inhibit Na, K and Cl co-transport in the ascending loop of Henle and increase venous capacitance	Ototoxicity Hypochloraemic alkalosis K ↓, Mg ↓, Na ↓ Impaired glucose tolerance Gout (urates ↑) Myalgia Allergic nephritis Hypercalciuria, with renal stone formation or nephro–calcinosis in neonates
Thiazide diuretics eg. bendrofluazide	Inhibit Na and K reabsorption in the early portion of the distal tubule and decrease peripheral resistance	K ↓, Mg ↓ Na ↓ (used in DI) Gout (urates ↑) Impaired glucose tolerance Serum Ca ↑
Potassium-sparing diuretics **a. Aldosterone antagonists** eg. spironolactone	Competitive inhibitors of aldosterone at the distal tubule	Na ↓ Gynaecomastia Gastrointestinal disturbance Impotence

b. Other potassium-sparing diuretics

eg. amiloride	Inhibit sodium reabsorption at the collecting duct	Na $\downarrow$, K $\uparrow$ Dry mouth Gastrointestinal disturbance
Carbonic anhydrase inhibitors		
eg. acetazolamide	Interfere with H^+ excretion, resulting in increase in Na excretion in proximal tubule	Metabolic acidosis Cl $\uparrow$, K $\downarrow$
Osmotic diuretics eg. mannitol, urea glucose	Filtered at the glomerulus but not reabsorbed, creating an osmotic gradient into the tubules, with Na and water excretion	Chills, fever Used in cerebral oedema

CAUSES OF HAEMATURIA

adenovirus II

Urinary tract infection
Renal stones
Glomerulonephritis   Alport syndrome
                       IgA nephropathy (Berger's)
Congenital malformations
Trauma
Tumours
Haematological   Coagulopathy
                   Thrombocytopenia
                   Sickle cell disease
                   Renal venous thrombosis
Exercise induced
Drugs

CAUSES OF PROTEINURIA

Proteinuria may be mild or heavy. Microalbuminuria is defined as 20–200 mg/day and is not detectable on dipsticks. Proteinuria may also be detected by measuring the albumin:creatinine ratio on a spot urine (normal = <0.1).

Physiological	Orthostatic Exercise induced Febrile	
Pathological	Tubular disease	Hereditary tubular dysfunction Acquired tubular dysfunction
	Glomerular disease	Glomerulonephritis Nephrotic syndrome
	Other	Tumours Drugs Stones, infection

RENAL RADIOLOGICAL INVESTIGATIVE TECHNIQUES

Ultrasound scan (USS)

The standard imaging procedure generates information on renal size and growth, structure and obstructions. No information obtained on renal function.

Intravenous urography (IVU)

Used to check detailed anatomy (ie. renal pelvis, calyces, ureters, stones and obstruction). Rarely needed.

Micturating cystourethrography (MCUG)

Radiolabelled scanning with urethral catheter in place and infant voiding. A sensitive technique to detect and grade reflux and outline urethral obstruction on voiding with the catheter removed. This is a relatively invasive procedure due to the necessity to place a catheter.

Static nuclear medicine scan (DMSA)

Static renal scanning with technetium-labelled 2,3-dimercaptosuccinic acid (DMSA). DMSA is taken up by proximal tubules and the functional cortical mass is outlined. Normal results range from >45% one kidney and <55% the other kidney. The scan is used to detect renal scarring and pyelonephritis (though a single scan cannot differentiate acute from chronic).

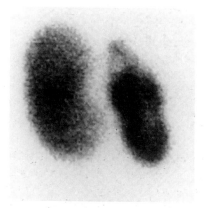

Figure 8.3 A 6-year-old girl presenting with urinary incontinence, both daytime and night-time wetting. Final diagnosis is that of a duplex right kidney with ectopic opening of the upper moiety urter below the bladder neck and VUR into the lower moiety with damage. Figure 8.3 is the right posterior oblique projection of the ^{99m}Tc-DMSA scan showing a defect in the upper pole of the right kidney. In addition, there is a focal defect on the lateral aspect of the lower portion of the right kidney, better seen in the oblique projection

Dynamic nuclear medicine scanning (DTPA and MAG 3)

Radioisotope scanning with technetium-labelled diethylenetriaminepentaacetic acid (DTPA) or mercaptoacetylglycine (MAG3). DTPA and MAG3 are freely filtered through the glomerulus. In a normal scan the isotope is quickly excreted, but with pathology the excretion is delayed. Frusemide is then given to differentiate an obstructed system (where delay continues) from an unobstructed system. Used to detect renal blood flow, function and drainage disorders and reflux in an older child who can control micturition on demand.

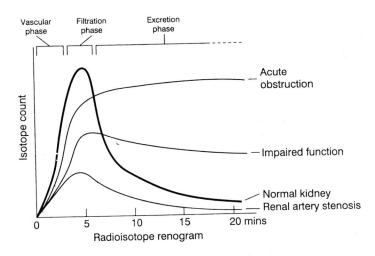

Figure 8.4 Normal and abnormal DTPA scans

Urinary tract infection (UTI)

This occurs in 3% of girls and 1% of boys; 50% of these children have a structural abnormality.

A urinary tract infection can present as acute cystitis, acute pyelonephritis, asymptomatic bacteriuria or septicaemia. Acute pyelonephritis may lead to renal scarring and changes of chronic pyelonephritis. UTI associated with reflux can cause scarring in a *growing kidney* and this can lead to hypertension and chronic renal failure.

Causes

Predisposing factors	Common bacteria
Female	*Escherichia coli*
Urinary tract abnormality	Proteus (boys particularly, triple phosphate stones)
Immunosuppression	Pseudomonas (common in structural abnormalities)

Clinical manifestations

Asymptomatic bacteriuria or:

Infant   Sepsis (PUO)

          Systemic infection

          Failure to thrive

Older child   Dysuria, frequency, nocturia, abdominal pain, incontinence of urine, haematuria, smelly urine

          Systemic infection (PUO)

Diagnosis

1. *Urine sample:*
   - *suprapubic aspiration (SPA) – in infants <1 year. Standard in sick infants*
   - *clean-catch urine – infants. Three samples collected prior to treatment*
   - *bag urine – infants. Contamination common. Three samples collected prior to treatment*
   - *catheter sample*
   - *midstream urine (MSU) – children >3 years (or younger with patience)*

   Signs of infection (on urinalysis, microscopy and culture):
     - *proteinuria, haematuria*
     - *pyuria (almost always)*   } Supportive
     - *organisms on microscopy*
     - *single species growth > 10^5/ml* – Diagnostic
2. *In unexplained fever and sick infants/children–urine culture, U&Es, creatinine, ESR, blood cultures*
3. *Urgent USS if there is a known structural abnormality and concern of obstruction or severe localised flank pain (looking for obstructed, infected kidney), or infant (PU valves?)*

Management

- *Antibiotic therapy:*   If unwell/infant – intravenous
                    If well child – oral therapy
- *Optimise hydration*
- *Commence prophylactic antibiotics until further investigations complete*
- *Drainage procedures if required .*

Further investigation in proven UTI

(This is a baseline protocol, individual units may vary in the detail.)

Prevention of UTI

- *High fluid intake*
- *Girls to wipe from front to back*
- *Empty bladder properly*
- *Avoid constipation*

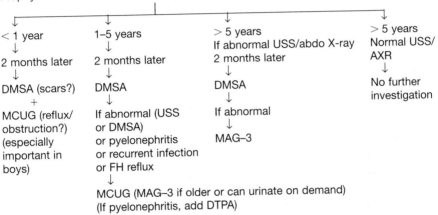

Proven UTI
↓
USS (and abdo X-ray if stones, obstruction, bladder or spinal anomaly suspected)
IVU if concern on USS (rarely needed)
↓
Prophylactic antibiotics until investigations are complete

< 1 year	1–5 years	> 5 years If abnormal USS/abdo X-ray	> 5 years Normal USS/AXR
↓	↓	↓	↓
2 months later	2 months later	2 months later	No further investigation
↓	↓	↓	
DMSA (scars?)	DMSA	DMSA	
+	↓	↓	
MCUG (reflux/obstruction?) (especially important in boys)	If abnormal (USS or DMSA) or pyelonephritis or recurrent infection or FH reflux	If abnormal ↓ MAG–3	
	↓		
	MCUG (MAG–3 if older or can urinate on demand) (If pyelonephritis, add DTPA)		

Figure 8.5 Further investigation in proven UTI

Vesicoureteric reflux

This is detected on renal investigation usually following UTI. It is reflux of urine from the bladder into the ureters ± renal pelvis, due to incompetence at the vesicoureteric junction or abnormality of the whole ureter.

Reflux can result in renal scarring (reflux nephropathy) because:

1. *renal pelvis exposed to high pressures*
2. *facilitates passage of bacteria to renal pelvis.*

- *10% is familial*
- *10% improvement in reflux per year*
- *20% of adult CRF is a result of reflux nephropathy*

Classification

Grades I–V.

- *Grades I and II – spontaneous resolution in 80%*
- *Grades III and IV – spontaneous resolution in 15%*

Management of reflux, recurrent UTIs or scarring

1. *Long-term prophylactic antibiotic therapy (trimethoprim 2 mg/kg/night or nitrofurantoin)*
2. *Routine MSU 3–4 monthly or when symptomatic*
3. *BP check six-monthly for life*
4. *Consider circumcision in boys if recurrent UTIs*

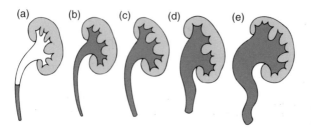

Figure 8.6 The simplest classification is by Scott who divided the types into those with normal calibre or dilated ureters

5. *Surgical reimplantation of the ureters (rarely needed) if medical management of reflux fails*
6. *If bilateral scarring, regular renal growth and function tests.*

Reinvestigate every two years, looking at:

1. *renal growth (USS)*
2. *if condition has resolved (DMSA, DTPA)*
3. *new scars (DMSA).*

Congenital urinary tract obstruction

NB. Ureteral dilatation does *not* always signify obstruction (congenitally abnormal ureters could be present).

Congenital obstruction may occur at the sites shown in Figure 8.7.

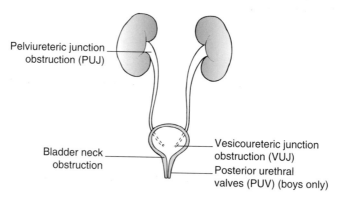

Pelviureteric junction obstruction (PUJ)

Bladder neck obstruction

Vesicoureteric junction obstruction (VUJ)

Posterior urethral valves (PUV) (boys only)

Figure 8.7 Urinary tract obstruction sites

Obstruction results in dilatation of the urinary tract proximal to the obstruction, ± hydronephrosis and hydroureter. Intrauterine detection of dilatation on antenatal ultrasound scan is possible.

POSTERIOR URETHRAL VALVE (PUV) OBSTRUCTION

This condition is seen in male infants and is important to recognise early as prompt surgical treatment may prevent rapid progression to renal failure (though irreversible

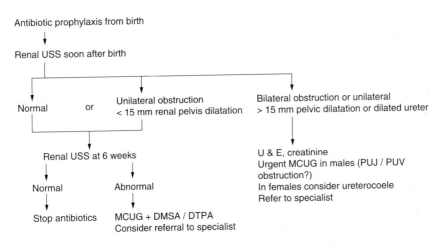

Figure 8.8 Management of an infant with antenatal urinary tract obstruction (individual protocols may vary)

damage may have already occurred prior to birth). It may present as sepsis during the first few weeks of life.

Nocturnal enuresis

Incidence: 5% 5 years
2–3% 10 years
<1% 15 years

It may be primary (always present) or secondary (occurs after continence was achieved).

Causes
Psychological
Organic   UTI
Constipation
Polyuria (eg. diabetes insipidus, IDDM, polyuric renal failure)
Neurological
Renal structural abnormality (eg. ectopic ureter)

Initial investigations
Urine sample Check for glycosuria, proteinuria
Microscopy and culture
Early morning urine osmolality
Renal USS (± AXR)

NB. The history is most important and guides investigations.

Management options

- *Bladder training*
- *Star charts (positive reinforcement)*
- *Alarm pads (negative reinforcement)*
- *Drugs:*
  1. *anticholinergics, eg. oxybutinin*
  2. *adrenergics, eg. ephedrine*
  3. *ADH analogue (desmopressin) for short-term relief*

Renal calculi

Incidence 1.5:1 000 000 children.

Clinical features

- *None*
- *UTI*
- *Haematuria, abdominal pain, renal failure (if bilateral)*
- *Family history*

Classification

Type	Causes
Calcium 80% (oxalate or phosphate) (m>f) (Radioopaque)	Idiopathic hypercalciuria, primary hyperparathyroidism, vitamin D excess, sarcoidosis, distal RTA, malignancies, immobilisation, juvenile rheumatoid arthritis, frusemide
Calcium oxalate (Radioopaque)	Type I and II hyperoxaluria Ileostomies, Crohn's disease (intestinal hyperoxaluria)
Uric acid 4% (Radiolucent)	Tumours, ileostomies, gout, hyperuricosuria Lesch–Nyan syndrome, G6PD
Mixed (struvite) 15% (staghorns) (Radioopaque)	Infection with urease-splitting bacteria (especially proteus in boys)

Type	Causes
Cystine 1% (Weakly radioopaque)	Cystinuria
Xanthine, very rare (Radiolucent)	XO deficiency

Investigations

Urine	M, C+S (NB. Proteus)
	Urinalysis for pH (distal RTA?)
	Amino acid screen (cystinuria?)
	Calcium/creatinine ratios or 24 hour collection
Blood	Renal function tests (creatinine, HCO_3 especially)
	Calcium, phosphate, alkaline phosphatase
	PTH if concern of hyperparathyroidism
Imaging	Abdo X-ray, renal USS, IVU
Stone analysis	

Management

- *High fluid intake*
- *Alkalinise the urine to pH >7.5 (cystine, uric acid stones)*
- *Stone removal via lithotripsy or cystoscopically*
- *Treat cause if possible*

Nephrotic syndrome

Incidence 1:50 000. Male:female 2:1. Typical age 1–6 years.
This condition is characterised by:

1. *proteinuria >40 (mg/hr/m^2) (child), >3.0 g/day (adult)*
2. *hypoalbuminaemia <25 mg/l*
3. *oedema*
4. *hyperlipidaemia – LDL ↑, triglycerides ↑*

Cause

Histology:
Minimal change 78%
Focal segmental glomerulosclerosis 10.5%
Proliferative: membranoproliferative ⎫
         diffuse mesangial   ⎬ 10.5%
         crescentic   ⎭
Membranous 1.5%
Nephrotic syndrome is usually idiopathic.
Secondary causes of nephrotic syndrome include any nephritis with sufficiently heavy proteinuria, eg. poststreptococcal, malaria, HSP, SLE, anaphylactoid, heavy metals, drugs (eg. penicillamine), tumours (eg. lymphomas).

Clinical features

Preceding URTI	
Oedema	Periorbital in mornings (first sign, often misdiagnosed as allergy)
	Scrotal, sacral, leg and ankle later in the day.

Ascites
Lethargy, anorexia, abdominal pain (eg. secondary to peritonitis or venous thrombosis), diarrhoea
Pleural effusions with SOB (uncommon)

Initial investigations

Urine	Dipstick for proteinuria (+3 or +4)
	Albumin:creatinine ratio (>200 mg/mmol)
	Na concentration (<20 mmol/l is an indication of hypovolaemia)
	M, C + S (microsopic haematuria and casts)
	Selective protein clearance (research only):
	IgG (large molecule): albumin (small molecule)
	Low ratio = selective protein leak. Seen in minimal change disease
Serum	FBC, ESR
	U&E, creatinine, albumin (<25 g/l), cholesterol and triglyceride ($\uparrow$)
	Complement factors C3 ($\downarrow$) (not in minimal change) and C4
	ASOT
	Hep B SAg (membranous)
Throat swab	M, C + S
Renal biopsy	Only if no response to steroids or atypical features of disease (ie. high creatinine, hypertension, older children or <1 year)

Management

1. *Oral corticosteroids – 60 mg/m^2/day (2 mg/kg/day) until no proteinuria for three days, then 40 mg/m^2 alternate days for four weeks. If no response to steroids <4–6 weeks, a renal biopsy should be considered*
2. *Oral penicillin prophylaxis*
3. *Monitor intravascular volume (see below)*
4. *Daily weight, electrolytes and albumin*
5. *Diuretics as needed (in hospital only)*
6. *Monitor proteinuria at home when recovered to assess for a relapse*

Features of hypovolaemia
Orthostatic hypotension, cool peripheries, capillary refill time $\uparrow$, oliguria, abdominal pain, tachycardia, significant core–periphery temperature difference, urine sodium <10 mmol/l, high or rising haematocrit.

Give albumin if hypovolaemic (4.5% albumin if in shock, 20% albumin 1 g/kg with diuretics over at least four hours if not in shock)

Complications

1. *Hypovolaemia (as above)*
2. *Infection, classically pneumococcal peritonitis, or gram-negative infection due to low immunoglobulins*
3. *Intravascular thrombosis, particularly renal vein thrombosis and deep vein thrombosis (DVT) (due to hypovolaemia and hypercoagulable state with a low antithrombin III.)*

4. *Hypercholesterolaemia*
5. *Acute tubular necrosis if severe hypovolaemia*

Prognosis

Steroid-sensitive disease: $\frac{1}{3}$ no relapses
$\frac{1}{3}$ occasional relapses
$\frac{1}{3}$ regular relapses

If regular relapses, alternative immunosuppression may be necessary, such as cyclophosphamide or cyclosporin.

Steroid-resistant disease: Alternative immunosupression. 50% progress to chronic renal failure

If well, follow up yearly, checking particularly BP and growth.

CONGENITAL NEPHROTIC SYNDROME

This is the development of nephrotic syndrome presenting antenatally or within the first month after birth.

Causes

Autosomal recessive, Finnish type, gene testing available, microcystic changes in the renal cortex.

Other causes   Congenital syphilis, toxoplasmosis
Diffuse mesangial sclerosis, Denys–Drash syndrome

Clinical features

- *Large oedematous placenta*
- *Proteinuria*
- *Clinical deterioration with oedema in the first week of life due to the increase in GFR (and therefore protein excretion)*

Management options

1. *Supportive therapy until large enough for renal transplantation (>10 kg)*
2. *Reduce the GFR with NSAIDS and ACE inhibitors, then unilateral nephrectomy, or bilateral nephrectomy with dialysis as necessary. Transplant when big enough (>10 kg).*

Death may occur from the complications (CRF, peritonitis, respiratory infections and strokes). Antenatal diagnosis is possible looking for AFP elevation in amniotic fluid and genetic analysis if mutation known.

Glomerulonephritis

A term covering several diseases involving inflammation of the glomerular capillaries. It is thought to be an immune-mediated disease. There are two major mechanisms of immunological injury:

1. *deposition of circulating antigen-antibody immune complexes (95% of GN)*
2. *deposition of antiglomerular basement membrane antibody (anti-GBM, 5% of GN, eg. Goodpasture syndrome).*

HISTOLOGICAL CLASSIFICATION OF GLOMERULAR PATHOLOGY

This may be asked about in exams.

	Histology	Common presentation	Common cause
1. Predominantly presenting as glomerulonephritis			
Proliferative GN			
Diffuse	Endothelial and mesangial cell proliferation Glomerulus packed with cells. Deposits of C3 and Ig	Acute nephritis	Poststreptococcal
Focal segmental	Some glomeruli normal, some have proliferative changes	Haematuria Proteinuria	Berger, SLE, HSP, shunt nephritis, SABE, PAN
With crescents (rapidly progressive GN)	Crescents (macrophages and epithelial cells) in most glomeruli	Renal failure	Goodpasture, PAN, Wegener's
Membranoproliferative (mesangiocapillary, MCGN)	Type I Mesangial cell proliferation Subendothelial immune complex deposits, BM splitting, C3 $\downarrow$, C4 N. Type II Mesangial cell proliferation Intramembranous immune complex deposits. C3 stain only.	Haematuria, proteinuria Nephritic, nephrotic, CRF	Idiopathic, Shunt nephritis
2. Predominantly presenting as nephrotic syndrome			
Membranous GN	Thickening of GBM due to immune deposits	Nephrotic in adults	Idiopathic Penicillamine Hepatitis B SLE, malaria
Minimal change nephropathy NB. Not a true GN	Fusion of podocytes of epithelial cells on EM (normal glomerulus on LM)	Nephrotic in children	Idiopathic
Focal segmental glomerulosclerosis	Glomerulosclerosis	Proteinuria Nephrotic CRF in 50%	Idiopathic Diabetes

ACUTE NEPHRITIC SYNDROME

This has three major characteristics:

1. *haematuria*
2. *oliguria*

3. *hypertension (secondary to fluid overload)*

Other features are:

- *red cell casts*
- *proteinuria*
- *oedema*

General investigations

Urine	Urinalysis (protein, blood, casts)
	M, C + S
Serum	FBC, ESR
	U&E, creatinine, LFTs
	Complement levels
	Viral titres and ASOT
	ANA
	HepB S antigen
Throat swab	M, C + S

Management

This is supportive.

1. *Fluid restriction:*
   insensible loss (3–400 ml/m^2/day) + urine output
2. *Sodium restriction, if necessary*
3. *Hypertension management. NB. Diuretics useful here (eg. frusemide)*
4. *Penicillin if positive throat swab or nephrotic picture*
5. *Dialysis if necessary (hyperkalaemia)*

POSTSTREPTOCOCCAL GLOMERULONEPHRITIS

Typically this presents as the nephritic syndrome 6–10 days after a Lancefield group A β-haemolytic streptococcal URTI or 21 days after streptococcal skin infection.

Investigations

General investigations for glomerulonephritis and specifically: antistreptolysin O titre (ASOT) (positive), anti-DNase B antibodies ($\uparrow$), C3 ($\downarrow$), C4 (N), throat swab (M, C + S)

Management

- *Ten-day course of penicillin if positive throat swab*
- *Supportive therapy as for nephritic syndrome (NB. steroids unhelpful)*

Prognosis

- *Spontaneous resolution in >95%. NB. Haematuria can continue for up to a year, but **not** proteinuria*
- *Renal biopsy only if atypical (ie. severe BP $\uparrow$, rising creatinine)*

HENOCH–SCHÖNLEIN PURPURA (HSP)

This is a vasculitic syndrome of small vessels. Male:female 2 : 1, 3–10 years. Mostly in late winter and early summer. Often there is a preceding URTI.

Clinical features

The four classical features are rash, joint involvement, abdominal pain and haematuria.

Rash Often the first sign. Vasculitic (macular, becoming purpuric). Typically on buttocks, extensor surfaces of lower limbs and pressure points (eg. sock line). Recurs over weeks

Joints Non-destructive arthritis of weight-bearing joints (hips, knees, ankles)

Abdominal pain Bloody stool due to intussusception. Pancreatitis, ileus, protein-losing enteropathy

Renal Glomerulonephritis (focal segmental) in 80%

Oedema Forehead, genitalia, hands and feet, periarticular

Other organs CNS, testis, pancreas, parotids, muscles, lungs (haemoptysis)

Renal disease

1. *Microscopic haematuria in 80%*
2. *Nephritic syndrome*
3. *Nephrotic syndrome*

Investigations to consider

- *Routine tests for nephritic and/or nephrotic syndrome*
- *ESR (↑)*
- *IgA (↑ in >50%)*
- *Clotting and platelet screen*

Management

- *Treat any suspected infection (particularly streptococcal disease)*
- *Supportive therapy for arthralgia, rash, fever and malaise*
- *Renal disease* Standard treatment of nephritis or nephrotic syndrome
  Renal biopsy if severe hypertension or increasing creatinine
  If crescentic disease, plasma exchange is used
- *Abdominal disease* Early use of steroids

Prognosis

Generally good. Although 5–10% progress to chronic renal disease. Low albumin is a sign of a poor prognosis.

IGA NEPHROPATHY (BERGER NEPHROPATHY)

This condition is *not* inherited. Male:female 2 : 1. A disease of focal segmental glomerulonephritis with IgA deposits in the mesangium.

Clinical features

- *Microscopic haematuria*
- *Macroscopic haematuria **during** infections (NB. not after)*

Specific investigations

- *Complement (underline: normal C3)*
- *Serum IgA (↑ in 20%)*
- *Renal biopsy*

anti - GBM nephritis
occur in transplanted
kidney.

Management

- *No specific therapy*
- *Follow-up for life essential*

Tx → ACEi
→ Immunsuppresants

Prognosis

- *Chronic renal failure develops in 25%*
- *Poor prognosis is associated with BP ↑ and proteinuria*

SYSTEMIC LUPUS ERYTHEMATOSUS NEPHRITIS

This is a systemic vasculitis with protean manifestations (see p. 334). Renal disease may involve various types of nephritis, classified by the WHO into five classes. They include focal and diffuse disease, and proliferate and membraneous disease.

Characteristically both C3 and C4 levels are depressed in active disease, ESR is high and CRP normal. Renal biopsy should be considered if haematuria and proteinuria develop in SLE.

Immunosuppressive therapy (steroids, cyclophosphamide and plasma exchange if necessary) is used in the management.

The renal disease may burn out.

GOODPASTURE DISEASE

Rare before teenage years. This disease may follow an upper respiratory tract infection and involves:

- *pulmonary haemorrhage in smokers (intermittent haemoptysis, anaemia, massive bleeding)*
- *severe progressive glomerulonephritis*
- *antibodies to lung and glomerular basement membrane (GBM)*

NB. *Goodpasture syndrome* is the clinical picture of pulmonary haemorrhage and glomerulonephritis seen in a systemic disorder (eg. SLE, PAN).

Diagnosis is confirmed by renal biopsy.

Therapies include immunosuppression, pulsed methylprednisolone and plasmapharesis. Patients may die in the acute stage of pulmonary haemorrhage or commonly progress to chronic renal failure.

ALPORT SYNDROME

X-linked dominant, autosomal dominant, spontaneous mutation (20%), worse in males. This syndrome involves:

Hereditary nephritis Microscopic haematuria (macroscopic with infections), protein-
uria, renal failure (by 20–30 years)
Sensorineural deafness High frequency, progressing to the whole speech range
Ocular defects (15%) Cataracts, anterior lenticonus, macular lesions.

The disease generally presents as haematuria and a young patient may show none of the above features. Parents and siblings of an affected individual should be screened for disease.

Typical 'basket weave' appearance (splitting of the BM) on electron microscopy of renal biopsy. Anti-GBM nephritis can occur in a transplanted kidney in these patients.

Haemolytic uraemic syndrome (HUS)

The commonest cause of acute renal failure in children in the UK. This is a disease involving:

1. *acute renal failure*
2. *microangiopathic haemolytic anaemia*
3. *thrombocytopaenia.*

Causes

E.coli Verotoxin producing *Escherichia coli* 0157 (10% of these infections develop into HUS).

Other bacteria eg. shigella (shigatoxin), salmonella, campylobacter
Familial Poor prognosis, presents <1 year, recurrent episodes
Viral eg. coxsackie, echovirus, varicella
Drugs eg. cyclosporin induced (post transplant), oral contraceptive pill
Other eg. SLE, postpartum

The most common causes are diarrhoea-positive disease and familial, the progno-
sis of the former being much better. Features and management of diarrhoea-positive disease are outlined.

Clinical features in diarrhoea-associated disease

- *Usually <5 years*
- *Bloody diarrhoea with 5–10 days later oliguria, pallor, lethargy and petechiae*
- *NB. Hypertension and hyperkalaemia are major causes of mortality*
- *Other organ damage – CNS (fits, coma), colitis, pancreatitis*
- *A high presenting WCC is associated with a poor prognosis*

Investigations

Serum U&E, creatinine, calcium, phosphate (changes of acute renal failure)
FBC and film (microangiopathic haemolytic anaemia, platelets ↓)
Coagulation screen (normal)
Urine Urinalysis (mild haematuria and mild proteinuria)
Stool M, C + S

Management

Therapy is supportive, as needed.

Fluid status	Careful assessment
	Frusemide may be needed
Hyperkalaemia	Salbutamol nebulisers or IV, insulin and dextrose, etc.
Dialysis	
Transfusions	Blood and rarely platelets
Cerebral involvement	Consider plasma exchange

NB. Long-term follow-up is essential, looking for hypertension or chronic renal disease.

Renal venous thrombosis

Causes

Neonate/Infant Asphyxia, dehydration, sepsis, maternal IDDM, hypercoagulable state eg. protein S or C deficiency
Older child Nephrotic syndrome, cyanotic CHD, contrast angiography
Hypercoagulable state

Clinical features

Infant Gross haematuria and unilateral or bilateral flank masses
Older child Micro/macroscopic haematuria and flank pain

Bilateral thrombosis will also result in acute renal failure.

Investigations

USS IVC (to check extension) and renal (renal enlargement)
Radionucleotide imaging Reduced renal function
Doppler flow studies

Differential diagnoses

Causes of haematuria IgA nephropathy, Alport syndrome, glomerulonephritis
Causes of renal enlargement Cystic kidneys, Wilms tumour, abscess, haematoma, hydronephrosis

Management

Unilateral   Supportive therapy with fluids, electrolyte management and treatment of infection

Bilateral   Fibrinolytic agents (eg. heparin, urokinase, TPA) and consider thrombectomy

Prognosis

The kidney becomes atrophic and should be removed if:

1. *hypertension develops*
2. *repeated UTIs occur*

Disorders of tubular function

RENAL TUBULAR ACIDOSIS (RTA)

This is a condition of *systemic acidosis* caused by renal tubular dysfunction. Three types of RTA exist: types I, II and IV (type III was reclassified as a variant of type I).

- *Types I and II result in a* **hypokalaemic** *hyperchloraemic metabolic acidosis*
- *Type IV results in a* **hyperkalaemic** *hyperchloraemic metabolic acidosis*

The urine pH should be measured within 20 minutes with a glass electrode and not dipsticks. Ammonium chloride loading can help distinguish between types I and II in mild acidosis, by accentuating the defect by increasing the serum acidification (type II *can* then acidify the urine).

Type I – distal RTA

This is due to a *failure of H^+ excretion* by the distal tubule (and urine pH *cannot* be <5.8). Loss of bicarbonate occurs and results in Cl $\uparrow$. There is a normal anion gap because chloride is increased to compensate for the acidosis.

Causes

Isolated   Autosomal dominant, autosomal recessive, sporadic

Secondary Interstitial nephritis   Obstructive nephropathy

                                              Pyelonephritis

                                              Medullary sponge kidney

                                              Transplant rejection

                                              SLE nephritis

                                              Ehlers–Danlos and Marfan syndrome

                                              Cirrhosis

                                              Nephrocalcinosis

                                              Sickle cell nephropathy

            Toxins   Lithium

                                              Amphotericin B

Biochemical findings

Serum	$HCO_3 \downarrow, K \downarrow, Ca \downarrow, Cl \uparrow$

Metabolic acidosis (Normal anion gap)

Urine	pH *cannot* be <5.8
	Hypercalciuria (stones)

Clinical findings

- Growth failure
- Nephrocalcinosis
- Renal stones
- Osteomalacia (no clinical rickets)
- Underlying disease

Management

- Bicarbonate supplements as sodium citrate solution or bicarbonate tablets
- Potassium supplements

Type II – proximal RTA

This is due to a *failure of proximal tubular bicarbonate reabsorption*. It is more severe than distal RTA. The serum bicarbonate falls until the bicarbonate threshold is reached (15–18 mmol/l) where no more HCO_3 loss occurs (because less HCO_3 is filtered and this level can all be reabsorbed distally). Because the distal tubular acidification mechanisms are intact, the urine *can* be acidified (pH <5.5) when there is acidosis or when given ammonium chloride.

Causes

Isolated	Autosomal dominant, sporadic
Secondary	Fanconi syndrome:
	Primary
	Secondary

Biochemical findings

Serum	$HCO_3 \downarrow, K \downarrow\downarrow, Cl \uparrow$

Metabolic acidosis (Anion gap normal)

Urine	pH may be <5.5
	$HCO_3 \uparrow$

Renal loss of other substances in Fanconi syndrome

Clinical findings

- Growth failure
- Rickets, polyuria, polydipsia (in Fanconi)
- Underlying disease
- No renal calcification

Management

- *Bicarbonate supplements* $+++$
- *Potassium supplements*

Type IV

In type IV there is hyperkalaemia plus acidosis secondary to failure of bicarbonate reabsorption $\pm$ aldosterone deficiency.

Causes

- *Adrenal disorders (A $\downarrow$, R $\uparrow$, renal function N)*
  Addison, CAH,
- *Hyporeninaemic hypoaldosteronism (A$\downarrow$, R$\downarrow$, renal function $\downarrow$)*
  Interstitial nephritis (commonest cause)
  Obstruction
  Pyelonephritis
  Diabetes mellitus
- *Pseudohypoaldosteronism (A$\uparrow$, R$\uparrow$)*
  Distal tubule unresponsive

  Key: A = aldosterone, R = renin

Biochemical findings
Serum   K $\uparrow$ Cl $\uparrow$
                 Renin $\downarrow$ or $\uparrow$, Aldosterone $\downarrow$ or $\uparrow$

Metabolic acidosis (Anion gap normal)
Urine   Ammonium $\downarrow$
                 pH may be <5.5

Clinical findings
Features of:
    primary renal disease
    adrenal disease

Management

- *Bicarbonate supplements*
- *Potassium reduction eg. diuretics*

FANCONI SYNDROME

This is a generalised defect in proximal tubular function. A hyperchloraemic hypokalaemic metabolic acidosis results (a type II proximal RTA).

Causes

Congenital	Acquired
Idiopathic (primary)	Heavy metals
Cystinosis	Drugs
Lowe syndrome	Chemotherapy eg. ifosfamide
Galactosaemia	Hyperparathyroidism
Tyrosinaemia type I	Vitamin D deficiency
Hereditary fructose intolerance	Interstitial nephritis
Wilson disease	Glue sniffing
Cytochrome C oxidase deficiency	

Clinical features

- *Underlying disease*
- *Failure to thrive*
- *Rickets*
- *Polyuria, polydipsia, dehydration*

Investigations

Urine   There is excessive urine loss of:
glucose, amino acids, PO_4, HCO_3, Na, Ca, K, urate.

Plasma   Cl $\uparrow$, K^+, $PO_4\downarrow$, hypouricaemia
Metabolic acidosis with normal anion gap

Management

1. *Diagnose and treat underlying disease*
2. *Rickets – large doses of vitamin D, phosphate supplements*
3. *Acidosis – bicarbonate supplements*
4. *Dehydration – extra salt and water, especially in hot weather*

CYSTINOSIS

Autosomal recessive. Condition due to cystine accumulation in lysosomes of the kidneys, bone marrow, liver, spleen, lymph nodes, leucocytes, cornea and fibroblasts.

Clinical features

Infantile form   Fanconi syndrome from three months of age
CRF by 10 years
Blond hair, fair skin
Photophobia (eye crystals) and decreased acuity
Hypothyroidism, diabetes
Growth retardation
Dementia (later)

Adolescent form   Milder and later onset renal disease

Adult type   No renal disease

Diagnosis

1. *Fibroblast or leucocyte cystine concentration ($\uparrow \times 100$)*
2. *Cystine crystals in bone marrow, rectal mucosa, lymph nodes*
3. *Slit-lamp examination of the eyes (corneal cystine crystals)*
4. *Genetic studies*

Management

1. *Phosphocysteamine (lowers intracellular cystine)*
2. *Phosphocysteamine eye drops*
3. *Fanconi treatment*
4. *Renal transplantation (when in ESRF)*

Long-term complications

These include CNS problems, myopathy, swallowing difficulty and pancreatic dysfunction (endo- and exocrine).

Antenatal diagnosis

- *Cystine $\uparrow$ in amniotic fluid cells*
- *DNA analysis (the gene is now known)*

CYSTINURIA

Incidence 1 : 650. This is an inborn error of reabsorption at the proximal tubule of the dibasic amino acids, resulting in increased renal excretion of them: **c**ystine, **o**rnithine, **a**rginine, **l**ysine (COAL).

NB. There is no systemic amino acid deficiency because they are synthesised in the body.

Clinical features

- *None*
- *Renal stones (<3% people affected) leading to haematuria, obstruction, CRF*

Diagnosis

- *Urine and stone analysis.*

Management

- *Alkalinise the urine*
- *High water intake*
- *D-penicillamine may help if the above methods are failing*

BARTTER SYNDROME

Autosomal recessive. This is a condition of renal potassium wasting with hypokalaemia, alkalosis, aldosterone $\uparrow$, but normal BP. The pathophysiology is defective chloride transport channels (NaK$_2$Cl channels) in the ascending limb of the loop of Henle. There are elevated renin and aldosterone levels with juxtaglomerular apparatus (JGA) hyperplasia.

Clinical features

- *Growth failure*
- *Weakness*
- *Vomiting, constipation*
- *Polyuria, polydipsia, salt craving*
- *Dehydration*
- *Normal BP*

Investigations

Serum	K $\downarrow$, Cl $\downarrow$, Mg $\downarrow$, (Na $\downarrow$ in severe cases)
	Ca $\uparrow$
	Metabolic alkalosis
	Aldosterone $\uparrow$, renin $\uparrow$, prostaglandin E2 $\uparrow$ (occasionally)
Urine	Excess K and Cl loss (sometimes Na and Ca loss also)
Renal biopsy	Hyperplasia of JGA

Management

1. *Oral potassium supplements*
2. *NaCl supplements*
3. *Indomethacin (reducing the GFR reduces the sodium delivery)*

GITELMAN SYNDROME

A similar condition often confused with Bartter syndrome, involving hypomagnesaemia, hypokalaemia and hypocalciuria, with normal growth. Caused by a defect in thiazide-sensitive NaCl channels in the distal tubule. Treatment includes magnesium supplements.

Congenital structural malformations

POTTER SEQUENCE

This involves:

1. *pulmonary hypoplasia*
2. *typical facies – widespaced eyes, epicanthic folds, broad flat nose, low-set ears, small chin*
3. *limb abnormalities*

It is due to severe oligohydramnios from:

- *renal agenesis (20%)*
- *autosomal recessive polycystic kidney disease (ARPKD), renal hypoplasia, medullary dysplasia, renal obstruction*

RENAL AGENESIS

Bilateral   Incidence 1 : 3000 births. Incompatible with extrauterine life

Unilateral Incidence 1 : 1000 live births. Incidental finding, normal renal function if other kidney normal.

HYPOPLASIA

Small kidneys with a decreased number of nephrons. This may be unilateral or bilateral. There is an increased risk of hypertension and, if bilateral, CRF.

DYSPLASIA

This is a development disorder with few or no nephrons in the kidney, cysts, abnormal ducts and non-renal elements (metaplasia). It may present as an abdominal mass at birth.

ECTOPIC KIDNEY (PELVIC)

Due to defective ascent of the kidney during development. Normal function usually but increased risk of UTI.

HORSESHOE KIDNEY

Incidence 1 : 500. Due to a fusion of the lower poles of the kidneys in the midline. Increased risk of Wilms tumour.

URETERIC DUPLICATION

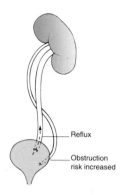

Figure 8.9 Ureteric duplication

PRUNE BELLY SYNDROME (EAGLE–BARRETT SYNDROME)

Incidence 1 : 40 000 births. An association of:

1. *deficient abdominal wall muscles*

2. *undescended testes*
3. *urinary tract abnormalities (typically dilated ureters, large bladder, patent urachus)*

The condition is thought to be due to severe urethral obstruction early in intrauterine life. Other organ abnormalities may be present.

The infants may have severe oligohydramnios and pulmonary hypoplasia and be still-born. Of those who survive, 50% develop renal failure from reflux and dysplastic kidneys.

BLADDER EXSTROPHY

Incidence 1: 40 000 births. Male > female. This condition is very variable in its features and severity.

Classical features

- *Bladder protrudes from the abdominal wall and its mucosa is exposed*
- *Pubic rami and recti muscles separated*
- *Umbilicus displaced downwards*
- *Epispadias (with undescended testes in boys and clitoral duplication in girls)*
- *Anteriorly displaced anus, rectal prolapse*

The condition results in urinary incontinence, increased incidence of bladder cancer, broad-based gait and sexual dysfunction. Management involves complex surgery.

AUTOSOMAL RECESSIVE POLYCYSTIC KIDNEY DISEASE (ARPKD) (INFANTILE POLYCYSTIC DISEASE)

Incidence 1: 20 000. Antenatal diagnosis possible. Autosomal recessive condition characterised by:

Renal   Cysts (dilatations of collecting ducts) may present as *enormous kidneys at birth*
            Haematuria, hypertension, polyuria
            CRF develops in 5–10 years
Liver   Cysts, hepatic fibrosis and portal hypertension
Lungs   Pulmonary hypoplasia ± Potter phenotype

Either the renal disease or the liver disease is the main feature.

AUTOSOMAL DOMINANT POLYCYSTIC KIDNEY DISEASE (ADPKD) (ADULT POLYCYSTIC DISEASE)

Incidence 1: 600. Autosomal dominant. Genetic defect on chromosome 16p (PKD1, 85%) or 4q (PKD2). Condition may be encountered in childhood, but commoner cause of ESRF in adults. Features include:

Renal   Bilateral enlarged kidneys with multiple cortical and medullary cysts
            Initial presentation usually >20 years with loin pain, haematuria and renal masses

Hypertension
Progresses to CRF by 40–70 years
Renal stones
Renal neoplasms
Other cysts   Liver (30%), pancreas, spleen, ovary
Other   Berry aneurysms

Urate metabolism

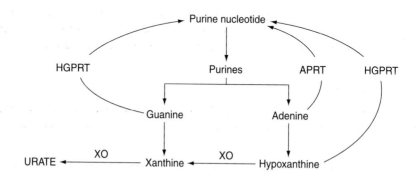

Key:
XO   = Xanthine oxidase
HGPRT = Hypoxantheine-guanine phosphoribosyl transferase
APRT   = Adenine phosphoribosyl transferase

Figure 8.10 Urate metabolism

HYPERURICAEMIA

Urates are poorly soluble and precipitate in the tissues. Joint crystallisation causes classic painful gouty arthritis, subcutaneous tissue precipitation results in gouty tophi (ears, bursae, tendons). Plasma urate is usually normal during acute gout attacks. Kidney precipitation causes renal stones and disease.

Causes
Synthesis ↑   Primary gout
Turnover ↑   Tumour lysis syndrome
            Psoriasis
            Starvation
            Polycythaemia
Excretion ↓   Renal dysfunction
            Thiazide diuretics
            Acidosis

Low-dose salicylates
Glycogen storage disease type 1
G6PD deficiency

Management

Acute High fluid intake, then colchicine and NSAIDs if necessary
Chronic XO inhibitors, eg. allopurinol
Uricosuric drugs, eg. probenicid, high-dose salicylates

LESCH–NYHAN SYNDROME

X-linked recessive. This is a condition where purines cannot be recycled due to a deficiency of HGPRT, with consequent raised uric acid levels. It results in mental deficiency, self-mutilation, gouty tophi and arthritis, athetosis and spasticity.

XANTHINURIA

Autosomal recessive, uncommon. This condition of XO deficiency results in decreased plasma urates and xanthine renal stones because xanthine is insoluble in acid urine.

Renal failure

This is a failure to maintain adequate fluid and pH balance due to renal insufficiency. Other features include impaired erythropoietin production, impaired vitamin D hydroxylation, and hypertension.

ACUTE RENAL FAILURE

Causes

These may be *prerenal* due to local or general circulatory failure, *renal* due to renal parenchymal damage or *postrenal* due to outflow obstruction. Prerenal will convert to intrinsic renal failure if not promptly treated.

Prerenal	Renal	Postrenal
Circulatory failure	HUS	Bilateral obstruction,
Hypovolaemic	GN eg. HSP, post-streptococcal	eg. tumour, stones
(burns, haemorrhage,	Interstitial nephritis	Neurogenic bladder
dehydration)	Drugs eg. anticancer	Trauma
Septic	Pyelonephritis	
Cardiac	Vasculitis	
Renal artery or vein occlusion	Myoglobinuria	
	Tumour lysis syndrome	
	Untreated prerenal failure	
	progressing to ATN	

Clinical features

Acute renal failure (ARF) presents as oliguria (<1 ml/kg/h or <300 ml/m^2/day) with oedema, hypertension, vomiting, lethargy, electrolyte disturbance and metabolic acidosis. (NB. Oliguria is <0.5 ml/kg/h in neonates.)

Acute tubular necrosis (ATN)

This is the most common pathophysiological finding in established ARF. It is the result of ischaemic tubular damage secondary to hypoperfusion.

Oliguria Initially

Polyuria During the recovery phase

The prognosis for full renal recovery is good, though it depends on the severity of the underlying cause.

Acute cortical necrosis (ACN)

Cortical necrosis is irreversible loss of renal function with glomerular damage that heals with scarring (glomerulosclerosis). Any cause of ATN, if severe, can lead to ACN.

Criteria to distinguish prerenal from renal causes

	Prerenal	Renal
Urine osmolality (mosmo/l)	>500	<350
Urine Na (mmol/l)	<20	>40
Urine specific gravity	>1.020	<1.010
Urine:plasma urea ratio	>4.1	<4.1
Urine:plasma osmo ratio	>1.2	<1.2
Fractional excretion filtered Na	$<1\%$	$>1\%$

(The normal response in normal kidneys is to retain sodium and water if the BP or renal perfusion falls.)

Management

Fluids	In oliguric phase, restrict to insensible loss (300 ml/m^2/day) + ongoing losses
	In polyuric phase maintain input and electrolytes (as above)
	Daily weight, electrolytes
Hyperkalaemia	An emergency if ECG changes are present. (See below)
Hyperphosphataemia	Give a phosphate binder (eg. calcium carbonate)
Hypocalcaemia	Give calcium and α-calcidol
Metabolic acidosis	Give bicarbonate or dialyse if pH <7.25
Hypertension	Correct for fluid overload, antihypertensives
Nutrition	Restrict protein, K, Na and PO$_4$
Anaemia	Transfuse as necessary (but watch K carefully)
Dialysis	Indicated if severe hyperkalaemia, hyponatremia, fluid overload, symptomatic uraemia or medical management not tolerated

Management of hyperkalaemia

Drug	Onset	Mechanism
10% calcium gluconate	Immediate	Stabilises cardiac membrane
Salbutamol (nebulised or IV)	5 min	Shifts potassium into cells
8.4% $NaHCO_3$ (IV)	5 min	Shifts potassium into cells
Fluid bolus with frusemide (IV)	minutes	Renal excretion of potassium
Glucose (I± insulin)	30 min	Shifts potassium into cells
Calcium resonium (oral or rectal with lactulose)	30 mins (rectal) 2 hours (oral)	Potassium excretion through gut
Dialysis	Rapid (haemodialysis) Slower (peritoneal)	Removes potassium

CHRONIC RENAL FAILURE

This occurs with decline in renal function over months or years.

Causes

- *Congenital malformations*
- *Glomerulonephritis*
- *Inherited nephropathy*
- *Systemic illness*

Clinical features

- *Malaise*
- *Growth failure*
- *Polyuria, nocturia, oliguria (if late or acute on chronic), proteinuria*
- *Uraemia   Itching, anorexia, nausea, vomiting, skin colour change, polyneuropathy (paraesthesia), restless legs syndrome, myoclonic twitching, mental slowing, coma. Rare in children*
- *Symptoms of anaemia*
- *Oedema (peripheral and pulmonary)*
- *Renal bone disease (osteodystrophy)*

Investigations

Urine   Urinalysis, M, C + S, osmolality
24-hour electrolytes and protein

Plasma   U&E, creatinine ($\uparrow$), phosphate ($\uparrow$), ionised calcium ($\downarrow$), bicarbonate ($\downarrow$), PTH ($\uparrow$)
FBC and film

Radiology Left wrist (bone age and osteodystrophy), renal USS, renal function tests

GFR   Estimate from creatinine or measure formally

Management

Diet	High energy, low protein (<1.5 g/kg/day)
	NG or gastrostomy feeds may be needed (nausea)
Osteodystrophy	This is manifest as PO_4 ↑, Ca↓ and secondary hyperparathyroidism
	The aim is for the PTH to be in the normal range
	Use dietary phosphate restriction
	Calcium carbonate (lowers PO_4)
	Vitamin D supplements (1-α-OH-cholecalciferol)
Sodium and acidosis	Sodium supplements (unless low urine output)
	Bicarbonate supplements (2 mmol/kg/day)
Anaemia	Erythropoietin therapy (subcutaneous)
Hormones	GH given to overcome GH resistance
Dialysis	
BP↑	Diuretics, nifedipine, β-blockers, etc.

DIALYSIS

This is necessary in endstage renal failure (ESRF). There are two methods.

Peritoneal dialysis

Peritoneal membrane used as a semipermeable membrane. The dialysate is run through a tube into the peritoneal cavity and the fluid changed regularly to repeat the process.

- *CAPD (continuous ambulatory peritoneal dialysis); 2–4 cycles per day done manually*
- *CCPD (continuous cycling peritoneal dialysis); dialysis occurs only at night with 6–10 exchanges done by machine*

Major complication is peritonitis.

Haemodialysis

This is technically more difficult. Access is obtained using an indwelling main venous catheter or by creating an A-V fistula (more common in adults).

RENAL TRANSPLANTATION

This is a preferable option to dialysis as lifestyle is markedly improved.

Transplant	Cadaveric or live related donor (HLA-matched)
	In the iliac fossa (attached to the common iliac vessels)
	Intra-abdominally in a small child
Immunosuppression	Cyclosporin, prednisolone and azathioprine
Complications	Rejection (acute or chronic)
	Infection (CMV, varicella)
	Hypertension
	Drug side-effects (weight gain, hirsuitism)
	Post-transplant tumours eg. post-transplant lymphoproliferative disease PTLPD) which is EBV driven

CYCLOSPORIN

Cyclosporin is a fungal derivative and inhibits the release of IL-2 from T helper cells. Levels must be monitored.

Side-effects   Gum hyperplasia, hypertrichosis
Nephrotoxicity, hypertension, hyperkalaemia, HUS , neurotoxicity , tremor

Hypertension

This is persistent elevation of BP (systolic or diastolic) >95th centile and is present in 1–3% of children.

Causes

Essential   (Rare in children, v. common in adults)
Secondary   Renal – parenchymal disease or renal vascular disease
Cardiovascular – coarctation, renal artery stenosis
Hormonal – Conn syndrome, phaeochromocytoma, CAH, Cushing syndrome
Drugs '

Clinical features

- *Usually asymptomatic*
- *May have headaches and blurred vision if severe*
- *Examine for renal masses, bruits, coarctation and eye changes (papilloedema, retinal haemorrhages)*

Investigations

Urine   Urinalysis, M,C+S
HVA and HMA
Plasma   FBC, U&E, creatinine, Ca, PO_4, fasting lipids
Renin, aldosterone level
Radiology   CXR, renal USS with Dopplers, renal function tests (DMSA ? scars), echocardiogram
ECG
Ophthalmological examination

Management options

Emergency

Nifedipine   Oral (sublingual may cause precipitant fall)
Sodium nitroprusside   Infusion ⎫
Labetalol   Infusion ⎬ with care to avoid precipitious BP fall.
Hydralazine   Slow IV bolus ⎭

Long term

- *Treat underlying cause*
- *Drug therapy eg. vasodilators, diuretics, β-blockers, ACE inhibitors*

FURTHER READING

Barratt TM, Avner ED, Harmon W *Pediatric nephrology* 4th Ed, Williams & Wilkins, Baltimore, 1999

Posthlethwaite RJ *Clinical paediatric nephrology* 2nd Ed, Butterworth-Heinneman, London 1994

9

Endocrinology, Growth and Puberty

- *Hypothalamus and pituitary*
- *Adrenal glands*
- *Thyroid gland*
- *Parathyroid glands*
- *Glucose metabolism*

- *Polycystic ovary syndrome (PCOS)*
- *Endocrine syndromes*
- *Growth and puberty*
- *Endocrine tests*

Hypothalamus and pituitary

PHYSIOLOGY

The anterior lobe of the pituitary develops from the Rathke pouch from an invagination of the oral endoderm. The posterior pituitary is part of a single functional unit called the neurohypophysis which comprises the neurons of the hypothalamus, the neuronal axons (the pituitary stalk) and the neuronal terminals in the posterior lobe of the pituitary.

PITUITARY TUMOURS

Pituitary tumours are the commonest cause of pituitary disease, and they include the following conditions:

1. *Craniopharyngioma*
2. *Pituitary gigantism/Acromegaly*
3. *Prolactinoma*
4. *Cushing disease (see p. 254)*
5. *Nelson syndrome*
6. *Non-functioning tumour*

They present with symptoms of one or both of:

1. *Space-occupying lesion*
   - *Raised intracranial pressure symptoms and signs (headache, papilloedema, etc.)*
   - *Visual field defects (bitemporal hemianopia)*
   - *Hydrocephalus (if CSF flow is interrupted)*
   - *Pressure on hypothalamic centres (appetite, thirst, somnolence/wakeful, precocious puberty)*

- *Cavernous sinus thrombosis (III, IV, VI cranial nerve lesions)*
- *Diencephalic syndrome*

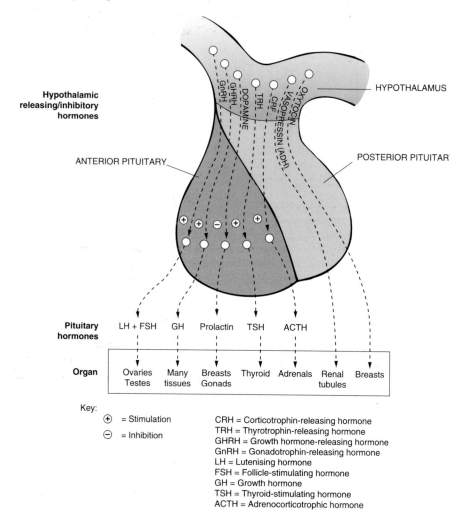

Figure 9.1 Hypothalamic and pituitary hormones

2. *Hormonal excess or deficiency.*

The following investigations and examinations are useful.

- *Visual field testing*
- *Cranial nerve testing*
- *MRI or CT scan (demonstrating a mass)*
- *Hormonal investigations (showing a deficiency or an excess)*

Treatment is with drugs, radiotherapy and/or surgery.

CRANIOPHARYNGIOMA

This is one of the most common supratentorial tumours in children. It arises from a remnant of the connection between the Rathke pouch and the oral cavity. It is often large and cystic and 50% occur under the age of 20 years. Calcification is seen in most cases on skull X-ray.

Presentation

- *Headaches, visual field defects and hydrocephalus (compression of the third ventricle)*
- *Hormonal effects of hypopituitarism:*
    growth failure, pubertal delay
    diabetes insipidus
    hypothyroidism
    adrenocortical deficiency

Essential examination and investigations are as above for pituitary tumours.

Treatment

This is with surgical removal (transfrontal or transsphenoidal). Postoperative radiotherapy is used if resection is incomplete or recurrence occurs. Postoperative hormonal deficiency is common and treated with supplementation as necessary.

PITUITARY GIGANTISM AND ACROMEGALY

This is usually caused by an acidophil adenoma of the pituitary producing excess growth hormone (very rarely due to excessive GHRH). The tumour is medium-large and most skull X-rays are abnormal. If the epiphyses are open, pituitary gigantism results, and if they are closed, acromegaly results.

Presentation

- *Space-occupying effects*
- *Hormonal effects (all, except tall stature, mainly seen in acromegaly):*
    tall stature with delayed epiphyseal fusion
    change in appearance (coarse facies, large tongue, frontal bossing, large jaw, large hands and hypogonadism)
    hyperprolactinaemia (30%)
    IDDM (25%)
    hypopituitarism (partial or complete of the anterior pituitary)
- *Others:*
    hypercalciuria, hyperphosphataemia (10%), recurrent infections, hypertension, atheroma and large bowel carcinoma

Essential examination and investigations

As for pituitary tumours. Specific hormonal tests are:

- *prolactin levels (raised in 30%)*
- *GH levels (↑)*

- *glucose tolerance test (fail to supress GH <2 μ/e, 25% have a diabetic result)*
- *Insulin-like growth factor IGF-1 levels ↑*
- *pituitary function tests (anterior pituitary)*

Treatment

- *Surgery*
- *Radiotherapy*
- *Octreotride (a somatostatin analogue)*
- *Bromocriptine*

PROLACTINOMA

This is the most common pituitary tumour that occurs in adolescence. They are mostly large tumours (macroadenoma) but may be small (microadenoma, <10 mm) producing excess prolactin. They are mostly postpubertal and twice as common in girls.

Presentation

- *Space-occupying effects (headache, visual field defects, etc.)*
- *Hormonal effects:*
    galactorrhoea, amenorrhoea
    hypogonadism, impotence, delayed puberty (a few cases only)
    hypopituitarism

Investigations are those of pituitary tumours in general, plus serum prolactin level. Prolactin levels of 2000–15 000 ng/ml are seen with a prolactinoma.

Treatment

- *Medical (Bromocriptine or Carbagoline)*
- *Surgical removal of tumour*

Other causes of hyperprolactinaemia

- *Stress*
- *Primary hypothyroidism*
- *Hypothalamic disease (acromegaly, craniopharyngioma)*
- *Polycystic ovaries*
- *Drugs (cimetidine, metoclopramide, oestrogens, opiates)*
- *Pregnancy, suckling*
- *Liver failure, cardiac failure, renal failure*

HYPOPITUITARISM

This can be a deficiency of either hypothalamic or pituitary hormones. It may also be selective or multiple, with growth hormone being the most common hormone affected. Panhypopituitarism is the deficiency of all anterior pituitary hormones. Vasopressin (ADH) and oxytocin will only be affected significantly if the hypothalamus is involved or there is a very large pituitary lesion.

Causes

Congenital   Anencephaly, holoprosencephaly
Septo-optic dysplasia (absence of septum pellucidum and optic nerve hypoplasia)
Kallman syndrome
Genetic deficiency (several types)
Empty sella syndrome

Destructive   Neoplastic (pituitary/hypothalamic, eg. craniopharyngioma, meningioma, glioma, secondary deposits)
Infective (meningitis, encephalitis, TB, toxoplasmosis)
Traumatic (postsurgery or radiotherapy, child abuse, traumatic delivery)
Infiltration (sarcoidosis, Langerhans cell histiocytosis, haemochromatosis)

Functional   Emotional deprivation, anorexia nervosa, starvation

Clinical features

These are dependent on the extent of the disease. Growth hormone is the most common deficiency, resulting in growth failure. Secondary hypothyroidism and ACTH deficiency (leading to adrenal failure) may be present. Hyperprolactinaemia, diabetes insipidus and deficiency of gonadotrophins may also be present.

If congenital, it may present as an emergency with apnoea, hypoglycaemia and cyanosis and male infants may have a microphallus. The child has a distinctive facies. When long-standing, there is 'alabaster skin' which is pale and hairless. Sexual maturation is delayed or absent and symptomatic hypoglycaemia with fasting occurs in 10–15%.

Investigations

Pituitary function tests need to be done, with each axis being investigated separately.

Treatment

This involves treating any underlying disease and replacing hormones as necessary.

DIABETES INSIPIDUS

This is characterised by polyuria and polydipsia and is due to a deficiency of vasopressin (ADH) or a renal insensitivity to it.

Clinical features

- *Polydipsia, polyuria, nocturia*
- *Anorexia, dehydration, lack of perspiration and production of large quantities of pale urine*
- *Rapid weight loss with collapse in infants*

Investigations

These show a *mismatch* between urine and plasma osmolalities.

1. *Plasma osmolality normal or high, and plasma Na high*
2. *Urine osmolality low: EMU osmolality <280 (normal >600)*
   Specific gravity 1.001–1.005
3. *Formal water deprivation test:*
   - *Deprive patient of water until either a mismatch between urine and plasma osmolality is demonstrated or >5% wt. loss or urine osmolality >700 mmol/kg*
   - *Observe failure to concentrate urine*
     Then give DDAVP and observe urine osmolality is raised
4. *A failure of response to exogenous ADH (DDAVP) indicates nephrogenic diabetes insipidus*
5. *Plasma ADH measurement is possible, and if inappropriately low for plasma osmolality indicates DI*
6. *Cranial MRI scan*

Causes

Cranial		Nephrogenic
Congenital	Aut dominant DIDMOAD	Congenital (X-linked recessive)
Tumour	Craniopharyngioma	Renal tubular acidosis
Infection	TB meningitis	Hypokalaemia
Infiltration	Sarcoidosis	Nephrocalcinosis
Ablation	Surgery, DXT	Drugs: demeclocycline
Newborn	Asphyxia, IVH	glibenclamide
	Listeria, meningitis	lithium
	Langerhans cell histiocytosis	

DIDMOAD = diabetes insipidus, diabetes mellitus, optic atrophy and deafness. Also known as Wolfram syndrome

Treatment

Cranial diabetes insipidus	DDAVP (desmopressin = ADH analogue) given IM or oral, or intranasal
Nephrogenic diabetes insipidus	Sensitise the renal tubules with thiazides, carbamazepine or chloramphenicol

NB. 5 yearly cranial MRI scans are necessary to detect cause, as this may be delayed by many years.

Differential diagnosis

Psychogenic polydipsia (compulsive water drinking). Here the urine will concentrate on water deprivation testing; however, there may be a decreased ability to concentrate urine if the condition is prolonged.

Water intoxication (deliberate/Munchausen by proxy).

SYNDROME OF INAPPROPRIATE ADH SECRETION (SIADH)

In this condition plasma levels of ADH are *inappropriately high* for the osmolality of the blood.

Clinical features

- *Often vague features*
- *Appetite loss (early), nausea, vomiting, confusion, irritability, fits and coma*
- *No evidence of dehydration, no oedema, normal blood pressure*

Investigations

1. *Plasma electrolytes:* Na ↓ *(115–120 mmol/l)*
   Cl↓
   Bicarbonate (N)
2. *Plasma osmolality low (<280 mmol/l)*
3. *Urine osmolality normal*
4. *Urine Na >30 mmol/l (ie. sodium excretion continues)*
5. *Hypouricaemia*

Causes

CNS	Head injury, meningitis, subdural haematoma, SLE vasculitis, brain tumour, Guillain–Barré syndrome, brain abscess
Tumours	Lymphoma, Ca. pancreas, Ca. duodenum, Ca. thymus, Ewing sarcoma
Lungs	Pneumonia, TB, lung abscess, cystic fibrosis, IPPV
Metabolic	Acute intermittent porphyria
Drugs	Chlorpropramide, carbamazepine, vincristine, cyclophosphamide, morphine
Infections	eg. Rotavirus

Treatment

1. *Fluid restrict*
2. *Daily weight, sodium and osmolality measurements*
3. *Demeclocycline (dimethylchlortetracycline) therapy to desensitise the kidney*
4. *If severe: hypertonic saline with frusemide is given under close observation*

Adrenal glands

THE GLUCOCORTICOID AXIS

Relative strength of glucocorticoids	
Cortisol (hydrocortisone)	1
Prednisolone	4
Dexamethasone	25

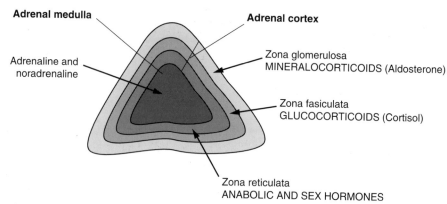

Figure 9.2 Adrenal gland

CUSHING SYNDROME

This results from a state of increased circulating glucocorticoids.

Causes

ACTH dependent	Pituitary tumour (basophilic adenoma (20%) or microadenoma (80%). NB. This is *Cushing disease*
	Ectopic ACTH production (extremely rare)
ACTH independent	Adrenal adenoma or carcinoma (most often <3 years)
	Exogenous steroids – the *commonest* cause

Clinical features

1. *Appearance:*
   Round face, large red cheeks – 'moon face'
   Truncal obesity – 'buffalo hump', 'lemon on sticks'
   Striae and bruises due to protein breakdown
   Masculinisation signs due to androgen production (acne, hypertrichosis and clitoral hypertrophy)
2. *Growth impairment*
3. *Osteoporosis*
4. *Impaired glucose tolerance, diabetes (glycosuria)*
5. *Hypertension*
6. *Pubertal delay*
7. *Weakness, headache, mental disturbance*
8. *Hyperpigmentation – seen with high ACTH only*

Investigations

These are divided into those investigations to establish the *diagnosis* and those to establish the *cause* of Cushing syndrome. NB. Random cortisol is of *no* benefit.

Diagnosis	Underlying cause

1. Serum – Na $\uparrow$, K $\downarrow$, alkalosis
2. Cortisol circadian rhythm:
   –0900 and 2400 cortisol
   –normal = pronounced rhythm
   –Cushing = high midnight levels
 	
3. Urine 24h free cortisol
4. Overnight dexamethasone
   suppression test
	1. ACTH level <10ng/l = ACTH
	   independent, 20–80 ng/l = normal/high
	   in ACTH dependent, >100–1000 ng/l =
	   high in ectopic ACTH
	2. Low and high-dose dexamethasone
	   suppression test
	3. CRF test (exaggerated ACTH response =
	   pituitary-dependent *Cushing disease*)
	4. Adrenal CT scan
	5. Pituitary MRI scan

Treatment

The options available include surgical removal of a pituitary lesion, radiotherapy to the pituitary, bilateral adrenalectomy (rarely done now), resection of adrenal adenoma and reduction of exogenous steroids where possible. Medical therapy with inhibitors of adrenal steroid biosynthesis (eg. ketoconazole).

NB. *Nelson syndrome* is the occurrence of a pituitary tumour after bilateral adrenalectomy, causing high ACTH levels and hyperpigmentation. It is very rare.

PRIMARY HYPERALDOSTERONISM

This is due to an adenoma of the zona glomerulosa in 60% of cases (known as Conn syndrome) and an adrenal cortical carcinoma in a minority. Approximately 30% are due to bilateral adrenal hyperplasia (secondary aldosteronism). *Secondary aldosteronism has several causes:*

- *Ascites – nephrotic syndrome, liver cirrhosis, CCF*
- *Hypovolaemia secondary to diuretic abuse*
- *Renal artery stenosis, Wilm's tumour*

Clinical features

- *Proximal muscle weakness, polyuria, polydipsia, nocturnal enuresis (all due to hypokalaemia)*
- *Hypertension with no oedema (due to hypernatraemia)*

Investigations

- *Plasma electrolytes – K $\downarrow$ Na $\uparrow$, metabolic alkalosis (20% have normal potassium at presentation)*
- *Plasma renin $\downarrow$ (NB. secondary aldosteronism-renin $\uparrow$)*
- *Urine aldosterone metabolites*
- *Urine Na:K ratio $\downarrow$ (normal = 2 : 1 mmol/kg/24hr)*

Treatment options

1. *Prednisolone (suppresses the hyperaldosteronism)*

2. *Spironolactone (aldosterone antagonist)*
3. *Surgical resection*

ADRENOCORTICAL INSUFFICIENCY

This is deficiency of all the adrenal cortical hormones, but cortisol causes the main effects.

Causes

Acute	Steroid withdrawal	
	Severe hypotension	
	Birth asphyxia	
	Sepsis NB. *Waterhouse-Freidrichson syndrome* of adrenal haemorrhage secondary to meningococcaemia	
	Trauma	
	Congenital causes	
Chronic	Primary (ACTH↑)	Destruction of adrenal cortex (*Addison disease*), due to autoimmune disease or TB
		Leukaemia, HIV infection, haemochromatosis
		Drugs eg. ketoconazole
		Adrenoleukodystrophy (adrenocortical insufficiency, with demyelination in CNS)
	Secondary (ACTH↓)	Pituitary or hypothalamic disease
		Long-term steroid therapy

Clinical features

Acute disease

Presents as an adrenal crisis: peripheral shutdown, cyanosis, tachycardia, tachypnoea, hypotension, drowsiness and coma. Fatal if not rapidly treated.

Chronic disease

In a baby, presentation is with apathy, vomiting, failure to thrive, hypoglycaemia and dehydration leading to circulatory collapse and coma.

In an older child, presentation is with weakness, fatigue, anorexia, nausea, vomiting, abdominal pain, diarrhoea and failure to thrive. Postural hypotension and salt craving. Hyperpigmentation of buccal mucosa, scars and skin creases occurs with primary disease (secondary to ACTH ↑).

Investigations

Serum electrolytes	Na↓, K↑, glucose ↓
Serum hormones	Cortisol ↓ (*no diurnal change*)
	ACTH ↑ (primary disease)
Synacthen test	Short and long if necessary

Treatment

Adrenal crisis   IV fluids and salt replacement
                   Hydrocortisone IV
                   Antibiotics if necessary

Long-term therapy This is with daily hydrocortisone and fludrocortisone

CONGENITAL ADRENAL HYPERPLASIA

Autosomal recessive, incidence 1 in 10 000. This condition results from deficiency of an enzyme involved in the cortisol synthetic pathways. The most common cause is 21-hydroxylase deficiency. The genetic defect is on chromosome 6 near the HLA region. The deficiency causes the steroid pathway to be deflected from cortisol synthesis down the alternative androgenic pathways.

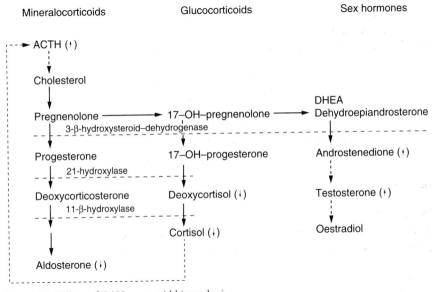

Figure 9.3 Effects of CAH on steroid biosynthesis

Clinical features

- *Masculinisation of a female baby*
- *Adrenal crisis at 2–3 weeks*
- *May present later with advanced bone age, tall stature (eventual short stature), precocious puberty, hypertension, skin pigmentation, hirsutism*

Investigations

Essential investigations

1. *Plasma 17-OH-progesterone ($\uparrow$)*
2. *Urine pregnanetriol ($\uparrow$)*
3. *Serum electrolytes: Na $\downarrow$, K $\uparrow$, glucose $\downarrow$*

4. *Karyotype*
5. *Pelvic ultrasound scan (looking for female organs in a masculinised female)*

Other investigations

1. *ACTH* ($\uparrow$)
2. *Cortisol* $\downarrow$, *testosterone* $\uparrow$, *aldosterone* $\downarrow$, *androstenedione* $\uparrow$

Treatment

Drugs Hydrocortisone 20 mg/m^2/day
          Fludrocortisone 150 μg/m^2/day
          Sodium chloride in infants
Surgery If necessary for masculinised females
Monitor Growth and skeletal maturity
          Androgens, 17-OH-progesterone, ACTH

During illness, give extra cortisol.

   NB. Antenatal diagnosis is possible. Dexamethasone is given to the mother in order to decrease fetal ACTH if baby is female.

Other variants

1. *11β-hydroxylase deficiency (5–8%)*
      Non salt-losing, Na $\uparrow$, *K* $\downarrow$, *BP* $\uparrow$
      Virilisation
      Diagnosis: 11-deoxycortisol $\uparrow$
2. *3β-hydroxysteroid dehydrogenase deficiency (<5%)*
      Salt-losing, Na $\downarrow$, *K* $\uparrow$
      Virilisation of girls, incomplete virilisation of boys
      Diagnosis: elevated pregnenolone, DHEA, 17-OH-pregnenolone

PHAEOCHROMOCYTOMA

This is a sympathetic nervous system tumour arising from chromaffin cells, secreting catecholamines. Mostly noradrenaline is released but some adrenaline is also released. Boys:girls = 2:1.

- *90% adrenal medulla tumour*
- *10% along the sympathetic chain*
- *25% multiple*
- *10% malignant*
- *10% recur*

Associations   MEN II, neurofibromatosis

Differential diagnosis
Autoimmune disease, renal artery stenosis.

Clinical features

The symptoms are frequently intermittent.

General   Palpitations, sweating, tremor, headaches, panic attacks, nausea and vomiting, weight loss

Cardiovascular instability   Tachycardia, bradycardia, hypertension, orthostatic hypotension

Investigations

1. *24-hour urine catecholamines increased (vanillymandelic acid (VMA) and metanephrins). NB. Dietary vanilla interferes with this test*
2. *MIBG scan (metaiodobenzylguanidine – a specific chromaffin tissue isotope scan)*
3. *Abdominal CT scan*
4. *Serum catecholamines*

Management

Surgical resection of the tumour under α (phenoxybenzamine) and β (propranolol) blockade.

Thyroid gland

PHYSIOLOGY

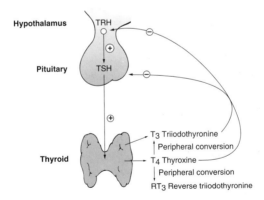

Figure 9.4 Thyroid axis

In plasma 99% of T4 and T3 is bound to thyroid binding globulin (TBG), and thyroid binding pre-albumin (TBPA) and albumin. Only the free form is active; 0.05% is in the free active form.

In acute or chronic illness, thyroid function is affected, with RT3↑, TBG↓, TSH↓. This results in low total and free T4 and T3 with a normal or low TSH, known as *sick euthyroid syndrome*.

Thyroxine (T4) and antithyroid drugs cross the placenta.

GUTHRIE TEST FOR HYPOTHYROIDISM

This is a measurement of TSH, taken as a capillary blood sample on day 6. An elevated level (>20 mU/l) is abnormal and indicative of hypothyroidism. False-negative results occur with:

- *prematurity or sick euthyroid syndrome*
- *TBG deficiency (congenital or acquired)*
- *secondary or tertiary hypothyroidism*

If the result is repeatedly equivocal (TSH 20–30 mU/l), thyroxine should be commenced and at a later date the thyroid function reassessed with a repeat TSH measurement and thyroid imaging.

HYPOTHYROIDISM

Causes

Primary   (Thyroid gland dysfunction – TSH ↑, thyroxine ↓)
Congenital
Atrophic autoimmune thyroiditis – thyroid microsomal antibodies
Hashimoto thyroiditis – goitre, microsomal antibodies, associated with Turner syndrome
Iodine deficiency – goitre, occurs in mountainous areas
Treatment of hyperthyroidism or radiotherapy for lymphoma, leukaemia
Drugs – amiodarone, iodine-containing medications

Secondary or   (TSH ↓, thyroxine↓)
tertiary   Pituitary disease (secondary)
Hypothalamic disease (tertiary)

Congenital Hypothyroidism
Incidence 1 in 4000

Causes

90% thyroid dysgenesis   Aplasia (1/3)
Ectopic (2/3) – lingual, sublingual or subhyoid thyroid

10% dyshormonogenesis   eg. Pendred syndrome (goitre, sensorineural deafness and hypothyroidism)

Transient disease   Due to placental transfer in maternal autoimmune thyroid disease or antithyroid drugs

Diagnosis usually on Guthrie test with TSH>100, confirmed with low serum T4.

Clinical features

Physical features   Macroglossia, umbilical hernia, wide-spaced eyes, flat nasal bridge, swollen eyelids, large fontanelles, dry skin, short broad fingers

Other   Prolonged neonatal jaundice (unconjugated)
Hypotonia, somnolence, feeding difficulties, hoarse cry, constipation, sluggishness, noisy respirations, apnoeas, cutis marmorata

Bradycardia, cardiomegaly, cardiac murmurs, low-voltage ECG with prolonged PR interval

Mental retardation

Clinical features of acquired hypothyroidism

NB. Thyroid dysgenesis and ectopic thyroid can present later, as acquired.

- *Deceleration of growth*
- *Delayed ossification*
- *Skin and hair – dry, lateral third eyebrow missing, hair dry and thin*
- *Cold intolerance*
- *Low energy levels*
- *Constipation*
- *Proximal myopathy, ataxia, slow reflexes*
- *Mental slowness at school often occurs late*
- *Headaches, precocious puberty and galactorrhoea (seen in secondary and tertiary disease)*

Investigations

Thyroid function tests are performed and enable differentiation of primary from secondary and tertiary disease. Other abnormalities seen on blood testing are hypercalcaemia, hypercholesterolaemia and hyperprolactinaemia.

Treatment

This is with thyroxine replacement, giving oral thyroxine 10–15 µg/kg/day.

HYPERTHYROIDISM

Causes

Graves' disease	Most common childhood cause
	Diffuse toxic goitre. Thyroid eye signs and pretibial myxoedema occur only in Graves' disease
	Female > male 5 : 1. HLA-B8, DW3 association
	TRSAb (thyrotrophin receptor stimulating antibodies)
	Autoimmune association (vitiligo, IDDM, RhA, ITP, Addison)
Solitary nodule/adenoma	Plummer disease, toxic uninodular goitre
de Quervain's thyroiditis	Acute disease with tender goitre
	Viral origin (mumps, coxsackie, adenovirus)
Reidel's thyroiditis	Dense thyroid fibrosis including neck vessels and trachea
Thyrotoxicosis facticia	Ingestion of thyroxine
Tumours	Ovarian teratoma, choriocarcinoma, hydatidiform mole
Transient neonatal	Secondary to maternal Graves disease, lasts 6–12 weeks

Clinical features

Usually of gradual onset

- *Hyperactivity, emotional lability, short attention spans*
- *Increased appetite with no weight gain*

- *Smooth skin, increased sweating, tremor*
- *Goitre (usually)*
- *Tachycardia, palpitations, dyspnoea, hypertension, cardiomegaly, atrial fibrillation (rare)*
- *Eye signs: exophthalmos, lid retraction, lid lag, impaired convergence*

Thyroid crisis

This is acute-onset hyperthyroidism and presents as tachycardia, hypertension and restlessness, progressing to delirium, coma and death if not rapidly treated.

Neonatal hyperthyroidism

These babies are classically premature, have IUGR, goitres, exophthalmos, microcephaly. They are irritable, hyperalert and may have tachycardia, tachypnoea, hyperthermia, jaundice, hypertension and progress to cardiac decompensation.

Investigations

1. *Free T4 and T3 elevated*
2. *TSH decreased*
3. *TRSAbs found in Graves' disease*

Treatment options

Medical	Antithyroid drugs (propylthiouracyl or carbimazole)
	Symptomatic control with β-blockers (propranolol)
	Radioactive Iodine
Surgery	Subtotal thyroidectomy
	Complications: hypoparathyroidism (transient or permanent), vocal cord paralysis

GOITRE

Goitre = an enlargement of the thyroid gland.
Child may be euthyroid, hypothyroid or hyperthyroid. Infants may have respiratory difficulties due to the large gland. Assess the goitre for size, consistency, diffuse/nodular. Check thyroid status. Additional investigations may include USS thyroid, thyroid scan and fine needle aspiration. Causes are listed below and include both congenital and acquired disorders.

Causes

Congenital	Maternal antithyroid drugs (hypothyroid usually)
	Maternal iodine-containing drugs eg. amoidarone (hypothyroid usually)
	Dyshormonogensis
	Congenital hyperthyroidism
	Iodine deficiency (rare)
	Thyroid teratoma
Older child	Colloid goitre (euthyroid, unknown cause, prepubertal girls)
	Autoimmune eg. Hashimoto's thyroiditis
	Graves disease

Thyroiditis
Iodine deficiency or iodine-containing drugs
Antithyroid drugs
Multinodular goitre (seen in McCune-Albright disease)
Thyroid tumour

THYROID TUMOURS

These are rare in children and are associated with previous thyroid irradiation as an infant. They present as solitary thyroid nodules ± cervical lymph node metastases. Girls > boys, 2:1.

Types			
Papillary	70%	Young people, slow growing, local	Good prognosis
Follicular	20%	Early metastases (lungs, bone)	Good prognosis
Medullary	5%	Often familial (eg. Marfan), MEN II, calcitonin ↑	Poor prognosis
Anaplastic	<5%	Aggressive	Very poor prognosis

The investigations necessary are lymph node biopsy, thyroid I^{131} scan (carcinoma usually appears as 'cold' nodules, ie. decreased concentration of isotope) and thyroid function tests. Treatment is with subtotal or near-total thyroidectomy with or without radiotherapy.

Parathyroid glands

CALCIUM PHYSIOLOGY

See Figure 9.5.

PTH
This results in ↑ plasma calcium, ↓ plasma phosphate by increasing gut absorption and renal tubular reabsorption of calcium, increasing $1, 25(OH)_2D_3$ synthesis, renal PO_4 excretion and bone absorption.

Calcium
50% albumin bound: 50% free ionised calcium (available). Correct plasma calcium for albumin (if albumin >40 g/l – corrected level is *lower*).

Calcitonin
32 amino acid polypeptide, secreted by the C-cells of the thyroid gland.

- *Decreases serum calcium (inhibits osteoclasts, ↑ renal calcium excretion)*
- *Decreases serum phosphate (↑ renal phosphate excretion)*

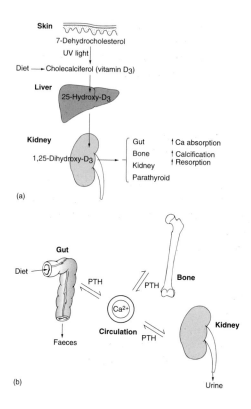

Figure 9.5 Calcium physiology. (a) Vitamin D metabolism and actions. (b) Calcium exchange

Vitamin D
- *Vitamin D* = *calciferol (D3)*
- *Alphacalcidol* = *1-α hydroxycholecalciferol*
- *Calcitriol* = *1, 25-dihydroxycholecalciferol (1,25(OH)₂D₃)*

HYPOCALCAEMIA

Causes

$PTH\downarrow$ (Ca $\downarrow$, PO_4 $\uparrow$)   Autoimmune (vitiligo, candidiasis)

DiGeorge (parathyroid and thymus hypo or aplasia, cardiac abnormalities, auricle hypoplasia, T cell immune defect, abnormal facies – see p. 12)

Surgical (post-thyroidectomy)

Pseudohypoparathyroidism

NB. Pseudo-pseudohypoparathyroidism (phenotype of pseudohypoparathyroidism with *normal* calcium)

$PTH\uparrow$ $(Ca\downarrow, PO_4\downarrow)$ Rickets/osteomalacia due to:

> intake vitamin $D\downarrow$
> metabolism vitamin $D \downarrow$ (renal, liver)
> excretion calcium $\uparrow$

Clinical features

- *Muscle cramps, paraesthesia, stiffness*
- *Laryngeal and carpopedal spasm, tetany*
- *Seizures*
- *Cataracts, soft teeth, horizontal lines on toe and finger nails*
- *Chovsteck's sign (facial muscle twitching on tapping facial nerve)*
- *Trousseau's sign (tetanic spasm of hands and wrist with BP cuff > above diastolic pressure for 3 mins)*
- *Long QT interval, papilloedema*

Investigations

Serum   Calcium $(\downarrow)$
        Phosphate $(\downarrow$ or $\uparrow)$
        Alkaline phosphatase $(\downarrow$ or $\uparrow)$
        Magnesium level (should be normal but necessary to exclude hypo-magnesaemia as cause of hypocalcaemia)
        PTH $(\downarrow, N$ or $\uparrow)$

Treatment

Emergency therapy   10% calcium gluconate IV stat dose, then 0.5–1 ml/min
                 NB. Calcium gluconate $= 8.9$ mg/ml
                        Calcium chloride $= 27$ mg/ml
Long term   Oral calcium supplements and oral vitamin D supplements (calcitriol or alfacalcidol)

PSEUDOHYPOPARATHYROIDISM

This is due to end-organ resistance to PTH, secondary to a G-protein receptor defect. Autosomal dominant.

Clinical features

- *Short, stocky with a round face*
- *Short 4th metacarpal*
- *Brachydactyly, bow legs, dimples on dorsum of hand*
- *Subcutaneous calcium deposits*
- *Mental retardation, calcification basal ganglia, cataracts*
- *Tetany, stridor, convulsions*

Investigations
Serum   Ca $\downarrow$, PO$_4$ $\uparrow$, alkaline phosphatase $\uparrow$
        PTH$\uparrow$

Diagnosis on decreased response in urine cAMP and phosphate after PTH infusion.

RICKETS

This is a failure in mineralisation of growing bone. In fully developed bone this is called osteomalacia. Daily vitamin D requirement is 400 IU.

Causes

Vitamin D intake inadequate   Nutritional (breastfed, poorly fed, prematurity)
                Malabsorption (coeliac disease, steatorrhoea, cystic fibrosis)
                Inadequate sunlight exposure (especially dark-skinned)
Metabolism of vitamin D   Renal disease NB. PO$_4$ $\uparrow$
                Liver disease
                Anticonvulsants eg. phenytoin (metabolises vitamin D)
Phosphate excretion increased   Familial hypophosphataemic rickets
                Vitamin D-dependent rickets: type I
                                type II (receptor defect)
                Fanconi syndrome

Clinical features

- *Craniotabes (ping-pong ball skull), frontal bossing, large anterior fontanelle with delayed closure (>2 years)*
- *Rachitic rosary (enlargement of costochondral junctions), Harrison groove or sulcus, pigeon chest*
- *Thickened wrists and ankles*
- *Dwarfism, kyphosis, bow legs, knock knees, small pelvis, coxa vara, late dentition with enamel defects, greenstick fractures*
- *Muscular weakness, pot belly*

Investigations

1. *Biochemical investigations (see table). NB. Classic nutritional rickets: check alk.phos, calcium, phosphate and PO$_4$-Ca product (low).*

	Ca	PO$_4$	PTH	Alk.phos	25(OH)D$_3$	1,25(OH)$_2$D$_3$
Nutritional	N,$\downarrow$	$\uparrow$ or $\downarrow$	$\uparrow$,N	$\uparrow$	$\downarrow$	$\downarrow$
Hypophosphataemic	N,$\downarrow$	$\downarrow$	N	$\uparrow$	N	$\downarrow$
Vit. D-dependent type I	$\downarrow$	$\downarrow$	$\uparrow$	$\uparrow$	N	$\downarrow$
Vit. D-dependent type II	$\downarrow$	$\downarrow$	$\uparrow$	$\uparrow$	N	$\uparrow$

2. *X-ray of left wrist (or left knee if <2 years). The X-ray findings are:*
   - *widened epiphyseal plate*
   - *cupping and fraying of the metaphysis*
   - *increased joint space*
   - *line of calcification seen when healing*
   - *also: cysts, subperiosteal erosions, fractures, Looser's zones osteopenia, if severe.*

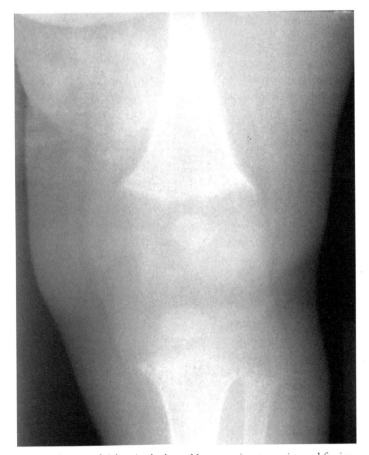

Figure 9.6 X-ray changes of rickets in the knee. Note prominent cupping and fraying

Treatment
This is with vitamin D in the necessary form.

Nutritional rickets Calciferol (D_3)
Renal disease Alphacalcidol ($1\alpha OHD_3$) or calcitriol ($1,25(OH)_2D_3$)

Familial hypophosphataemic rickets (= vitamin D-resistant rickets)
X-linked dominant

Underlying problem   1. Defective proximal tubular reabsorption of phosphate
2. Reduced $1,25(OH)_2D_3$ synthesis

Treatment is $1,25(OH)_2D_3$ and oral phosphate supplements.

Vitamin D-dependent rickets

Autosomal recessive. Characterised by a calcium deficiency with secondary hyper-parathyroidism and a renal tubular acidosis. There are two types:

- *type I – low $1,25(OH)_2D_3$ levels*
- *type II – $1,25(OH)_2D_3$ receptor defect*

Treatment is with $1,25(OH)_2D_3$. (Type 1 have good response).

HYPERCALCAEMIA

Causes

$PTH \uparrow (Ca \uparrow, PO_4 \downarrow)$ Primary hyperparathyroidism (hyperplasia or adenoma. NB. MEN I and II)

Tertiary hyperparathyroidism (PTH $\uparrow$ after long-standing secondary hyperparathyroidism now treated)

Ectopic (other tumours)

$PTH \downarrow (Ca \uparrow, PO_4 \uparrow)$ Vitamin D $\uparrow$ (sarcoidosis, TB, lymphoma, berylliosis, excess vitamin D)

Williams syndrome (7q-, hypercalcaemia, supravalvular aortic stenosis, AVSD, peripheral pulmonary stenosis, stellate iris, cocktail party manner, typical facies – see p. 12)

Malignancy (leukaemia, lymphoma, neuroblastoma)

Hypothyroidism (vitamin D metabolism decreased)

Hyperthyroidism

Familial hypocalciuric hypercalcaemia (PTH inappropriately normal, autosomal dominant, usually asymptomatic)

Clinical features

- **Stones** *(renal)*, **bones** *(pain)*, **abdominal moans** *(ulcers)*, **psychiatric groans**
- *Anorexia, vomiting, constipation, peptic ulcers, pancreatitis*
- *Corneal calcification, conjunctival injection, polyuria (nephrogenic DI from nephrocalcinosis), hypertension*
- *Chondrocalcinosis (30%), subperiosteal bone erosions, hypokalaemia*
- *Cardiac arrest with high calcium levels (>3.75) and convulsions*

Investigations

Serum   Calcium, phosphate, alkaline phosphatase and renal function PTH levels. Hand X-ray.

Management

Severe   IV biphosphonates (etidronate, pamidronate)
Hydration with frusemide

Mild   Oral phosphates (diarrhoea)
           Calcitonin
           Steroids (sarcoidosis)

Hypoparathyroidectomy if necessary (primary hyperparathyroidism).

Glucose metabolism

Blood glucose is generally maintained in the non-fasted state between 3.5 and 8.0 mmol/l. Glucose is consumed by the brain as a primary source of energy. Muscle may utilise glucose for energy or store it as glycogen. Adipose tissue is also a store for glucose and uses glucose for triglyceride synthesis. The liver is the principal site for glucose storage, where it is kept as glycogen. Glucose may be manufactured from glycogen, fat or protein by a process called gluconeogenesis.

The maintenance of a constant blood glucose level is under the control of the hormone insulin. High insulin levels cause the blood glucose level to fall by increasing glucose utilisation and decreasing glucose production. Low insulin levels have the converse effect. Other hormones are involved and have the opposite effect to insulin: these are glucagon, adrenaline, cortisol and growth hormone. Insulin is produced by the pancreatic β-cells as proinsulin. Proinsulin is broken down into C peptide (biologically inert) and insulin during the secretory process. The insulin then travels in the portal circulation to the liver where it exerts its main action.

DIABETES MELLITUS

Diabetes mellitus is a syndrome characterised by a chronic state of hyperglycaemia due to a deficiency of insulin or of its action. It is the most common endocrine disorder in childhood and adolescence. There are two types of diabetes mellitus: type I and type II.

Type I (IDDM, juvenile–onset diabetes)

This is characterised by a dependence on exogenous insulin for the maintenance of life, hence the name IDDM (insulin-dependent diabetes mellitus). Prevalence is 1 in 300 in the UK and rising. Presentation most commonly in spring and autumn.

Cause is unknown, though there is evidence of genetic, autoimmune and viral factors contributing.

Genetic   30% identical twin concordance
              HLA-B8, DR3, DR4
              Father has IDDM – 1 in 20 risk for child
              Mother has IDDM – 1 in 40 risk for child
              Sibling has IDDM – 1 in 20 risk
Autoimmune 80% have ICA (islet cell antibodies) on presentation
              Association with other autoimmune disease and HLA antibodies
Viral

Type II (NIDDM, maturity-onset diabetes)

These are not insulin dependent although insulin may be required to correct hyperglycaemia and ketosis is uncommon but occurs. There is 100% concordance in identical twins. It may present at any age but is unusual in children, mostly occurring over the age of 40 years and therefore will not be discussed further.

Clinical presentation

1. *Short history (2–4 weeks) of polyuria (osmotic diuresis), polydipsia (dehydration) and weight loss (fluid depletion and muscle and fat breakdown)*
2. *Ketoacidosis*
3. *Asymptomatic glycosuria*

Diagnosis

Symptomatic   Random venous plasma glucose $> = 11.1$ mmol/l or
Fasting plasma glucose $> = 7.0$ mmol/l or
2 hour plasma glucose $> = 11.1$ mmol/l 2 hours post 75 g glucose load (in OGGT)

Asymptomatic   Venous plasma sample in diabetic range and confirmation with repeat glucose test in diabetic range on another day (fasting, random or 2 hours post-glucose load)

NB. Whole blood glucose differs from plasma glucose. The whole blood glucose measures 10% lower than plasma glucose. Glycosuria occurs in 1% of the population (secondary to low renal threshold).

Impaired glucose tolerance: during a formal 75 g oral glucose tolerance test (OGGT), fasting plasma glucose <7.0 mmol/l and 2 hour venous plasma glucose >7.8 mmol/l but <11.1 mmol/l)

Treatment

Diet   This should be high in unrefined carbohydrates (slow absorption therefore fewer glucose swings). Calories obtained approximately as 55% CHD, 35% fat and 15% protein.

Insulin   Subcutaneous insulin injections given in the thigh, arm or abdomen and rotated to prevent lipoatrophy.

- *Twice-daily regime*   am *before breakfast, 2/3rds daily dose, short-acting (1/3) and medium-acting (2/3)*
pm *before tea, 1/3rd daily dose, short-acting (1/3) and medium-acting (2/3)*
- *Multiple-dose 'pen injection' regime. Used in older children. More convenient*

Insulin types

- Ultra-short acting insulin analogues eg. Humulog, Novorapid
- Short-acting (crystalline, soluble), eg. Actrapid, Humulin S
- Medium- or long-acting (mixed with zinc or protamine), eg. Monotard, Humulin I
- Soluble, protamine mixture, eg. Humulin M1 (10% soluble), Humulin M2 (20% soluble), Mixtard 30/70

Blood glucose monitoring Regular BM Stix done at home to assess control. Urine glucose unreliable due to variable renal threshold and inability to detect hypoglycaemia. Glycosylated Hb (HbA1c) or fructosamine give an indication of blood glucose levels over the previous six weeks.

Problems

1. *Hypoglycaemia. Symptoms usually occur with plasma glucose levels <3 mmol/l (sweaty, dizzy and irritable). Treat with oral glucose (drink or gel) or glucagon injection. NB. The 'dawn phenomenon' – hypoglycaemia at night from too much insulin given to counteract the 4am growth hormone surge (called 'somogyi')*
2. *Weight increase*
3. *Behavioural problems – common in adolescence, often non-compliant. Labelled 'brittle diabetes'*
4. *Insulin resistance – usually due to obesity*
5. *Illness – insulin must be continued during illness*
6. *Lipoatrophy/lipohypertrophy*

Long-term complications

1. *Microvascular disease – diabetic eye disease, renal disease, neuropathy*
2. *Macrovascular disease – stroke, myocardial infarction, limb amputation*

Diabetic ketoacidosis

A state of uncontrolled catabolism associated with insulin deficiency, resulting in hyperglycaemia, osmotic diuresis and dehydration. Lipolysis resulting in free fatty acids broken down to ketone bodies which cause a metabolic acidosis. It may result from an intercurrent illness or interruption of insulin therapy or be a new presentation.

Clinical features

Hyperventilation (Kussmaul respiration), dehydration, nausea, vomiting, abdominal pain.

Management

1. *General resuscitation if necessary*
2. *Blood for blood glucose, urea and electrolytes, FBC and PCV and arterial blood gas*
3. *Fluid and insulin therapy under close observation of state and blood parameters:*

Fluid Circulating volume expansion with a bolus of 10–20 ml/kg 0.9% saline
Rehydrate calculated volume deficit over 48 hours with 0.9% saline initially, adding potassium with careful monitoring (risk of hypokalaemia as K pushed back into the cells)
Change fluid to 0.18% saline 4% dextrose when blood glucose <12 mmol/l
Bicarbonate infusion in severe acidosis

Insulin Insulin infusion of soluble insulin 0.05–0.1 units/kg/h to reduce blood glucose at a rate of <5 mmol/l/h
When able to eat, transfer to subcutaneous insulin regime of 0.5–0.7 units/kg/day

HYPOGLYCAEMIA

Hypoglycaemia is currently defined as a blood glucose level of less than 2.6 mmol/l. As glucose levels fall, the insulin concentration falls and lipolysis and ketogenesis are activated. With a blood glucose level of <2.2 mmol/l, the plasma insulin should be undetectable.

Clinical features

Neonate   Apnoea, cyanosis, hypotonia, lethargy, poor feeding and seizures

Older child Pallor, anxiety, nausea, tremor, sweatiness, headache, diplopia, decreased acuity, dizziness, seizures, poor concentration, behavioural change, coma

Causes

Transient neonatal hypoglycaemia	
1. Substrate deficiency	Premature, SGA (low levels of liver glycogen, muscle protein and body fat and poorly developed enzyme system for gluconeogenesis)
2. Hyperinsulinaemia	Infant of diabetic mother
Persistent hypoglycaemia	
1. Hyperinsulinism	Nesidioblastosis
	Insulinoma
	Beckwith–Wiedemann syndrome
	Deliberate exogenous administration
2. Hormone deficiency states	Growth hormone, ACTH and adrenaline deficiency, Addison disease, hypopituitarism
3. Substrate deficiency	Ketotic hypoglycaemia
4. Metabolic	Glycogen storage disease (types I, III, VI, IX)
	Carbohydrate metabolism disorder eg. galactosaemia, hereditary fructose intolerance
	Fructosaemia
	Fatty acid oxidation defect, eg. carnitine deficiency (primary or secondary), LCAD
	Organic acidaemia, eg. MSUD (maple syrup urine disease)
5. Other	Poisoning (aspirin, alcohol, insulin)
	Liver failure, Reye syndrome
	Shock

Nesidioblastosis

This is a developmental disorder where there are hyperplastic, abnormally dispersed β-cells, resulting in inappropriately high levels of plasma insulin. See below for management.

Ketotic hypoglycaemia

This presents between 18 months and five years and resolves spontaneously by 8–9 years. It occurs when a child misses an evening meal or is unwell, causing a relatively prolonged fast, and they are difficult to arouse in the morning or may have a seizure. They have hypoglycaemia, ketonaemia, ketonuria and plasma insulin levels are appropriately low. It may represent the low end of the spectrum of a child's ability to tolerate a fast. These children have low alanine levels (a substrate released from muscle during fasting), so may have a defect in this mechanism. They also have a low muscle bulk and therefore have a low supply of substrate.

Investigations
Essential investigations in the event of a hypoglycaemic episode (which may be induced by fasting):

- *blood glucose*
- *plasma insulin, cortisol, growth hormone, proinsulin (and C-peptide if exogenous administration is suspected)*
- *β-OH-butyrate, acetoacetate, FFAs, alanine*
- *ammonia, LFTs*
- *first urine sample for ketones, organic and amino acids, non-glucose-reducing substances*

Management
Episode of hypoglycaemia 10% dextrose 2 ml/kg (=0.2 g/kg) intravenous over 5 min (may need 20% dextrose 1–2 ml/kg (=0.2–0.4 g/kg) IV over 5 mins)
Then infusion of 10% dextrose 5–8 mg/kg/min

NB. Normal infants produce 5–8 mg/kg/min of glucose in the fasting state. This falls to 1–2 mg/kg/min in older children. A neonate with hyperinsulinism may require up to 10–20 mg/kg/min of glucose.

Hyperinsulinism (nesidioblastosis) is treated with diazoxide and a thiazide diuretic, followed by octeotride. Subtotal pancreatectomy is indicated if medical management fails.

Pancreatic tumours

These arise from APUD cells (amine precursor uptake and decarboxylation) in the pancreas.

GASTRINOMA (Zollinger–Ellison syndrome)
Always malignant and slow growing. It is a tumour of the G-cells of the pancreas, which produce gastrin.

Gastrin→Gastric acid→Peptic ulcers (stomach, duodenum, jejunum)

The symptoms are those of peptic ulcers plus diarrhoea secondary to abnormally low intestinal pH.

Diagnosis

- *Serum gastrin ↑*

- *Acid studies (high output)*
- *Ocreotide-labelled isotope scan*

Treatment

- *Omeprazole (proton pump inhibitor)*
- *Octreotide*
- *Surgery if possible*

VIPOMA

This is a pancreatic tumour, secreting VIP (vasointestinal polypeptide).

VIP→intestinal secretion→diarrhoea

Diagnosis

- *Serum VIP↑*
- *PHI (peptide histidine isoleucine) also raised*

Treatment

- *Octreotide*
- *Surgical resection (if possible)*

GLUCAGONOMA

This is a pancreatic tumour of the α-cells producing glucagon. The result is diabetes mellitus. A necrotic migratory erythematous rash is characteristic.

Diagnosis
Serum glucagon ↑
NB. Enteroglucagonoma = glucagon-secreting tumour of the right kidney and jejunal villi hypertrophy.

INSULINOMA

This is an islet cell adenoma that secretes insulin. It presents insidiously with recurrent fasting hypoglycaemia.

Diagnosis
Failure to suppress insulin with fasting hypoglycaemia
MRI scan, coeliac angiography (v. difficult in infants) to locate tumour.

Treatment
Surgical excision

Polycystic ovary syndrome (PCOS)

This is a very common condition involving large, polycystic ovaries (in arrested follicular development) and increased circulating androgens. It is also known as the

Stein–Levanthal syndrome. The onset is usually around puberty and the cause is not well understood.

Clinical features

- *Secondary amenorrhoea, irregular menstruation*
- *Obesity*
- *Hirsutism*
- *Mild virilisation, with acne*
- *Anovulatory infertility*
- *Insulin resistance*

Investigations

USS showing enlarged ovaries with multiple 3–5 mm cysts arranged circumferentially and increased stroma

Hormones   Raised LH:FSH ratio (>2:1)

       Plasma LH ↑
       Free circulating androgens ↑
       Testosterone ↑ or normal
       Mild hyperprolactinaemia
       FSH normal or ↓

NB. Must rule out differential diagnosis of adrenal disorders.

Treatment options

(Treatment is symptomatic)

- *Ovarian suppression with the oral contraceptive pill or cyproterone (an antiandrogen)*
- *Pituitary ACTH suppression with prednisolone*
- *To improve fertility, ovarian wedge resection and clomiphene*

Endocrine syndromes

TYPE I POLYGLANDULAR AUTOIMMUNE SYNDROME

This is the association of:

1. *hypoparathyroidism*
2. *Addison disease*
3. *mucocutaneous candidiasis and*
4. *autoimmune thyroiditis (10%)*

SCHMIDT SYNDROME (TYPE II POLYGLANDULAR AUTOIMMUNE SYNDROME)

This is the association of:

1. *Addison's disease*

2. *IDDM*

3. *autoimmune thyroiditis*

AUTOIMMUNE ASSOCIATIONS

Thyroid disease, IDDM, Addison disease, pernicious anaemia, alopecia, vitiligo.

MULTIPLE ENDOCRINE NEOPLASIA

Autosomal dominant. The association of a number of endocrine tumours.

MEN I	MEN IIa
Parathyroid	Adrenal (phaeochromocytoma, Cushing)
Pituitary (prolactin or GH or ACTH)	Thyroid (medullary carcinoma)
Pancreas	Parathyroid hyperplasia
(Thyroid)	
(Adrenal)	
Fasting calcium level ($\uparrow$?)	Calcitonin level $\uparrow$ (medullary ca. thyroid)
	Look for phaeochromocytoma

MEN IIb is the same as MEN IIa, with Marfanoid features and multiple neuromas.

Prophylactic total thyroidectomy is performed if the child is known to carry the gene for MEN II.

Growth and puberty

GROWTH

Growth measurements

A child's height, weight (and head circumference if below the age of two years) are plotted on growth charts. Separate charts exist to plot growth velocity. The charts outline the centiles of children ranging from the 0.4th centile (equivalent to -2.67 standard deviations) to the 99.6th centile. If a child lies outside these centiles there is likely to be an organic cause (though four in 1000 normal children will be below the 0.4th centile). It is important to look at trends over six months to one year to assess the rate of growth, deviations from a centile and discrepancies between height, weight and head circumference.

Decimal age

This is used on certain growth charts. It is calculated by converting the month and day of the child's date of birth and the current date to three-figure numbers obtained from a table on the growth chart. The figure for the date of birth together with the year is then subtracted from the figure for the current date (together with the year) to give the decimal age.

Expected height

The mean parental height is calculated and taken into account when assessing a child's height potential. It is calculated as follows:

Boy: $\dfrac{(\text{mother's ht.} + 12.5 \text{ cm}) + \text{father's ht.}}{2}$ Girl: $\dfrac{(\text{father's ht.} - 12.5 \text{ cm}) + \text{mother's ht.}}{2}$

Bone age (skeletal maturity)

This is calculated from an X-ray of the left hand (left knee if <2 years). It is plotted on the growth chart and compared to the chronological age. A delayed bone age means that the child will have a greater final height potential than a child with a normal or advanced bone age. Familial delayed maturation causes a delayed bone age, and severe illness and hypothyroidism cause a severely delayed bone age. Androgens and thyroid hormones can accelerate the bone age.

'Catch-up' growth

This is seen for a few months in babies who had intrauterine growth retardation and after illness. NB. Premature babies should have their growth charts adjusted for age until the age of 2 years.

Velocity

This is a sensitive indicator of growth problems, and is the 'gold standard' for growth assessment. Two measurements are needed six months to one year apart. The difference between the two is measured in cm/yr and plotted at the midpoint in time.

Short stature

This is usually defined as a height below the 3rd centile, approximately two standard deviations below the mean. A height velocity measurement below the 25th centile is abnormal.

Causes

Familial	The most common cause. Expected height calculation from parental heights
Constitutional delay	Delayed puberty, delayed bone age and family history, good final height
Emotional deprivation	Small child (may also be underweight with delayed puberty). Biochemical picture of GH deficiency
Chronic illness	Any chronic illness, inadequate nutrition
Endocrine	Growth hormone deficiency: isolated pituitary deficiency/hypopituitarism Laron dwarfism (GH insensitivity) Hypothyroidism Pseudohypoparathyroidism Cushing syndrome or exogenous steroids
Chromosomal	Turner syndrome, Russel-Silver dwarfism, Bloom syndrome

Disproportionate	Limb–trunk discrepancy
	Seen in bone dysplasias eg. achondroplasia and hypochondroplasia

Investigations

These will be led by the clinical findings and history. Investigations to consider are:

1. *bone age*
2. *TFTs*
3. *FBC, ESR, bone profile*
4. *urinalysis*
5. *karyotype*
6. *IGF-1 and IGFBP 3*
7. *pituitary provocation tests*
8. *visual fields, CT or MRI brain*
9. *coeliac screen*
10. *skeletal survey*
11. *ultrasound scan of uterus and ovaries*

Treatment

Treat underlying cause.

Tall stature

This is usually defined as a height above the 97th centile and is much less common than short stature.

Causes

Familial	The most common cause
Hormonal	Pituitary gigantism (rare)
	Precocious puberty (final height short) from CAH, hyperthyroidism, excess sex steroids
Syndrome	Klinefelter syndrome (XXY)
	Marfan syndrome, homocystinuria
	Sotos syndrome ('cerebral gigantism' – learning difficulties, clumsiness, big hands and feet, large ears, prominent forehead)
	Beckwith–Weidemann syndrome (see p. 18)

Investigations

Those to consider are:

- *bone age*
- *growth hormone, IGF-1, IGFBP 3*
- *TFTs*
- *homocystine*
- *CT or MRI brain scan*
- *CAH investigations*

Treatment

It is possible to treat with high-dose oestrogen therapy in girls and testosterone therapy in boys, which cause premature fusion of the epiphyses.

PUBERTY

Pubertal staging

Pubertal stage is assessed using the sexual maturity rating devised by Tanner in 1962.

Boys G (1–5), P (1–5), A (1–3), testicular volume
Girls B (1–5), P (1–5), A (1–3), menarche

Puberty onset (timing variable)

Girls	(8–13 years)	Breast stage 2	Breasts first sign
Boys	(9–14 years)	Testes 4 ml	Testes first sign

Pubertal growth spurt timing

Girls   Breast stage 2–3 (12.2 years)
Boys   Testes volume >10 ml (13.9 years)

G Genitals (boys)

Stage 1	Preadolescent
Stage 2	Scrotum pink and texture change, slight enlargement of penis
Stage 3	Longer penis, larger testes
Stage 4	Penis increases in breadth, dark scrotum
Stage 5	Adult size

B Breasts

Stage 1	Preadolescent
Stage 2	Breast bud
Stage 3	Larger but no contour separation
Stage 4	Areola and papilla form secondary mound
Stage 5	Mature – papilla projects, areola follows breast contour

P Pubic Hair

Stage 1	Prepubertal
Stage 2	Few, fine hairs
Stage 3	Darkens, coarsens, starts to curl
Stage 4	Adult type, smaller area
Stage 5	Adult distribution

A Axillary Hair

Stage 1	No hair
Stage 2	Scanty hair
Stage 3	Adult hair pattern

Menarche

Occurs at breast stage 4, only 5–6 cm of growth left (<4% final height).

- **Thelarche** *is breast development*
- **Adrenarche** *is pubic and axillary hair development.*

Precocious puberty

True precocious puberty is the development of secondary sexual characteristics in a normal progression accompanied by a growth spurt, leading to full sexual maturity from activation of the central axis. False precocious puberty is gonadotrophin independent and there may be an unusual progression of sexual maturity. Isolated premature thelarche, adrenarche and menarche occur.

Girls	Development of secondary sexual characteristics <8 years is abnormal
	Mostly familial
Boys	Development of secondary sexual characteristics <9 years is abnormal
	Mostly pathological. NB. Intracranial tumours, dysgerminomas

Causes

True **Gonadotrophin dependent (hypothalamic–pituitary–gonadal axis activated) LH↑, FSH↑**

Familial

Central: congenital eg. neurofibromatosis, hydrocephalus
acquired eg. postsepsis, surgery, DXT '
tumours

Hypothyroidism

False **Gonadotrophin independent (excess sex steroids not driven centrally) LH↓, FSH↓**

Adrenal: tumour
congenital adrenal hyperplasia

Gonadal: ovarian tumour
testicular tumour (Leydig cell)

McCune–Albright syndrome

Primary hypothyroidism

Exogenous sex steroids

Examination and investigations

Always check:

1. *clinical staging*
2. *bone age*
3. *pelvic USS or orchidometer (normal puberty shows multicystic ovaries, ?ovarian tumour)*

In boys, have a low threshold for cranial imaging (?tumour) and hCG and AFP (?testicular tumour).

Treatment

If necessary, true precocious puberty is treated with GnRH analogues and false puberty with androgen or oestrogen inhibitors as appropriate.

McCune–Albright syndrome

This is a syndrome of endocrine dysfunction with hyperpigmentation and skeletal fibrous dysplasia. The underlying defect is in the G-protein controlling cAMP in cells.

This results in activation of receptors with a cAMP mechanism, causing autonomous glandular hyperfunction. The syndrome involves:

Skin Patchy hyperpigmentation with café-au-lait patches (of very irregular outline)
Bone Fibrous dysplasia (visible as radiolucent areas on X-ray), pathological fractures
Endocrine Overactivity of ovary, thyroid, adrenal glands, pituitary

Delayed puberty

This is failure of onset of puberty by 13 years in a girl and 14 years in a boy. Mainly boys are affected and the cause is usually constitutional delay (short, delayed bone age, family history).

Causes

Gonadotrophin secretion low

Constitutional	Familial
	Sporadic
Hypothalamic-pituitary	Panhypopituitarism
	GnRH deficiency
	⋆ Hypothyroidism
	Intracranial tumour
	Prolactinoma
	Kallman syndrome
Systemic disease	Severe disease eg. renal failure
	Emotional eg. anorexia nervosa

Gonadotrophin secretion high

Gonadal dysgenesis	Turner syndrome
Gonadal disease	Trauma, DXT, torsion
Steroid hormone enzyme deficiencies	CAH 3β-deficiency
Chromosomal	Klinefelter syndrome

Investigations

1. Pubertal staging and bone age
2. Thyroid function tests
3. Gonadotrophin, sex steroid hormone levels
4. Karyotype
5. Occasionally LHRH and testicular responsiveness to three injections of HCG

Treatment

This depends on the underlying condition. In males with constitutional delay, use androgenic anabolic steroids (oxandrolone) with low-dose testosterone only if necessary. In females use ethinyl oestradiol or oxandrolone.

Kallman syndrome

Syndrome of isolated hypogonadotrophism, causing secondary hypogonadism. Other features are anosmia, cleft palate, colour blindness, ichthyosis and renal abnormalities. Inheritance usually X-linked.

SEXUAL DIFFERENTIATION DISORDERS – AMBIGUOUS GENITALIA

Disorders of sexual differentiation can be due to overvirilisation of a female (female pseudohermaphrodite, 46 XX), undervirilisation of a male (male pseudohermaphrodite, 46 XY) or a true hermaphrodite (both ovarian and testicular tissue present). Affected patients will have a discrepancy between the morphology of the gonads and the morphology of the external genitalia.

Causes

Female pseudohermaphrodite (over masculinised)
46 XX + ovaries

Fetal	CAH 21-hydroxylase deficiency
	11β-hydroxylase deficiency
Maternal	Virilising tumours (adrenal, ovarian)
	Drugs

Male pseudohermaphrodite (under masculinised)
46 XY + testes

1. *Defect in testes differentiation* – gonadal dysgenesis/agenesis
2. *Defect in testicular hormones* – CAH-3β-hydroxylase deficiency
3. *Defect in androgen activity* – 5α-reductase deficiency, androgen insensitivity syndrome (complete or partial)

 True hermaphrodite
Ovarian + testicular tissue

1. *46 XX*
2. *46 XY*
3. *46 XX/XY chimera*

Investigations

1. *Chromosomes – karyotype*
2. *Pelvic and abdominal USS (internal genitalia and adrenal glands)*
3. *Adrenal steroids*

Endocrine tests

NB. These are outlined for exam reference only. Tests performed in expert centres.

GH STIMULATION TEST

GH secretion is stimulated by a variety of ways eg. fasting, insulin induced, glucogen, clonidine or arginine. Hypoglycaemia with a blood glucose <2.2 mmol/l is produced and samples collected as over on p. 283.

Time (min)	0	30	60	90	120	180
Glucose (mmol/l)	5	<2.2	★	★	★	★
Cortisol (nmol/l)	★	★	★	★	★	★
Growth hormone (mU/l)		★	★	★	★	★

★ indicates sample should be taken.
Normal response = GH >20 mU/l
              = Cortisol increase >200 nmol/l and/or peak >500 nmol/l

COMBINED PITUITARY PROVOCATION TEST

Clonidine test + TRH + LHRH stimulation tests.

TRH STIMULATION TEST

Give TRH and sample:

Time (min)	0	20	60
TSH mU/l	★	★	★

LHRH STIMULATION TEST

Give LHRH and sample:

Time (mins)	0	30	60
LH U/l	★	★	★
FSH U/l	★	★	★

NB. Absent response does not establish pituitary deficiency.

DEXAMETHASONE SUPPRESSION TESTS

Overnight suppression test

- Used to confirm normal suppression of adrenal cortex
- Dexamethasone 0.5 mg (or 10 μg/kg BW) given orally at 2200 hours
- Plasma cortisol measured at 0800 on the following day
- Normally plasma cortisol is suppressed to <100 nmol/l
- In Cushing syndrome there is failure to suppress

Low-dose suppression 48-hour test

- Confirmation of Cushing syndrome, where there is failure of suppression
- Dexamethasone given 0.5 mg/kg orally six hourly for 48 hours

Time	0	24h	48h	72h
Plasma cortisol	★	★	★	
ACTH			★	
24 h urine free cortisol	★			★

Normal = 48h plasma cortisol <140 nmol/l, ACTH <5 pmol/l, urine cortisol to less than half the baseline.

High-dose suppression

- *Used to differentiate pituitary-dependent Cushing syndrome (which will suppress in 90%) from ACTH-independent disease which will still not suppress. NB. This test can be hard to interpret*
- *Dexamethasone 2 mg given six hourly for eight doses from 0900 on day 1*
- *Plasma cortisol and 24 h urine steroids measured at 0900 on days 0 and 2*
- *Normally plasma cortisol is suppressed on day 2 to <50% of the value on day 0*

SYNACTHEN STIMULATION TESTS

Short synacthen test (ACTH analogue)

- *Purpose: this is used to detect primary adrenal failure, where the cortisol levels are below that expected*
- *Dose of 0.25 mg (250 μg) synacthen (tetracosactrin) given IM or IV (or 35 μg/kg BW) and cortisol levels measured as follows*

Time (min)	0	30	60
Cortisol nmol/l	★	★	★

Normal = cortisol increase >200 nmol/l, cortisol peak >500 nmol/l.
Peak value may occur at 30 or 60 minutes.

Long synacthen test

- *Purpose: differentiates primary from secondary adrenal failure (in secondary adrenal failure, cortisol production will be stimulated)*
- *Six 12-hourly tetracosactrin 0.5 μg/m^2 SA IM. Measure:*

Time (min)	0800h day 1	0800h day 2	0800h day 3
Cortisol (nmol/l)	★	★	★

Normal = cortisol peak >500 nmol/l.
Depressed response with elevated ACTH levels confirms primary adrenal failure.

GLUCOSE TOLERANCE TEST

A standard dose of glucose is given after an overnight fast. Blood glucose levels are taken at time 0 and 2 hours.

Time (min)	0	120
Plasma glucose (normal)	<7.8	<11.1
Plasma glucose (diabetes)	>7.8	>11.1
Plasma glucose (IGT)	<7.8	7.8–11.1

NB. Blood glucose measures 10% lower than plasma glucose. A blood glucose of 6.7 mmol/l corresponds to a plasma glucose of 7.8 mmol/l and a blood glucose of 10 mmol/l corresponds to a plasma glucose of 11.1 mmol/l.

FURTHER READING

Brook C *Clinical Paediatric Endicrinology* 3rd Ed, Blackwell Science, London, 1995
Brook C *A guide to the practice of paediatric endocrinology*, Cambridge University Press, Cambridge, 1993

10

Metabolic disorders

- *Metabolic disorders*
- *Amino acid metabolism disorders*
- *Organic acidaemias*
- *Urea cycle defects*
- *Carbohydrate metabolism disorders*
- *Lipid metabolism disorders*

- *Transport defects*
- *Peroxisomal disorders*
- *Mitochondrial disorders*
- *Lysosomal storage disorders*
- *Mucopolysaccharidoses*
- *The porphyrias*

Metabolic disorders

Inborn errors of metabolism are inherited biochemical disorders and are generally autosomal recessive conditions (though there are notable exceptions).

FEATURES SUGGESTIVE OF A METABOLIC DISORDER

The following are features to be aware of when considering a metabolic diagnosis.

Parental history

- *Consanguinous parents*
- *Previous unexplained neonatal deaths*
- *Particular ethnic group (certain diseases only)*

Clinical features

Neonatal presentation

- *Normal-appearing child at birth (some conditions are associated with dysmorphism)*
- *Poor feeding*
- *Vomiting*
- *Lethargy*
- *Seizures*
- *Coma*
- *Unusual odour*
- *Hypoglycaemia, acidosis (with some defects)*

Postneonatal presentation

- *Encephalopathy, developmental regression, Reye syndrome, motor deficits, seizures*
- *Intermittent episodes of vomiting, acidosis, hypoglycaemia and/or coma triggered by stress eg. infections, surgery*

Examination findings

- *Organomegaly (eg. hepatomegaly)*
- *Cardiac disease*
- *Ocular involvement (eg. cherry red spot)*
- *Skin manifestations*
- *Unusual odour*
- *Non-specific neurological findings*

FIRST-LINE INVESTIGATIONS AND METABOLIC SCREEN

Serum	Ammonia	↑ in urea cycle defects and some organic acidaemias (also ↑ in liver failure and sepsis)
	Glucose	May be ↓ in FAOD defects, mitochondrial defects and organic acidaemias
	Ketones	Prominent in organic acidaemias, inappropriately low in FAODs
	Urea and electrolytes	May be deranged, signs of dehydration, renal tubular dysfunction
	LFTs, coag. screen	May be abnormal (eg. tyrosinaemia, urea cycle defects, FAODs, mitochondrial defects and galactosaemia)
	Plasma amino acids	Diagnostic in aminoacidopathies, strongly suggestive in urea cycle defects
	Lactate	Classically elevated in mitochondrial defects, biotin disorders and some glycogen storage defects. May be elevated in organic acidaemias and liver failure
Blood gas	pH	Acidosis eg. organic acidaemias, lactic acidosis Resp. alkalosis early on in urea cycle defects
	Bicarbonate	Low eg. organic acidaemias
Urine	Organic acids	↑ in organic acidaemias
	Ketones	Prominent in organic acidaemias, inappropriately low in FAODs
CSF	Lactate	Mitochondrial disorders
	Glycine	↑ in some organic acidaemias and non-ketotic hyperglycinaemia

Amino acid metabolism disorders

PHENYLKETONURIA (PKU)

Incidence 1:10 000–20 000

Metabolic defect
Enzyme deficiency Phenylalanine hydroxylase (low or absent)
Biochemical result Phenylalanine and its alternative pathway metabolites accumulate in the tissues

Phenylalanine
hydroxylase
Pathway: Phenylalanine—x→Tyrosine

Clinical features
NB. The classic picture of disease described below is rarely observed now due to treatment.

Normal at birth

Odour Musty (classic, though in reality simply smells unusual)
General Early severe vomiting, seborrhoeic dermatitis (mild)
CNS Severe developmental delay from 4–6 months, hypertonia
Later: Neurological features of spastic cerebral palsy, athetosis, hyperactivity
Rocking motion, acquired microcephaly
Appearance Fair hair, fair skin and blue eyes (if not treated)

Specific investigations
1. *Guthrie test – blood phenylalanine levels (raised after protein feeds begin, 24–48 hours after birth)*
2. *Specific levels – blood phenylalanine ($\uparrow$) and tyrosine (normal)*

Management
Diet manipulation Low-phenylalanine diet for life. Especially important in the first five years
NB. *Some* phenylalanine must be given as it is not synthesised in the body.
Typical diet consists of 5–15 g of natural protein with remaining protein requirement given as phenylalanine free amino acid formula
Pregnancy Diet must be strictly adhered to because high phenylalanine levels result in foetal abnormalities (eg. CHD) and mental retardation

HEPATORENAL TYROSINAEMIA (TYPE 1)

Main features Hepatocellular degeneration and renal Fanconi syndrome, Aut. recessive
Enzyme deficiency Fumarylacetoacetase

Biochemical result Tyrosinaemia and succinylacetonuria
Associations French-Canadians (Quebequoise)

Clinical features

Acute form Symptoms <6 months of age
Vomiting, diarrhoea, irritability, failure to thrive, rickets
Hepatocellular dysfunction: acute liver failure, jaundice, bleeding tendency
Developmental delay, cabbage/sweet odour
Death <1 year

Chronic form Symptoms >1 year
Developmental delay, failure to thrive
Cirrhosis, splenomegaly, hepatocellular carcinoma
Renal tubular dysfunction (Fanconi syndrome), rickets
Polyneuropathy (episodes of severe leg pains, hypertonia, ileus)
Death by 10 years until recently but new treatments have improved this

Diagnostic investigations

Cultured fibroblasts Fumarylacetoacetase enzyme ($\downarrow$)
Plasma amino acids Tyrosine ($\uparrow$)
Urine organic acids Succinylacetone and tyrosine metabolites ($\uparrow$)
Serum α-FP$\uparrow$
Liver biopsy Features of cirrhosis

Management

1. *Diet—low tyrosine and phenylalanine amino acid formula*
2. *NTBC therapy (this compound results in an enzyme block above the defect. Essentially it turns tyrosinaemia type 1 into the relatively benign tyrosinaemia type 3)*
3. *Liver transplant early in disease (alternative treatment to NTBC)*

HOMOCYSTINURIA

Prevalence 1: 200 000, autosomal recessive.

Enzyme deficiency Cystathionine synthase
Biochemical result Homocysteine and methionine accumulation

Clinical features

General Marfanoid habitus, fair hair, fair skin, blue eyes, malar flush
CNS Mental retardation (common), seizures (20%)
Skeletal Osteoporosis, platyspondyly
CVS Arterial and venous thromboembolism
Eye Lens subluxation (*downward*)

Diagnostic investigations

Serum Free/total homocyst(e)ine ($\uparrow$), methionine ($\uparrow$)

Urine   Homocystinuria
Enzyme Assay in cultured fibroblasts, lymphocytes or liver biopsy

Management

- *May be responsive to high-dose vitamin B_6 (pyridoxine) therapy*
- *Betaine (alternative pathway for homocysteine metabolism)*
- *Diet – methionine restriction, cystine supplementation*

NON-KETOTIC HYPERGLYCINAEMIA

Hyperglycinaemia is seen in:

1. *ketotic hyperglycinaemia – seen in organic acidaemias (see below)*
2. *non-ketotic hyperglycinaemia*

Autosomal recessive
Enzyme defect   Defect in the glycine cleavage system involved in glycine degra-
                       dation
Clinical features Neonatal illness with vomiting, lethargy, seizures, coma and death
                       within hours if untreated
                       If survival occurs, severe mental retardation, myoclonic seizures
                       and spasticity are seen
                       A late-onset form is also described

Investigations

1. *Glycine levels Glycine increased in plasma, urine and CSF*
                    High CSF: plasma glycine ratio.
                    NB. Normal pH
2. *No demonstrable organic acidaemia*

Management
No effective long-term treatment.

Organic acidaemias

These involve elevation of one or more organic acids and patients often present in the
first few days of life severely unwell with acidosis, vomiting and neurological features.
If the initial period is survived, intermittent acute attacks occur triggered by stress.

Presentation

Clinical features Vomiting, lethargy, seizures, coma, hypertonia, opisthotonus,
                       hypoglycaemia, metabolic acidosis
Investigations   Metabolic acidosis, hypoglycaemia, ketosis and hyperammo-
                       naemia (>200)

Diagnosis is by characteristic urinary organic acid profile. Confirmation by enzyme analysis.

Management

Acute attacks are treated with rehydration and calories (to prevent a catabolic state), correction of acidosis and haemofiltration if necessary. Benzoate may be helpful to remove ammonia. Carnitine may also be beneficial. Seek expert help.

In MSUD the branched chain amino acids may be lowered by encouraging protein synthesis with branched chain free amino acid formula.

Long-term clinical features common to all organic acidopathies (depends on severity of acute attacks): mental retardation, seizures and movement disorders. Failure to thrive, anorexia, osteoporosis and renal impairment are also frequently seen.

Long-term treatment consists of a low-protein diet and avoidance of catabolism (ie. high carbohydrate feeds during intercurrent illness, low threshold for IV fluids). Carnitine may be beneficial in removing toxic metabolites and replacing free carnitine.

Disease	Enzyme defect	Specific treatments
Maple syrup urine disease (MSUD)*	Branched chain ketoacid dehydrogenase	MSUD protein formula
Methymalonic acidaemia	MM mutase or cobalamin (B_{12}) defect	B_{12} (if responsive), combined liver and renal transplant, Metronidazole
Isovaleric acidaemia	Isovaleryl CoA dehydrogenase	Glycine
Proprionic acidaemia	Propionyl CoA carboxylase	Metronidazole
*Also commonly known as an aminoacidopathy		

Biotinadase deficiency

Classically presents in infancy with developmental delay, lactic acidosis, seizures and an eczema-type rash. Angular stomatitis, alopecia, hearing loss and ataxia are also seen. There is a characteristic urinary organic acid picture with confirmation of the diagnosis by measuring biotinadase activity.

Urea cycle defects

These are defects in the metabolism of ammonia in the urea cycle and are therefore associated with high ammonia levels. They often present with overwhelming neonatal illness with hyperammonaemia (lethargy, poor feeding, convulsions, coma, respiratory failure). Late onset, either acutely or with a history of repeated attacks, is also well described. Alternatively, they sometimes present with developmental delay (*especially arginase deficiency*).

The five enzymes involved in urea synthesis are:

- *carbamylphosphate synthetase (CPS)*
- *ornithine transcarbamylase (OTC)*
- *arginosuccinate synthetase (AS) (citrullinaemia)*
- *arginosuccinate lyase (AL) (arginosuccinic acidaemia)*
- *arginase (argininaemia)*

N–acetylglutamate synthetase is required for the activation of the cycle. Deficiencies of all these enzymes occur, resulting in urea cycle defects.

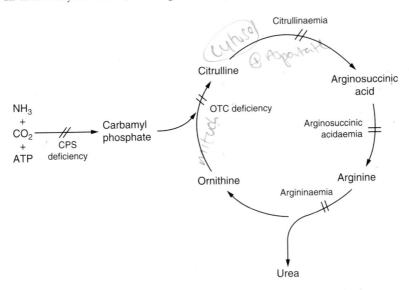

Figure 10.1 Urea cycle

All the urea cycle defects except OTC are autosomal recessive. OTC is X linked; boys tend to die as neonates.

Hyperammonaemia

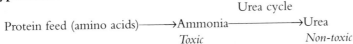

Protein feed (amino acids)———→Ammonia————————→Urea
Toxic   *Non-toxic*

Diagnosis

- *Serum ammonia ↑ (usually >200 μM)*
- *Acidosis is a late phenomenon in urea cycle defects (as opposed to organic acidaemias)*
- *Plasma amino acid glutamine raised*
- *Plasma amino acids and urine orotic acid usually enable one to make an initial diagnosis*
- *Enzyme assay is required to confirm diagnosis*

Treatment

Acute

1. *Remove ammonia*   *Increase waste nitrogen excretion using IV sodium benzoate, sodium phenylbutyrate and arginine*
Or dialysis if above ineffective
Seek expert help
2. *Increase calories to prevent protein breakdown*   *IV 10% glucose, lipids*
Nil by mouth, no protein
NG feeding with low-protein feed after 48–72 hours
3. *IV hydration and electrolyte balance*

Long-term

- *Dietary protein restriction*
- *Supplements of benzoate, phenylbutyrate and arginine (or citrulline in OTC deficiency)*
- *Avoid catabolic states*

Carbohydrate metabolism disorders

GALACTOSAEMIA

Incidence 1:60 000, autosomal recessive. Gene on Ch. 9 p. 13, various mutations seen. Enzyme deficiency: galactose-1-phosphate uridyl transferase (pnemonic = GAL-I-PUT). This results in inability to metabolise galactose or lactose (glucose + galactose). Accumulation of galactose-1-phosphate results in damage to the brain, liver and kidney.

Clinical features

Newborn/infant   Vomiting, hypoglycaemia, feeding difficulties
Seizures, irritability, developmental delay
Jaundice, hepatomegaly, liver failure, DIC
Cataracts, splenomegaly, *E. coli* sepsis (typical)

Diagnostic investigations

Diagnosis   Enzyme assay in red blood cells
Urine   Non-glucose reducing substances present when milk fed ie. Clinitest positive, Clinistix negative (specific for glucose)

Management

Lactose and galactose-free diet. Speech-language problems (especially dysarthria) and ovarian failure almost inevitable even with therapy.

HEREDITARY FRUCTOSE INTOLERANCE

Incidence 1:40 000, autosomal recessive. Enzyme deficiency: aldolase B. This results in inability to metabolise fructose or sucrose (glucose + fructose). Breast milk and most formulas do not contain fructose thus symptoms occur upon introduction of fruits and vegetables. Fructose-1-phosphate accumulates in hepatocytes.

Clinical features
Similar to those of galactosaemia on feeding fructose.

- *Abdominal pain, vomiting*
- *Proteinuria*
- *Liver disease results from chronic fructose ingestion*

Diagnostic investigations

- *Urine-reducing substance that is not glucose*
- *Enzyme analysis (liver)*
- *Genetic marker*

Management
Elimination of fructose from the diet.

GLYCOGEN STORAGE DISEASES

These are the result of several different enzyme deficiencies and cause glycogen accumulation in tissues. There are nine different types, the most common of which are outlined below.

Diagnosis is made by enzyme assay in blood, liver or muscle biopsy.

Treatment of GSD 1 and 3 includes avoidance of fasting with continuous overnight feeds and/or uncooked cornstarch.

Disease/enzyme	Features
GSD 1/glycogen-6-phosphatase	Hepatomegaly, short stature, hypoglycaemia (severe), lactic acidosis Urate and triglycerides elevated Liver adenoma and nephropathy late complications Type 1b has neutropenia
GSD 2/acid maltase (Pompe disease)	Cardiomyopathy, skeletal myopathy, macroglossia, death Late-onset form – myopathy
GSD 3/debrancher enzyme	Hepatomegaly, short stature, hypoglycaemia (moderate) May develop myopathy, liver disease
GSD 6/liver phosphorylase and GSD 9/liver phosphorylase kinase	Hepatomegaly, short stature, symptoms of hypoglycaemia (mild)

Lipid metabolism disorders

FATTY ACID OXIDATION DISORDERS

Fatty acids are oxidised to CO_2 and water in skeletal muscle and heart and to ketones in the liver. Fats are the main source of energy during starvation (carbohydrates usually being the main source). All the genetic disorders in the fatty acid oxidation pathway are autosomal recessive.

Examples
MCAD	Medium-chain acyl–CoA dehydrogenase deficiency
VLCAD	Very long-chain acyl–CoA dehydrogenase deficiency
LCHAD	Long-chain L-3-hydroxyacyl–CoA dehydrogenase deficiency
CPT1	Carnitine palmitoyl transferase 1 deficiency

Clinical features
Acute attack	Vomiting, hypoglycaemia, lethargy and coma induced by fasting
Cardiac	Cardiomyopathy
Muscles	Muscle weakness, acute rhabdomyolysis
Liver	Reye-like syndrome

NB. May present as sudden death following an intercurrent illness.

Investigations

- *During acute attack – hypoglycaemia with inappropriately low urinary ketones, ie.* hypoketotic hypoglycaemia
- *Urinary organic acids (often highly suggestive metabolic profile)*
- *Total and free carnitine levels may be low*
- Acylcarnitine profile of blood spot by tandem mass spectrometry is usually diagnostic
- *Confirmation by fibroblast FAOD studies, molecular genetics, eg. common MCAD mutation*

Management

- *Prevention of fasting stress*
- *Carnitine may be beneficial*

HYPERLIPIDAEMIAS

These are a range of inherited disorders that result in raised serum lipoproteins. Investigation is with a fasting blood lipid profile. Management is controversial. Guidelines are available. Children less than 10 years rarely require drug therapy.

1. *Diet (low fat, high fibre)*
2. *Drugs – bile acid binders eg. cholestyramine, and cholesterol biosynthesis (HMGcoA reductase) inhibitors*

Classification

Name	Cause	Lab. findings	Clinical
1. Hypertriglyceridaemias			
Lipoprotein lipase (LPL) deficiency	LPL mutations resulting in inability to hydrolyse triglycerides in chylomicrons and VLDLs	↑ Triglycerides (mainly chylomicrons)	Recurrent pancreatitis Xanthomata
Familial hypertriglyceridaemia	Heterogeneous	↑ Triglycerides	Asymptomatic in children Associated with IDDM, obesity, hypertension and coronary heart disease
2. Hypercholesterolaemia			
Familial hypercholesterolaemia	Low-density lipoprotein receptor deficiency	↑ Cholesterol (mainly LDL)	Usually asymptomatic in childhood Xanthomata and early atherosclerosis in adulthood
Polygenic hypercholesterolaemia	Heterogeneous	Moderate ↑ cholesterol	Increased risk of CHD in adulthood
3. Combined hyperlipidaemia			
Familial combined hyperlipidaemia	Heterogeneous	↑ Cholesterol and triglycerides (LDL and VLDL)	Increased risk of CHD in adulthood Xanthomata

Transport defects

HARTNUP DISEASE

Autosomal recessive

Defect Transport of neutral amino acids across the intestinal mucosa (absorption) and renal tubules (reabsorption)

Biochemical result Tryptophan deficiency (an essential amino acid). Tryptophan is used to manufacture nicotinamide and therefore a deficiency of this may occur, resulting in features of pellagra (see p. 178).

Clinical features
Asymptomatic (most children)

Skin Photosensitivity (pellagra-type rash), eczema

CNS Episodic cerebellar ataxia, headaches, developmental delay, emotional instability

Other Muscle pain, weakness

Diagnostic investigations
Urine Aminoaciduria of neutral amino acids

Plasma   Amino acid screen (neutral amino acids $\downarrow$ or N)

Management
Diet   Nicotinic acid supplements and high-protein diet
            Possible dietary supplementation of neutral amino acid esters

Avoid sunlight.

Peroxisomal disorders

Incidence 1:25 000 to 50 000.

Peroxisomes are intracellular organelles containing at least 40 enzymes. They are involved in long chain fatty acid oxidation, plasmalogen biosynthesis and bile acid synthesis. Many of the disorders result from a failure to transport the enzymes into the peroxisome (peroxisomal biogenesis disorders). All are autosomal recessive except X-linked adrenoleukodystrophy.

Examples

1. *Peroxisomal biogenesis defects: features as below, also known as (although in reality part of one clinical spectrum):*
   - *Zellweger syndrome (severe)*
   - *neonatal adrenoleucodystrophy*
   - *infantile Refsum disease*
2. *X-linked adrenoleucodystrophy (see below)*
3. *Rhizomelic chondrodysplasia punctata: can be caused by enzyme deficiency or biogenesis defect*

Clinical features
The following may be evident:

General   Dysmorphism
CNS   Neuronal migration defects, sensorineural deafness
Liver   Cirrhosis
Eyes   Corneal clouding, congenital cataracts, glaucoma, retinopathy
CVS   CHD
Renal   Cysts
Skeletal Chondrodysplasia punctata (stippled appearance of epiphyses, apparent on X-ray)

Investigations
Serum   VLCFA, pyristinic and phytanic acid (elevated in peroxisomal biogenesis disorders and X-linked adrenoleukodystrophy only)
Red blood cell   Plasmalogens
Fibroblast   Peroxisomal enzyme analysis
X-ray   Chondrodysplasia punctata

Antenatal diagnosis possible with chorionic villous or amniotic fluid cell sampling.

NB. Chondrodysplasia punctata is seen in:

- *Zellweger syndrome*
- *rhizomelic chondrodysplasia punctata*
- *warfarin teratogenicity*
- *Conradi–Hunermann syndrome*

X-LINKED ADRENOLEUKODYSTROPHY

A disorder of peroxisomal VLCFA β-oxidation. This results in accumulation of VLCFAs, progressive adrenal cortex dysfunction and neuronal white matter degeneration. There are several phenotypes. Gene on Xq28.

Clinical features

Presentation at 5–15 years with academic deterioration, behavioural disturbance, difficulty walking, seizures, ataxia, progressing to spastic quadriplegia and pseudobulbar palsy, Addison's (may be presenting complaint). Death within 10 years. Some children have only Addison's disease with neurological features only occurring as adults.

Diagnostic investigations

- *Very long chain fatty acids* ↑
- *Adrenal cortical dysfunction*
- *CNS periventricular demyelination on MRI scan*
- *Neuropsychiatric assessment*

Management

- *Supportive therapy with adrenal steroid replacement, NG feeding or gastrostomy and anticonvulsants*
- *Dietary restriction of saturated very long chain fatty acids and supplements with monounsaturated fatty acids (Lorenzo's oil) is not curative but may be beneficial*
- *BMT is curative (doesn't reverse pathology, however)*

Mitochondrial disorders

These disorders may present at any age, in any organ and by any mode of inheritance. They include pyruvate dehydrogenase (PDH) deficiency and respiratory chain disorders (electron transport chain disorders). Alternatively called disorders of oxidative phosphorylation.

Clinical features

Features suggestive of mitochondrial dysfunction include (especially when in combination):

Muscle	Abnormal tone, weakness, exercise intolerance
Eyes	Ophthalmoplegia, optic atrophy, cataract, retinitis pigmentosa, cortical blindness

CNS	Developmental delay, seizures, movement disorders, coma, stroke
Cardiac	Cardiomyopathy, conduction defects
Hepatobiliary	Liver failure, pancreatic dysfunction
Haematological	Anaemia (sideroblastic in Pearson's), pancytopenia
Renal	Tubulopathy
Gastrointestinal	Dysfunction
Other	Growth retardation

Diagnosis

An elevated 'free-floating' blood lactate, *in the absence* of sepsis, hypoxia, poor tissue perfusion or another metabolic disorder known to cause high lactate, in a child with a combination of the above symptoms is highly suggestive of a mitochondrial disorder. An elevated CSF lactate is probably even more specific.

Diagnosis is confirmed by enzyme analysis of fibroblasts, muscle or liver. A successful molecular diagnosis is currently uncommon in children but will probably become the investigation of choice in the near future. Most disorders are probably of autosomal recessive inheritance.

Well-known phenotypes include:

Congenital lactic acidosis	Floppy neonate, often with cardiomyopathy, liver dysfunction and renal tubular dysfunction. Lactate very high. Death in infancy
Leigh syndrome	Initially normal child, progressive basal ganglia and brainstem dysfunction
MELAS	**M**itochondrial **E**ncephalomyopathy, **L**actic **A**cidosis and **S**troke-like episodes. Short stature, lactic acidosis, mitochondrial point mutations (maternal inheritance). Onset usually in late childhood or adulthood
Pearson syndrome	Transfusion-dependent sideroblastic anaemia, pancreatic dysfunction, short stature, myopathy, developmental delay, mitochondrial DNA deletions

Lysosomal storage disorders

These are diseases due to a deficiency of a specific hydrolase enzyme resulting in lipid being stored (usually as a glycosphingolipid) within the lysosomes. They may be stored only in the peripheral tissues or only in the CNS or in both, resulting in different clinical features.

The majority are heterogeneous, ie. there are infantile, juvenile and adult-onset forms. They are all autosomal recessive.

Diagnosis is by enzyme assay in cultured fibroblasts or leucocytes.

Disease	Enzyme	CNS	Hepatospleno-megaly	Skeletal dysplasia	Ophthalmic	Other features
G$_{M1}$ gangliosidosis	B-galactosidase	+++	+++	+++	Cherry red spot	Hurler-like features, can have features at birth
G$_{M2}$ gangliosidosis (Tay-Sachs)	Hexoaminidase A	+++	0	0	Cherry red spot	Hyperacusis, macrocephaly
G$_{M2}$ gangliosidosis (Sandhoff)	Hexoaminidase A & B	+++	0	0	Cherry red spot	Hyperacusis, macrocephaly
Neimann-Pick A	Sphingomyelinase	+++	+++	0	Cherry red spot	Vacuolated lymphocytes
Neimann-Pick B	Sphingomyelinase	+/−	++	0	+/−	Vacuolated lymphocytes
Neimann-Pick C	Abnormal cholesterol esterification	++	+	0	Ophthalmoplegia	Vacuolated lymphocytes
Krabbe	Galactosylceramide	+++	0	0	Optic atrophy	Irritability, ↓ nerve conduction, ↓CSF protein
Metachromatic leucodystrophy	Arylsulfatase A	+++	0	0	Optic atrophy	↓nerve conduction, ↓CSF protein
Gaucher, type 1	B-glucocerebrosidase	0	+++ (especially spleen)	++		Growth delay, pulmonary infiltration, thrombocytopenia
Gaucher, type 2	B-glucocerebrosidase	+++	++	++	Blindness	Early death, not responsive to enzyme replacement therapy
Gaucher, type 3	B-glucocerebrosidase	+	+++	+	Paralysis of lateral gaze	Myoclonus, defects in visual saccades
Mucolipidosis type II (I-cell disease)	GlcNAc phosphotransferase	+++	+	+++	Corneal clouding	Hurler-like. Type III mild phenotype

Mucopolysaccharidoses

These are a group of lysosomal disorders caused by defective degradation and storage in the lysosomes of mucopolysaccharides (glycosaminoglycans). These substances make up much of the intercellular substance of connective tissue.

The main mucopolysaccharides involved are dermatan sulphate, heparan sulphate and keratan sulphate.

General features ('Hurler' phenotype)

Features Progressive coarsening of features

Skeletal *Dysostosis multiplex* (X-ray changes seen: gibbus deformity, oval-shaped vertebrae, oar-shaped ribs, thickened skull, coxa valga, cortical thinning of long bones, tapered phalanges)

CNS Progressive cognitive regression

Other organs Hepatosplenomegaly, heart (cardiomyopathy, valvular lesions), corneal clouding, skin thickening

Diagnosis

1. *Urine glycosaminoglycans (GAGs)* ↑
2. *Specific enzyme deficiency on assay of leucocytes, cultured fibroblasts or serum*
3. *DNA analysis*

Treatment

- *Bone marrow transplant suitable in some patients*
- *Treatment of complications and anticipation of problems*
- *Often no specific treatment*

There is a wide variation within each disease so the same 'disease' can present as a neonate or in adulthood. Genotype-phenotype correlation exists in most. All are inherited in an autosomal recessive way apart from Hunter (X-linked).

Variations from the 'Hurler' phenotype include:

Type 1	Hurler
Type 1	Scheie: mild variant, normal intelligence
Type 2	Hunter: no corneal clouding
Type 3	Sanfilippo: severe cognitive and behavioural problems, less facial coarsening, no corneal clouding. Four different enzyme causes
Type 4	Morquio: severe skeletal deformity, less CNS involvement
Type 6	Maroteaux-Lamy: no CNS involvement, mild coarsening of features
Type 7	Sly: rare

The porphyrias

These are inherited or acquired disorders of the enzymes involved in haem biosynthesis. They may be acute or non-acute, depending on their presentation. The acute porphyrias are *all* characterised by acute attacks during which the urine ALA and PBG are raised. They may also be classified according to where the excess porphyrins are stored as *hepatic* (liver) or *erythropoietic* (bone marrow).

Classification

	Hepatic	Erythropoietic
Acute	Acute intermittent porphyria (AIP)	
	Variegate porphyria (VP)	
	Hereditary coproporphyria (HCP)	
Non-acute	Porphyria cutanea tarda (PCS)	Congenital erythropoietic porphyria (CEP)
		Erthyropoietic protoporphyria (EPP)

The haem biosynthesis pathway

Pathway intermediates	Enzyme	Porphyria
Succinyl CoA + glycine		
↓	ALA synthase	
ALA		
↓	ALA dehydrase	

PBG
↓   PBG deaminase   AIP
Uroporphyrinogen I
↓   Urocosynthase   CEP
Uroporphyrinogen III
↓   Urodecarboxylase   PCS
Coproporphyrinogen III
↓   Copro-oxidase   HCP
Protoporphyrinogen IX
↓   Proto-oxidase   VP
Protoporphyrin IX
↓   Ferrochelatase   EPP
Heme

Key: ALA = δ-*aminolaevulinic acid*
         PBG = *Porphobilinogen*

THE PORPHYRIAS

Clinical features	Investigation/Diagnosis	Management
Acute intermittent porphyria (AIP)		
Aut.dominant. Female > male		

Presentation 20–30 years with *acute attacks* precipitated by:
  Drugs eg. OCP, barbiturates
  Calorie reduction, menstruation
  Stress, eg. illness, psychological
	Urine – Red-brown on standing
	– ALA and PBG (↑during attacks – may be normal in between)
	– uroporphyrin and coproporphyrin↑
		Acute attacks:
		– Identification and removal of precipitant, analgesia, sedation
		– Glucose and haematin infusion to remove the porphyrins

Acute attacks: 1. *Abdominal* – pain, vomiting, constipation, may mimic acute abdomen 2. *Neurological* – motor or sensory polyneuropathy, cranial nerve lesions 3. *Cardiovascular* – Tachycardia, hypertension 4. *Neuropsychiatric* – anxiety, depression, psychosis No skin disease	*Serum* ALA and PBG (↑during attacks) *Stool* Uroporphyrin and coproporphyrin↑ **Diagnosis:** RBC PBG deaminase↓	

Variegate Porphyria (VP)

Aut.Dominant
Acute attacks as for AIP
Bullous photosensitive rash

Stool Protoporphyrin↑★
Urine Red-brown on
standing
ALA and PBG↑ during
attacks, coproporphyrin↑
Plasma Fluoresces

Treatment as for AIP

Diagnosis: Proto-oxidase↓

Hereditary Coproporphyria (HCP)

Aut.Dominant
Acute attacks as for AIP
Photosensitive rash similar to
PCS (about 30%)

Urine and stool
Coproporphyrin↑↑↑★
Urine Red-brown on
standing
ALA and PBG↑ during
attacks

Treatment as for AIP

Diagnosis: Coproporphyrin
oxidase↓ (liver, leucocytes,
fibroblasts)

Non-Acute

Porphyria Cutanea Tarda (PCS, porphyria cutanea symptomatica

Inherited or acquired
Sporadic type – male
predominantly, onset 45–50 years,
medication and alcohol related
Familial type – prepubertal, equal
sex incidence

Urine Uroporphyrin↑
coproporphyrin(↑)
Serum Transferrin(↑)
TIBC↑
Liver biopsy iron overload
features (due to altered iron
metabolism)

1. Avoid precipitants
2. Regular venesection, or low dose chloroquine

Diagnosis:
Urodecarboxylase↓ (in all
tissues)

Skin Bullous (subepidermal),
photoensitive rash that scars,
pigmentation of sun-exposed
areas. Facial and arm hypertrichosis
Skin fragility
Liver Chronic liver disease,
tumours

Congenital Erythropoetic Porphyria (CEP)

Autosomal recessive
Urine Red, pink nappies

Urine Uroporphyrins↑

Avoid sunlight

Skin Photosensitivity with bullae and scarring Brown teeth (*erythrodontia-pathognomonic*) Hypertrichosis, scarring alopecia, nail dystrophy	Coproporphyrins↑ *Stool* Coproporphyrin↑↑ *RBC* Uroporphyrins↑, coproporphyrins↑	Transfusions BMT may be helpful
Eyes Lenticular scarring, ulceration and cataracts leading to blindness *Other* Splenomegaly (secondary to haemolysis)	**Diagnosis:** RBC urocosynthetase↓	

Erythropoetic Proto Porphyria (EPP)

Autosomal dominant Variable (mild to severe) *Skin* Burning sensation on sun exposure with erythema, purpura (vesicles rare) Facial skin normal Onset symptoms >3 years *Liver* May be affected Cirrhosis, cholelithiasis	*RBC, stool, serum –* protoporphyrin↑ *RBC's* fluoresce **Diagnosis:** Ferrochetolase (hemesynthetase)↓ in all tissues	Avoid sun exposure, sunscreen β-carotene (photoprotection) Liver disease – Cholestryamine, bile salts and liver transplant if necessary

FURTHER READING

Scriver CR *Metabolic and molecular basis of inherited disease*, McGraw Hill, New York, 1995

Nyhan WL, Ozand PT *Atlas of metabolic disease*, 1st Ed. Chapman and Hall Medical, London, 1998

Fernandes J, Saundubray JM, van den Berghe G Eds. *Inborn metabolic diseases*. Springer-Verlag, Berlin, 1995

11

Dermatology

- *Terminology of common lesions*
- *Neonatal conditions*
- *Nappy rash*
- *Rashes associated with systemic disease*
- *Infections*
- *Atopic eczema*
- *Acne (vulgaris)*
- *Psoriasis*
- *Vascular birthmarks*

- *Naevi*
- *Alopecia*
- *Disorders of pigmentation*
- *Congenital ichthyoses*
- *Vesiculobullous disorders*
- *DNA fragility syndromes*
- *Ectodermal dysplasias*
- *Mastocytosis*
- *Cutis laxa*

Terminology of common lesions

Lesion	Description	Example
Macule	Flat disc with alteration in colour or texture	Freckle
Papule	Circumscribed palpable elevation <0.5 cm diameter	Wart
Nodule	Solid mass in the skin >0.5 cm diameter	Erythema nodosum
Plaque	Elevated area >2 cm diameter	Psoriasis
Scale	A flake of stratum corneum	Ichthyosis, psoriasis
Wheal	A transient area of dermal oedema	Urticaria
Vesicle	Visible fluid accumulation <0.5 cm diameter	Herpes
Bulla	Visible fluid accumulation >0.5 cm diameter	Burns, chronic bullous dermatosis of childhood
Ulcer	Loss of dermis and epidermis	Aphthous ulcer

Neonatal conditions

ERYTHEMA TOXICUM NEONATORUM

Benign condition of unknown cause occurring around day 2 in up to 50% of full-term neonates. Eruptions of yellow papules or pustules (containing eosinophils) with surrounding erythematous flare. May be widely dispersed. Self-limiting condition (2–4 days).

MILIA

Epidermal inclusion cysts, containing keratin. White papules common in neonates on the face and gingiva (Epstein pearls). Resolve <6 weeks. Sebaceous gland hyperplasia is similar, with small yellow papules mostly over the nose and forehead, due to maternal androgens.

SUCKING BLISTER

Bulla on the finger, lips or forearms caused by *in utero* sucking of the affected area. NB. *Sucking pad* on the lips is an area of hyperkeratosis.

SALMON PATCH

A common vascular malformation, present as small pale pink vascular macules (due to dilated superficial dermal capillaries) on eyelids, glabella, forehead or nape of the neck. They tend to fade during first few months of life, except the nuchal lesions which generally remain. These are 'stork bites'.

MONGOLIAN BLUE SPOT

Blue macular lesions on sacral area, back, shoulders and legs. Common in dark-skinned races. Due to deep dermal melanocytes. Generally fade during first few years (though they may persist).

SEBACEOUS NAEVUS

A small yellow oval plaque with no hair, on the head or neck of babies. They are composed of sebaceous glands and may become malignant after adolescence. They should be removed before adolescence.

APLASIA CUTIS CONGENITA

Developmental absence of skin, usually solitary or multiple small ulcers on the scalp. May be associated with malformation syndromes, embryological defects or intrauterine infection.

Nappy rash

The main causes of nappy rash are:

Irritant dermatitis	Due to irritant effect of urine and faeces. *The creases are spared* Treat with a barrier ointment, regular nappy change and a topical combined antifungal and hydrocortisone ointment
Candida infection	No sparing of the skin creases, satellite lesions seen Treat with antifungal or combined antifungal and hydrocortisone ointment Occasionally requires oral antifungal treatment

Seborrhoeic dermatitis	Rash of unknown cause; may also present as cradle cap and elsewhere on the body. Red moist rash with fine yellow scales. Not pruritic. Onset 2–6 weeks age
	Treat with combined antifungal and hydrocortisone ointment and emollients
	Can clear spontaneously after 6–8 weeks but often evolves into typical atopic dermatitis
Atopic eczema	May present as nappy rash due to superimposed local irritation
	Treat with emollients and combined antifungal and hydrocortisone ointment
Psoriasis	May present as an intractable nappy rash. Well-defined, red, dry and scaly

Rashes associated with systemic disease

ERYTHEMA NODOSUM

Females >males. Usually >6 years. Painful, shiny, hot, red elevated oval nodules (1–3 cm) over the shins. May occur on calves, thighs, upper limbs. They become purple and then fade over 2–4 weeks. Other features are fever, malaise, arthralgia and hilar lymphadenopathy.

Causes

Infections	Bacterial – streptococcus, mycoplasma, TB
	Enteric infections – salmonella, yersinia
	Viral – EBV, HBV, chlamydia
	Fungal – histoplasma, coccidiomycosis
Inflammatory bowel disease	Crohn's disease, ulcerative colitis
Autoimmune disease	Sarcoidosis, SLE, Behçet disease
Drugs	Sulphonamides, oral contraceptive pill

ERYTHEMA MULTIFORME

A reaction involving skin ± mucous membranes. Erythematous macules cover extensor surfaces, palms, soles and trunk and may then become bullous.

Target lesions are pathognomonic (erythematous border, dusky centre and middle paler ring).

Stevens–Johnson syndrome

A severe form of the disease with systemic upset. Conjunctivitis, uveitis corneal ulceration and corneal scarring may occur. Oral and genital ulcers. Treatment is supportive (eg. IV fluids and intensive therapy) as needed. Ophthalmological consultation essential. (Considered on a spectrum with TEN).

Causes

Infections	Bacterial – group A streptococcus, mycoplasma
	Viral – HSV, EBV
	Fungal – histoplasmosis
Drugs	Penicillin,sulphonamides,aspirin,anticonvulsants,barbiturates
Connective tissue disease	SLE, sarcoidosis
Malignancy	Leukaemia, lymphoma
Other	Vaccinations, radiotherapy

TOXIC EPIDERMAL NECROLYSIS (TEN)

A condition triggered by many different insults, involving a reaction with damage to the basal cell layer of the epidermis and large sheets of epidermis coming off. It is more common in adults. It is thought to be part of the same spectrum of disease as Stevens–Johnson syndrome.

Causes

Drugs	eg. sulphonamides, penicillin, NSAIDs, anticonvulsants, allopurinol
Other	GVHD, viral infections, measle immunization, radiotherapy, leukaemia, lymphoma

Clinical features

Prodrome	Fever, malaise, diffuse erythema and *skin tenderness*
Skin	Inflammation of eyes (corneal scarring may result), mouth, genitalia
	Loss of sheets of epidermis, flaccid bullae
	Nikolsky sign positive (epidermis separates with gentle shearing pressure)
	Loss of hair and nails
Systemic	Dehydration, secondary infection, septicaemia, liver derangement, glycosuria, pulmonary oedema, renal failure, anaemia, neutropenia

Management

Remove cause	
Treat as a burn	Intensive care, IV fluid therapy, ventilation may be necessary, antibiotics as necessary
	Skin care (eg. paraffin dressings)
	Strong analgesia
Eye care	As for Stevens–Johnson syndrome

Prognosis

Most cases survive but there is significant mortality.

NB. Toxic shock syndrome (TSS) is a condition seen most commonly in menstruating women, involving erythema and desquamation, but there are no bullae and no skin tenderness (see p. 63).

Infections

IMPETIGO

Common condition presenting as *honey-coloured crusts* usually around the mouth and nose, though may be widespread. Highly contagious.

Causes	*Staphylococcus aureus* (may become bullous)
	Streptococcus
	Secondary staphylococcal infection of atopic eczema or scabies
Treatment	Topical antibiotics if minor and treat any underlying cause
	Systemic antibiotics if widespread

STAPHYLOCOCCAL SCALDED SKIN SYNDROME (SSSS)

Generally children <5 years. An exfoliative dermatitis caused by exfoliative toxins of a staphylococcal infection (phage group II, including strains 55 and 71).

Clinical features

Systemic	Severe malaise, fever, dehydration, irritability, sepsis, electrolyte imbalance
Skin	Brightly erythematous skin, fissuring and crusting around eyes, nose and lips, blistering, skin tenderness
	Desquamation – peeling sheets of epidermis 2–3 days later
	Nikolsky sign positive (epidermis separates with gentle shearing pressure)
Other	Pharyngitis, conjunctivitis

Investigations

Cultures	Skin and blood
Skin biopsy	Intraepidermal splitting (between the granular and spinous layers)
	Frozen section of peeled skin can give a rapid diagnosis if necessary
Serum	FBC (features of sepsis), electrolytes (features of dehydration)

Management

Antibiotics	Systemic antistaphylococcal antibiotic therapy
Skin	Emollient application
General	Care of systemic state (fluid and electrolyte balance, protein loss, temperature control). IV fluids may be necessary

RINGWORM (DERMATOPHYTOSES)

This is due to dermatophyte fungi which invade the keratin layer. The ringworm fungi include Trichophyton, Epidermophyton and Microsporum. 'Tinea' = moth-eaten.
Infections include:

- *Tinea capitis* = scalp
- *Tinea pedis* = feet (mainly soles and toe webs)
- *Tinea ungium* = nails

- *Tinea corporis = body (trunk and limbs)*
- *Tinea cruris   = groin*

Clinical features

A ringworm lesion is annular, scaling and erythematous with an active, raised border and central clearing.

In tinea capitis, the hairs are broken just above the scalp, producing a black dot appearance. A 'kerion' is an inflamed, pustular scalp lesion.

Investigations

Woods light	Some fungi fluoresce (with spores outside the hair shaft ie. ectothrix)
Fungal identification	(Skin scrapings, nail clippings, hair) Fungal hyphae may be seen on microscopy but fungal culture is essential for confirmation and identification of the fungus

Management

Topical antifungals	Tinea pedis and localised skin lesions
Systemic antifungals	Scalp and nail infections and widespread lesions

PITYRIASIS VERSICOLOR

Common yeast infection of adolescence with *Pityrosporum orale* (*Malassezia furfur*) (a skin commensal). Presents as macules usually on the neck, upper chest, upper arms and back. In whites they are reddish-brown and in dark-skinned races they may be hypo- or hyperpigmented.

Investigations

Woods light	Lesions become more apparent
Skin scrapings	Microscopy and culture

Management

Topical imidazoles (eg. ketoconazole)

WARTS (VERRUCAE)

These are caused by the human papillomavirus (HPV). Types include:

Common warts	Papules with rough surface, typically on fingers, hands, face, knees and elbows, HPV type 2
Plantar warts	Flat painful warts on soles, HPV type 1
Plane warts	Slightly elevated, HPV type 3. Koebnerise. Resistant to treatment
Filiform warts	Protruberant warts, around nose and mouth. Refractory to topical therapy
Genital warts	*Condylomata accuminata* (occur on mucous membranes) Papillomatous in perianal area, labia, vaginal introitus and penis Also occur on the lips, tongue and conjunctivae

NB. May indicate sexual abuse
If <3 years, may be transferred from the birth canal

Management
Spontaneous regression occurs in 50% within two years. Treatment options include:

- *cryotherapy, lactic acid and salicylic acid applications with paring of the wart (common, plantar)*
- *podophyllin applications used in genital warts.*
- *topical retin A (plane warts)*
- *oral cimetidine (multiple refractory common warts)*

MOLLUSCUM CONTAGIOSUM

Common infection in school children with a pox virus. Spread by contact and scratching lesions. Widespread infection in immnuosuppression and atopic dermatitis.

Clinical features
Pearly papules with a central umbilicus. If squeezed, the central cheesy core of cells infected with viruses is extruded.

Clinical diagnosis, though central plug material may be identified on microscopy.

Management
Spontaneous resolution within 6–9 months (can last years). Advise to use separate towel and baths. No treatment is usually necessary. Occasionally they may need to be treated, which can be done with cryotherapy.

PITYRIASIS ROSEA

Probable viral cause (?HHV 7). Common in children and adolescents.

Clinical features

Prodrome (rare) Fever, malaise, arthralgia

Skin *Herald patch* – a large (1–10 cm) round erythematous lesion with raised border; 5–10 days later a maculopapular rash, lesions with a peripheral scale, sometimes pruritic. Rash follows cutaneous cleavage lines and hence has a 'Christmas tree' pattern on the back. Resolves in 2–12 weeks

Management
Non-specific. Emollients and antihistamines and topical steroid if necessary.

SCABIES

An irritative skin reaction to the female mite, *Sarcoptes scabiei*. Transmission by direct contact.

Clinical features

Scabies burrows Curved erythematous tracts with the mite in a vesicle at one end
Occurs in finger webs, wrists, elbows, ankles, genitalia and breasts
In infants it occurs on palms, soles and axillae

Rash Widespread, intensely itchy eruption after 4–6 weeks due to sensitivity to the mite and its products. Erythematons papules, pustules,
excoriation and burrows

Investigations

- *Clinical diagnosis*
- *Removal of the mite or its eggs with a needle, and identification under the microscope*

Management

Treat patient and all close contacts.

The whole body is covered in lotion (eg. malathion or permethrin), especially the webs between the fingers and toes: In children <2 years the face,
scalp, neck and ears must also be covered. The lotion is washed off after eight
hours. In young children medical supervision is advised and certain lotions are
not recommended.

All bed linen and clothes must be washed.

Atopic eczema (Atopic dermatitis)

An inflammatory condition of the skin.

Incidence 10% children
Associations Family/personal history of atopy (ie. asthma, hayfever, eczema)

Generally begins from 3 months–2 years and improves with age.

Clinical features

- *Pruritis*
- *IgE ↑ (80%)*
- *Dry skin, lichenification post-inflammatory pigmentation changes (chronic eczema)*
- *Erythema, vesicles, weeping and crusting of excoriated areas (acute and subacute eczema)*
- *Lymphadenopathy in widespread disease*
- *Distribution: generalised, in infants especially face and extensor surfaces*
  tendency to flexural involvement in older children
  other forms include discoid (annular lesions) and pompholyx (tiny vesicles, very pruritic)

Complications

1. *Secondary staphylococcal or streptococcal infection*
2. *Eczema herpeticum – HSV infection in a child with atopic eczema. Widespread, potentially serious infection, must be treated with antivirals (acyclovir IV if concern).*

Management
Several therapies are available. In order of increasing disease severity:

Avoid irritants	Soap and biological detergents; use cotton clothing
	Avoid contact with cats and dogs if other measures fail
	House dust mite reduction (no carpets, hoovering, mattress cover)
Emollients	eg. emollients in baths and as soap and moisturiser
Topical steroids	Use the minimum effective dose:
	Mild (class IV), eg. hydrocortisone 1%
	Moderate (class III), eg. clobetasone butyrate 0.05%
	Potent (class II), eg. betamethasone 0.1%
	Very potent (class I), eg. clobetasol propionate 0.05%
Occlusive bandages	Paste bandages with emollient, steroid or coal tar
	'Wet wraps' – wet dressings over applied emollient and steroid (NB. These increase the steroid potency by 10 times)
Antihistamines	To reduce itch, usually at night, orally

Oral beclomethasone
Chinese herbal treatment (tea, baths) (NB. Renal and liver toxicity reported)
Oral steroids
UVB or PUVA (psoralen with UV light)
Immunosuppressives (eg. azathioprine, cylosporin)

Note. Other eczematous conditions include: seborrheic dermatitis, irritant napkin dermatitis, pomphylox, pityriasis alba and allergic contact dermatitis.

Acne (vulgaris)

A common condition due to blockage of the pilosebaceous duct. Incidence high during puberty under the influence of androgenic hormones, generally improves by early 20s.

Propionibacterium acnes is associated with acne.

Clinical features
Areas most affected are the face, chest and back (sebaceous glands most numerous).

Lesions seen	Comedo (blackhead)
	Closed comedo (white head)
	Inflammatory papules and pustules and cysts

Treatment options
Topical therapy	Abrasives, exfoliatives (eg. products containing benzoyl peroxide)
	Antibiotics eg. erythromycin, clindamycin
	Topical retinoic acid lotion or gel
	UV light

Systemic therapy   Antibiotics eg. tetracycline (not <12 years)
Hormones eg. oral contraceptive pill containing cyproterone acetate
Retinoic acid (oral therapy for four to six months)

Psoriasis

A disease of rapid epidermal proliferation. Familial, rare <2 years.

Clinical features

- *Well-demarcated silvery-scaled, erythematous plaques, classically over extensor surfaces and scalp. In children the face and scalp are often first affected*
- *Nail pitting and onycholysis (rare in children)*
- *It may present as intractable nappy rash*
- *Psoriatic arthritis (rare in children)*

Types include:

- *Guttate psoriasis – many scattered small plaques. Commonest presentation in children, occurs after streptococcal sore throat. Check ASOT and throat swab*
- *Chronic plaque psoriasis*
- *Pustular psoriasis (if generalised, this is a serious life-threatening condition)*

Management options

- *Topical steroids*
- *Coal tar preparations (shampoo, soap, topical combined with steroids)*
- *Dithranol*
- *Calcipotriol*
- *In severe refractory cases oral retinoids, PUVA, UVB or cytotoxic therapy (eg. methotrexate, cyclosporin) may be used*

Vascular birthmarks

PORT-WINE STAIN (NAEVUS FLAMMEUS)

Permanent vascular malformation with ectasia of superficial dermal capillaries. Always present at birth. A macular erythema that gradually darkens with age.

Association: Glancoma with occular port wine stain (15–25%)

Treatment options

1. *Flashlamp-pumped pulsed dye laser*
2. *Cosmetic camouflage*

STURGE–WEBER SYNDROME

A syndrome involving:

1. *facial port-wine stain roughly in the distribution of V1 and V2 branch of the trigeminal nerve, almost always involving the forehead and upper eyelid*
2. *leptomeningeal angioma (on same side of the head) causing:*
   focal seizures
   and/or hemiparesis (slowly progressive)
   mental retardation

Glaucoma of the ipsilateral eye may be present (30–60%).

Investigations
SXR	Intracranial calcification, 'railroad track' appearance
CT brain scan	Intracranial calcification, cortical atrophy
MRI brain scan	Vascular anomaly outlined (with gadolinium enhancement)
Ophthalmology	Intraocular pressure measurement

Management
Seizures	Anticonvulsants
	Surgery (hemispherectomy or lobectomy) may be considered
Glaucoma	Regular intraocular pressure checks and any necessary treatment
Port-wine stain	Laser therapy and camouflage as above

KLIPPEL–TRENAUNAY SYNDROME

A syndrome involving:

1. *port-wine stain on a limb*
2. *soft tissue and bony hypertrophy*

There may also be:

- *venous varicosities, thromboses, ulceration*
- *A-V fistulas (described by Weber ie. Klippel Trenaunay Weber Syndrome)*

Complications
Cardiac failure, DVT, pain, haematuria (bladder lesions), rectal bleeding (bowel lesions).

Investigations
- *Angiograms, if needed*
- *MRI scan, if needed*

Management
- *Port-wine treatment as above*
- *Cardiac failure treatment*
- *Orthopaedic procedures (leg length discrepancies)*
- *Surgical treatment if necessary*

INFANTILE HAEMANGIOMA

These vascular proliferations are rarely present at birth, but appear during the first two months. Superficial lesions are bright red (= strawberry haemangiomas), deeper ones are bluish (= cavernous haemangiomas).

Incidence   1:20 infants

Association   Premature birth

The natural history is to enlarge until 6–12 months, then to slowly regress. Most have involuted by five years. Residual cosmetic defect in a few.

No treatment necessary unless:

- *large disfiguring lesion*
- *complications*

Complications

- *Ulceration/infection*
- *Haemorrhage*
- *Platelet consumption coagulopathy (Kasabach–Merritt)*
- *Heart failure (multiple haemangiomas with internal lesions)*
- *Visual impairment*
- *Airway obstruction (stridor, feeding difficulties)*

Management options

- *Systemic steroid course*
- *Intralesional steroid injection*
- *Laser therapy (early, ulcerated lesions)*
- *Interferon-α therapy*
- *Surgical excision*

KASABACH–MERRITT SYNDROME

A syndrome of:

1. *rapidly enlarging haemangioma*
2. *consumption coagulopathy (acute or chronic) – thrombocytopenia, consumption of clotting factors, petechiae, haemorrhage, anaemia*

High-output cardiac failure may result from AV shunting in large lesions.

Management

- *Platelet, blood and FFP transfusions*
- *Cardiac failure treatment*
- *Haemangioma therapy (as above); embolisation may be necessary*

NEONATAL HAEMANGIOMATOSIS

Multiple small haemangiomas of the skin, with internal haemangiomas of two or more organs (eg. liver, CNS, gastrointestinal tract and lung). USS and CT/MRI scans needed to detect extent of disease. High-output cardiac failure is seen from AV shunting, particularly if liver haemangiomas are present.

NAEVI

Naevi are skin lesions with a collection of cells that are normally found in the skin. Melanocytic naevi (moles) are benign tumours of melanocytes. They may be congenital or acquired.

CONGENITAL MELANOCYTIC NAEVUS (CMN)

Approximately 1% of infants. May be small, giant or intermediate. Giant CMNs (>20 cm diameter) incidence 1: 10 000. These are generally on the trunk or lower limbs (eg. 'bathing trunk naevus'). Associated with leptomeningeal melanosis (diagnosed on MRI scan) and increased risk of melanoma (exact risk unknown). May be treated early with dermabrasion or surgically by tissue expansion or left and observed.

ACQUIRED MELANOCYTIC NAEVUS

These appear mainly during childhood and adolescence. Average number is 25–50 per adult. Melanoma risk related to numbers of naevi, sun exposure and sunburn during childhood and immunosuppression. They are classified as *junctional* (flat, pigmented), *compound* (raised, pigmented with junctional component), *intradermal* (raised, skin coloured) or *blue naevus* (dark bluish colour) according to their depth.

SPITZ NAEVUS

Is a rapidly growing pigmented naevus in children, with histological features resembling a malignant naevus. It is benign, most commonly on the face, and is removed if there is doubt of the diagnosis.

INFLAMMATORY LINEAR VERRUCOUS EPIDERMAL NAEVUS (ILVEN)

An uncommon condition usually appearing in the first six months of life. A linear epidermal naevus that has a warty appearance and may be pruritic. It is generally refractory to treatments. Treatment options include steroids, cryotherapy, surgical excision and laser therapy. ILVEN may improve spontaneously.

Alopecia

This is hair loss to the extent that the scalp becomes abnormally visible.

DIFFUSE HAIR LOSS

Telogen effluvium   Hair loss in the telogen (resting) phase
Seen 3–4 months after an event or illness, recovers six months later, eg. severe illness, pregnancy, stress, sudden weight loss, blanket friction (babies)

Anagen effluvium   Hair loss in the anogen (growing) phase, eg. chemotherapy, radio-therapy

PATCHY HAIR LOSS

Trichotillomania   Hair loss due to pulling hairs, may be associated with obsessive com-pulsive disorder

Alopecia areata   Circular patches of hair loss developing rapidly. Cause unknown
Alopecia totalis – all the scalp
Alopecia universalis – all the scalp and body
'*Exclamation mark*' hairs seen (short new hairs the shape of exclama-tion marks under the microscope)
Associations: autoimmune disease, atopy, Down syndrome
Variable prognosis

Disorders of pigmentation

GENERALISED PIGMENTATION CHANGES

Albinism

This is due to a partial or complete failure of melanin production of which there are many types, mostly autosomal recessive.
Melanin production:

Phenylalanine $\rightarrow$ *Tyrosine* $\rightarrow$ *Melanin*

Tyrosinase catalyses three steps in this process.

Clinical features

A depigmentation of the skin, iris and retina (all or some affected).

Skin   Depigmentation of skin (pink) and hair (white) although they may have some pigment

Eyes   Blue–grey irises, nystagmus, photophobia, decreased acuity, prominent red reflex

Complications   Blindness, skin cancers

Oculocutaneous albinism

There are nine types including:

Type IA (tyrosinase negative)	Pale skin, white hair, red iris
Type II (tyrosinase positive)	Most common, some pigmentation. Gene defect on chromosome 15q11–13
	Seen in 1% of Prader–Willi and Angelman syndrome
Hermansky–Pudlack syndrome	A tyrosinase-positive albinism associated with:
	• *platelet storage pool deficiency and coagulation problem*
	• $\pm$ *pulmonary fibrosis, granulomatous colitis*
Chediak–Higashi syndrome	Tyrosinase-positive oculocutaneous albinism with abnormal leucocyte granules and increased infections (see p. 39)

Ocular albinism

There are four types. Only the eyes are affected. Sensorineural deafness may be associated.

Management

There is no specific management. Protection from sun exposure and ophthalmology follow up is important.

LOCALISED PIGMENTATION CHANGES

Incontinentia pigmenti

X-linked dominant (mostly lethal in males, functional mosaic in females). Gene locus has been demonstrated on Xq28 and Xp11.2.

Clinical features

There are three stages but the sequence is irregular and stages may overlap.

Skin	Stage 1	Vesicles in linear patterns on limbs, occur in crops (first weeks of life)
	Stage 2	Red plaques, papular, warty lesions in linear patterns (from four months)
	Stage 3	Classic picture, from 1–16 years. Hyperpigmentation in linear streaks and whorls (following Blashko's lines) in a 'splashed' or 'Chinese figure' distribution. This may be the only stage seen. These slowly fade to become hypopigmented, atrophic lesions
Teeth		Conical teeth, hypodontia
Hair (25%)		Cicatricial alopecia
Eye (30%)		Microphthalmos, optic atrophy, strabismus, cataracts, blindness
CNS (25%)		Seizures, microcephaly, mental retardation, spasticity, paralysis
Nails		Usually normal, may be dystrophic and small

Hypomelanosis of Ito

A clinical picture of hypopigmented lines and whorls following lines of Blashko usually present from birth, resembling (though unrelated to) the late stages of incontinentia pigmentii.

Clinical features

CNS	Mental retardation, seizures, microcephaly, hypotonia
Musculoskeletal	Scoliosis, limb deformities
Eyes	Strabismus, nystagmus
CVS	CHD

Piebaldism (white spotting)

Autosomal dominant. Localised patches of depigmentation due to absence of melanocytes, mostly on the upper chest, abdomen and limbs, and a white forelock. Bilateral involvement, though not symmetrical. The patches are present from birth and remain unchanged throughout life.

Waardenburg syndrome

Autosomal dominant, variable penetrance. Type I caused by mutations in PAX3 gene (ch. 2q), Type II by mutations in Ch. 3p. A syndrome of:

- *lateral displacement of inner canthi (type I only), inner third of the eyebrow is hyperplastic, brows may be confluent, broad nasal bridge*
- *white forelock, premature greying in the third decade*
- *deafness (25% type I, 50% type II)*
- *heterochromic iris (25%), hypopigmented fundus*
- *cutaneous depigmentation lesions resembling piebaldism*

Vitiligo

An acquired condition. Theories of aetiology include autoimmune, neurogenic and self-destructive mechanisms.

Associations	Thyroid disease, hypoparathyroidism
	IDDM, pernicious anaemia, Addison disease
	Myaesthenia gravis, alopecia areata, morphoea
	Malignant melanoma, halo naevus
	Raised autoantibodies
	Positive family history (40%)

Clinical features

Usually symmetrical hypomelanotic macules, especially around the eyes and mouth, in the axillae and groin (areas that are usually hyperpigmented) and trauma sites. Premature greying of hair associated. Presentation <20 years in half of cases.

Management

- *Drug treatments: topical steroids initially*
  oral psoralens with UV light
- *Camouflage make-up*
- *Sun protection for affected areas*

Prognosis

May repigment spontaneously (10–20%) but usually progresses.

Congenital ichthyoses

These are a heterogeneous group of conditions with rough, dry skin and scaling.

HARLEQUIN ICHTHYOSIS

A severe erythrodermic ichthyosis with a distinct appearance at birth. Features include the following.

- *Prematurity (occasionally stillborn)*
- *A rigid, hyperkeratotic covering of thick, yellow plaques at birth*
- *Cracks occur soon after birth leaving deep red fissures (like a harlequin)*
- *Ears are tethered, hands and feet encased, mouth open*
- *Severe ectropion (everted eyes) and eclabion (everted lips)*

These features result in limited chest expansion, temperature instability, potential dehydration and electrolyte imbalance, feeding difficulties and susceptibility to infections.

Initial management

- *Intensive care in a humidified incubator*
- *Regular application of paraffin oil*
- *High fluid intake (may need NG or IV) with careful electrolyte monitoring*
- *Early recognition and treatment of sepsis*
- *Oral retinoid therapy may be used*

With good general care and early retinoid therapy these babies now survive (mortality used to be high). The survivors have a distinct severe ichthyosis.

COLLOIDIAN BABY

A distinct appearance at birth with a tight, glistening membrane covering (like a sausage skin), with less severe features than harlequin ichthyosis. Everted lips and eyes may be present.

Initial general management is as for a harlequin ichthyosis (retinoids are not used).

These infants survive and generally develop an ichthyosiform erythroderma (non-bullous ichthyosiform erythroderma or lamellar ichthyosis). Occasionally skin is normal.

ICHTHYOSIS VULGARIS

Autosomal dominant. Incidence 1:300. Mild roughening and scaling of the skin.

X-LINKED RECESSIVE ICHTHYOSIS (XLRI)

X-linked, female carriers may have some features. A mild ichthyosis with dark skin scaling, corneal opacities. There is an underlying lipid defect of steroid sulphatase deficiency.

Prolonged labour in carrier mothers (due to placental steroid sulphatase deficiency).

Kallman syndrome

XLRI associated with anosmia, hypogonadotrophic hypogonadism and neurological defects.

LAMELLAR ICHTHYOSIS

Autosomal recessive, very rare condition. Brown, scaly skin ('lizard skin'), with thick soles and palms.

NON-BULLOUS ICHTHYOSIFORM ERYTHRODERMA (NBIE)

Autosomal recessive, rare condition. Fine white scales and erythroderma.

MANAGEMENT OF ICHTHYOSES

- *Emollients (bath oils, frequent application of paraffin oil)*
- *Oral retinoid therapy in severe types*

Vesiculobullous disorders

EPIDERMOLYSIS BULLOSA

A group of diseases involving blister formation with minor trauma. The main types (of which various subtypes exist) are as follows.

Epidermolysis bullosa simplex

Autosomal dominant, the most frequent form. Intraepidermal blisters of the arms, legs, hands, feet and scalp, palms and soles mainly affected in some types. Non-scarring. Improves with age. Mutations in keratin genes.

Junctional epidermolysis bullosa (epidermolysis bullosa letalis)

Autosomal recessive, several genes involved. Blisters within the lamina lucida. All areas of skin affected, nails are shed. Internal blistering of the respiratory and gastrointestinal tracts, mid-facial erosions, hoarse voice, stridor. Death usually in infancy, though a non-lethal form exists with survival into adulthood.

Dystrophic epidermolysis bullosa

Blisters below the lamina densa. Both types caused by mutations in the COL7A1 gene that encodes for the anchoring fibril protein, type VII collagen.

Autosomal dominant form	Scarring blisters mostly of the hands, feet and sacrum
	Nail loss. Generally less severe than recessive form
Autosomal recessive form	Severe disease with widespread atrophic scarring blisters with milia formation, *mitten hand* deformity (digital fusion), oesophageal strictures
	Poor nutrition, anaemia, sparse hair, dystrophic nails, corneal ulceration

CHRONIC BULLOUS DERMATOSIS OF CHILDHOOD (LINEAR IGA DERMATOSIS)

Usually occurs <10 years.

Associations   HLA-B8, DR3

Clinical features

Bullae	Multiple tense bullae on buttocks, genitals, trunk, perioral area, face and limbs
	Urticated plaques with blisters around the edge (*string of pearls* sign)
	Mucosal involvement. Blisters may form rosettes
	Pruritis sometimes present
	Usually of 3–4 years duration

Investigations

Skin biopsy   Subepidermal blister, linear IgA BMZ antibodies.

Management

Dapsone (steroids if no response).

DNA fragility syndromes

XERODERMA PIGMENTOSUM (XP)

Autosomal recessive. Disorder of defective DNA repair. Light in the wavelengths 280–340 nm results in DNA damage. Seven complementation groups (on different chromosomes) known.

Clinical features

Skin	Freckling, erythema, scaling, crusting and telangiectasia in sun-exposed areas (premature ageing)
	Skin cancers develop (BCC, SCC, malignant melanoma)
Eyes	Corneal opacities, blepharitis, photophobia, eventual blindness
CNS (20%)	Mental retardation, deafness

Management

- *Total sun protection (glasses, clothes, total sunblock)*
- *Antenatal diagnosis possible with amniocentesis*

Prognosis

Early death from developing cancers and neurological problems.

Ectodermal dysplasias

A group of many disorders involving a defect of teeth, hair, nails and skin. There are many subtypes.

EEC SYNDROME (ECTRODACTYLY-ECTODERMAL DYSPLASIA-CLEFTING SYNDROME)

Autosomal dominant.

1. *Ectodermal dysplasia (dry skin, wispy hair, no eyelashes)*
2. *Cleft lip ± palate*
3. *Lacrimal duct stenosis*
4. *Ectrodactyly (split hands and feet, 'lobster claw' deformity)*
5. *Peg-shaped teeth*

HYPOHIDROTIC ECTODERMAL DYSPLASIA

X-linked recessive. A syndrome of:

1. *decreased/absent sweat glands – discomfort in hot temperatures, unexplained fevers*
2. *hypotrichosis*
3. *hypodontia, conical teeth*

Other features include:

Facial dysmorphism	Large ears, flat nasal bridge, frontal bossing, thick everted lips
Hair	Sparse, dry, short scalp hair
Skin	Dry, hypopigmented, prematurely aged, brittle nails
CNS	Learning difficulties in approximately 30%

Investigations

Sweat pores	Absent or decreased in palmar ridges
Sweat test	Reduced or absent (pilocarpine iontophoresis)
Skin biopsy (palm)	Eccrine gland hypo/aplasia

HIDROTIC ECTODERMAL DYSPLASIA

Autosomal dominant.

1. *Small/absent dystrophic nails*

2. *Hyperkeratosis of palms and soles*
3. *Thin, pale, brittle hair*

NB. Normal sweating and teeth.

Mastocytosis

Disorder involving mast cell aggregates in the dermis. The clinical picture is variable with urticaria pigmentosa most commonly seen in children.

Clinical features

Skin	Pruritis, mastocytomas (solitary skin lesions that involute spontaneously)
	Urticaria pigmentosa: crops of maculopapular lesions during first two years (yellow to brown). Blisters seen in infants
	Darier sign on stroking a lesion (erythema and whealing)
Diffuse cutaneous mastocytosis	Yellow thickened skin, intense pruritis ± systemic involvement
Systemic	Features of histamine release (tachycardia, hypotension, syncope, wheezing) may rarely occur

Prognosis
Spontaneous resolution in 50% by puberty.

Cutis laxa

Autosomal recessive, autosomal dominant or acquired. Pathogenesis is due to defect(s) in elastin (exact mechanism unknown). *Acquired cutis laxa* appears during childhood and may follow a febrile illness, connective tissue disease (eg. SLE, amyloidosis), inflammatory skin condition (eg. erythema multiforme) or occur in babies from women on penicillamine.

Clinical features

Skin	Folds of lax skin from birth or later in childhood
	Premature ageing, facial appearance: '*bloodhound*' appearance.
Other features	(Seen in recessive types) Hernias, rectal prolapse, diverticular disease, pneumothoraces, emphysema, peripheral pulmonary stenosis, aortic dilatation, skeletal abnormalities, dental caries and growth retardation.

FURTHER READING

Harper J, Orange A, Prose N Textbook of paediatric dermatology, Blackwell Science, London, 2000

DuVivier A, Higgins EM Skin disease in childhood and adolescence, Blackwell Science, London, 1996

12

Rheumatic and musculoskeletal diseases

- *Autoantibodies*
- *Juvenile chronic arthritis*
- *Spondyloarthropathies*
- *Infective arthritis*
- *Systemic lupus erythematosus (SLE)*
- *Antiphospholipid syndrome*
- *Idiopathic inflammatory myopathies*
- *Scleroderma*
- *Mixed connective tissue disease (MCTD)*
- *Sjögren syndrome*
- *Ehlers–Danlos syndrome*
- *Vasculitis*
- *Amyloidosis*
- *Osteogenesis imperfecta*
- *Osteopetrosis*
- *Osteochondrodysplasias*
- *Other musculoskeletal conditions*

Autoantibodies

Non-organ specific autoantibodies associated with rheumatic disease are outlined.

Rheumatoid factors (RhF)
Antibody to the Fc portion of IgG (usually IgM detected, also IgG, IgA and IgE).
Positive in   Rheumatoid arthritis (80%), JCA (5–10%)
              Connective tissue disease, eg. SLE, Sjögren syndrome
              Chronic infectións, eg. HIV, hepatitis, TB, endocarditis
              Leukaemia, lymphoid malignancies
              Pulmonary fibrosis
              General population ($\leq$4%)

Antinuclear antibodies (ANA)
These are antibodies to nuclear components and include:
Anti-ds DNA   SLE (80%, specific)
Anti-ss DNA   SLE (90%, non-specific), drug-induced lupus, other connective tissue
                disease, normals
Anticentromere   CREST syndrome
Antihistone   SLE, drug-induced lupus particularly

Anti-extractable nuclear antigens (ENA)
These include:

Anti-Sm (Smith)	SLE (20%, very specific)
Anti-nRNP	MCTD (100%), SLE
Anti-SSA (Ro)	Congenital heart block, Sjögren syndrome, SLE
Anti-SSB (La)	Congenital heart block, Sjögren syndrome, SLE
Anti Jo-1	Myositis, fibrosing alveolitis

Antineutrophil cytoplasmic antibodies (ANCA)
Antibodies to antigens within the cytoplasm of neutrophils.

c-ANCA (cytoplasmic)	Wegener granulomatosis (specific), Kawasaki disease
p-ANCA (perinuclear)	Connective tissue disease, vasculitis

Antiphospholipid antibodies
Antibodies to phospholipid antigens. Associated with thrombosis *in vivo* but coagulation prolongation *in vitro*. Seen in SLE and antiphospholipid syndrome, eg. anti-β1-glycoprotein, anticardiolipin lupus anticoagulant test positive.

Juvenile chronic arthritis (JCA)

A group of disorders with chronic synovitis (> 6 weeks) ± extraarticular features occurring before age 16 years. Cause unknown: though immunological and infective mechanisms suspected. Involved joints show stiffness (early morning), swelling, limited painful movement, warm and tender to touch. Contractures may occur rapidly.

X-ray changes
Early Soft tissue swelling, periosteal new bone formation
Late Subchondral bone erosions, osteoporosis. Joint space narrowing, destruction of bones, deformity, fusion or subluxation

PAUCIARTICULAR-ONSET DISEASE
Involvement of ≤ 4 large joints in the first six months. Two types exist:

Type I
- *Predominately females, < 4 years*
- *Knees, ankles, elbows* — Bony overgrowth, leg length discrepancy and valgus deformity are very important features 20% develop polyarthritis and severe disease ("extended pauciarticular onset JCA")
- *Chronic iridocyclitis (30%)* — No early symptoms, detectable with slit-lamp only Untreated causes synechiae, glaucoma, cataracts and blindness
Slit-lamp examination imperative 3–4 monthly
Treatment with topical steroids and mydriatics

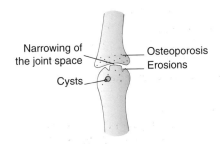

Figure 12.1 X-ray changes in JCA

- *ANA positive (90%)*
- *HLA-DR5, 8, DP0201 positive*
- *RhF and HLA-B27 negative*
- *ESR ($\uparrow$ or N)*

Type II (Juvenile-onset spondylarthropathy)

- *predominantly Males, >9 years*
- *Lower limb arthritis, sacroiliac pain, axial disease*
- *Progression to spondylarthropathy*
- *Acute iridocyclitis (10%)*
- *HLA-B27 (75%)*
- *RhF and ANA negative*
- *ESR ($\uparrow$ or N)*

POLYARTICULAR-ONSET DISEASE

Involvement of >4 joints
Female > male
  Two types exist:

RhF negative (30% of JCA)   Moderate to severe disease, <8 years, HLA-DR1
Asymmetrical, small and large joints, especially the TMJ
and cervical spine
Occasional iridocyclitis (5%)

RhF positive (10% of JCA)   More severe, >8 years, HLA-DR4
Symmetrical, hands and feet and hips
Rheumatoid nodules, tenosynovitis
Vasculitis

Particular joint problems seen due to distorted growth:

Cervical spine	Fusion or subluxation, anaesthetic difficulties
Temporomandibular joint (TMJ)	Micrognathia, dental hygiene and anaesthetic difficulties
Hips	Destruction, limb shortening
Knee	Overgrowth causing valgus deformity

Investigations

ESR ↑

ANA may be positive

SYSTEMIC–ONSET DISEASE

All ages. Females = males

A clinical diagnosis of exclusion

Differential diagnoses: Malignancy (eg. lymphoma, neuroblastoma)
                          Infection, vasculitis, other connective tissue disease

Clinical features

Fevers	39–40°C, intermittent, appears very unwell when febrile
Rash	Variable, salmon-pink, during febrile periods, may be urticarial
Myalgia, arthralgia	
Hepatosplenomegaly	
Lymphadenopathy	
Other	Pericardial effusions, pleuritis, abdominal pain
Joints	Polyarticular arthritis occurs within months of onset in 50% (associated with severe, destructive, chronic course), mild disease in others
Late features	Short stature, micrognathia, amyloidosis (invariable)

Investigations

FBC	Anaemia of chronic disease, WCC ↑ (neutrophilia), platelets ↑
ESR	↑
Autoantibodies	ANA and RhF negative

Management of JCA

1. Physiotherapy, splinting, occupational therapy, psychological therapy
2. NSAIDS
3. Steroids – oral or IV pulsed methylprednisolone
4. Intraarticular crystalline steroid injections
5. Disease-modifying drugs, eg. methotrexate, cyclosporin

Spondylarthropathies

These are HLA-B27 associated and RhF-negative disorders.

JUVENILE-ONSET SPONDYLOARTHROPATHY (See above)

JUVENILE ANKYLOSING SPONDYLITIS

Clinical features   Back pain and stiffness
Sacroiliac joints involvement (may progress to lumbar and cervical spine joints, though rarely <12 years)
Associations   HLA-B27 (95%)
Male > female, onset >8 years (peak 20–30 years)

Other clinical features

- *Peripheral lower limb arthritis*
- *Plantar fasciitis*
- *Enthesopathy (swelling at tendon and ligament insertions)*
- *Iridocyclitis*
- *Aortic incompetence (aortitis)*
- *Fever, anaemia, growth retardation, amyloid glomerulonephritis*

Investigations
ESR   ↑
FBC   Anaemia
X-ray   Erosion of sacroiliac joints, loss of lumbar lordosis, 'Bamboo spine', **tramline appearance** (calcification of interspinous ligaments and syndesmophytes forming between vertebrae)

Management

1. *Physiotherapy and posture exercises*
2. *NSAIDS*
3. *Sulphasalazine*

REITER SYNDROME

An acute reactive arthritis following gastrointestinal or venereal infection, involving:

1. *Arthritis (lower limbs, asymmetrical, may become chronic)*
2. *Ocular inflammation (uveitis, conjunctivitis)*
3. *Sterile urethritis*

Gastrointestinal infections   Shigella, salmonella, campylobacter, yersinia
Venereal infections   Chlamydia, non-specific urethritis (NSU)
Associations   HLA-B27 (80%)
Male > female

Other features

- *Fever*
- *Keratoderma blenorrhagica*
- *Plantar fasciitis*
- *Enthesopathy*
- *Nail dystrophy*
- *Sacroiliitis*
- *Mouth ulceration*

The disease may become chronic and transform into a spondylarthropathy.

Investigations

ESR	↑
FBC	Anaemia (of chronic disease), Hb may be normal, WCC ↑
Autoantibodies	ANA and RhF negative
Stool and urine	M, C and S

Management

1. *Antibiotics*
2. *Physiotherapy*
3. *NSAIDs*

REACTIVE ARTHRITIS

A sterile arthritis following an infection (eg. gastrointestinal, influenza, mycoplasma, EBV, streptococcal). The arthritis affects a few joints only, may be migratory and is self-limiting. Some children develop a chronic spondylarthropathy later.
NB. Rheumatic fever is a reactive arthritis.

ARTHRITIS OF INFLAMMATORY BOWEL DISEASE

Arthritis associated with ulcerative colitis or Crohn's disease. Male = female, >4 years.

Clinical features

- *Pauci- or polyarticular arthritis of large joints*
- *Onset before, during or after bowel disease*
- *Usually varies with bowel disease activity, though some cases (spondylitic) progress regardless of control of underlying bowel disease*

Investigations

FBC	WCC normal, Hb ↓
ESR	↑
Autoantibodies	ANA and RhF negative
HLA association	HLA-B27 positive in spondylitic group only

Management

1. *Physiotherapy*
2. *Treat IBD (sulphasalazine and steroids helpful for both IBD and arthritis)*
3. *NSAIDs*

JUVENILE PSORIATIC ARTHRITIS

Uncommon in childhood. Females > males. Psoriasis precedes arthritis in 50% and vice versa in 50%.

- *Asymmetrical arthritis of several joints*
- *Severe destructive disease occasionally (arthritis mutilans)*
- *Dactylitis (swollen, sausage-shaped fingers)*
- *Tendinitis*
- *Nail pitting*
- *Psoriatic skin lesions on extensor surfaces*

Investigations

FBC	Anaemia, WCC ↑
ESR	↑
Autoantibodies	ANA may be positive, RhF negative

Management

As for JCA.

Infective arthritis

Infection in the joint space, usually occurs <2 years, from haematogenous spread. Serious joint destruction if not promptly treated.

Causes

Bacterial	Staphylococcus, streptococcus, meningococcus, gonococcus, haemophilus (young children), yersinia (iron overload), TB, salmonella (sickle cell disease), *Borrelia burgdorferi* (Lyme disease)
Viral	Adenovirus, parvovirus, CMV, rubella, mumps, VZV, EBV
Fungal	Blastomycosis, coccidiomycosis, cryptococcus, *Histoplasma capsulatum*
Other	Mycoplasma, guinea worm

Clinical features

Joint	Hot, red, tender joint with markedly reduced range of movement
Child	Unwell, febrile, pseudoparesis of affected limb, very painful to move joint

NB. Osteomyelitis may have a sympathetic joint effusion, but tenderness is over the **bone**. Hip disease may present with referred pain to the knee.

Investigations

FBC	Neutrophils ↑
ESR, CRP	↑
Blood culture	
X-ray	Normal initially, helpful to eliminate trauma
Joint USS	Useful for hips
Bone scan	Hot spots in involved joint and periarticular area
Joint aspiration	M, C and S

Management

Antibiotics	Prolonged IV course (eg. flucloxacillin + third-generation cephalosporin)
Surgical	Athroscopic or arthrotomy joint washout (always necessary in hip disease)
Physiotherapy	Joint immobilisation initially, then mobilised to prevent deformity

Systemic lupus erythematosus (SLE)

A multisystem disease associated with serum antibodies against nuclear components. Females > males, usually >5 years.

Associations	HLA-B8, -DR2, -DR3
	African/Oriental > Caucasians

Clinical features

General (96%)	Malaise, weight loss, fever
Musculoskeletal	Arthralgia (80%), arthritis, aseptic necrosis hip and knee, myalgia, myositis
Skin (96%)	**Butterfly rash** (80%), papular, vesicular, purpuric, vasculitic lesions, Raynaud's phenomena, photosensitivity (33%), alopecia, oral ulcers **Discoid lupus:** Plaques and scarring, *skin only* involved, as a separate entity
Lungs (67%)	Effusions, pleurisy, fibrosis, pulmonary emboli rare
CNS (50%)	Depression, psychosis, CVA, cranial nerve palsies, ataxia, epilepsy, peripheral neuropathy, headache, transverse myelitis, blurred vision, chorea
Kidneys (80%)	Proteinuria, glomerulonephritis, BP ↑ (see p. 229)
Heart (40%)	Pericarditis, myocarditis, endocarditis (**Libman–Sachs endocarditis**), cardiomyopathy, aortic valve
Gastrointestinal	Hepatosplenomegaly, mesenteric arteritis, IBD
Blood (91%)	Platelets ↓, haemolytic anaemia, neutrophils ↓
Eyes (30%)	Cytoid bodies (retinal lesions), retinitis, episcleritis, iritis, Sjögren syndrome

Investigations

FBC	Anaemia (chronic disease or autoimmune), platelets ↓, WCC ↓

Acute phase proteins	ESR ↑ (with disease activity)
Autoantibodies	**dsDNA** (50%), anti–Sm (20%) **specific for SLE**
	ANA (positive)
	Anticardiolipin (antiphospholipid), lupus anticoagulant
	RhF (positive in 50%)
Immunology	Complement (↓ in active disease), IgG and IgM (↑)
Histology	Haematoxylin bodies (amorphous extracellular material staining with haematoxylin), vasculitis, granulomas. Immune complex, immunoglobulin and complement deposition

Management

- *NSAIDs (mild disease)*
- *Hydroxychloroquine, topical steroids (skin and discoid lupus)*
- *Steroids (IV or oral)*
- *Immunosuppressives (eg. cyclophosphamide, azathioprine)*

NEONATAL LUPUS

Usually occurs in infants of mothers with Ro/SSA ± SSB(La) antibodies (SLE or Sjögren syndrome), and is acquired transplacentally.

Clinical features
This presents with different combinations of clinical features.

1. *Congenital heart block*
2. *Neonatal lupus rash*
3. *Haematological abnormalities (Hb ↓, platelets ↓, WCC ↓)*

Investigations

Autoantibodies	ANA, anti-SSA (Ro), anti-platelet, Coombs' positive
FBC	Platelets ↓, Hb ↓, WCC ↓
ECG	Complete heart block

Management
Skin and blood features are transient
Cardiac disease permanent (see p. 115)

Antiphospholipid syndrome

A syndrome characterised by antiphospholipid antibodies which are involved in thrombosis. May be associated with SLE (hence the antibody is also known as lupus anticoagulant).

Clinical features

Thrombosis   Arterial and venous, strokes, Budd–Chiari syndrome

CNS disease   Epilepsy, migraine, strokes

Skin   **Livedo reticularis**, thrombophlebitis, splinter haemorrhages, fingertip ulcers

Other   Valvular heart disease, recurrent spontaneous abortions

Investigations

Coagulation   APTT prolonged and **does not correct** with added serum *in vitro*

Management

Anticoagulation   Aspirin if antibody positive, warfarin if serious thrombotic event

Treatment of SLE

Idiopathic inflammatory myopathies

These include:

- *dermatomyositis (commonest)*
- *polymyositis (no skin involvement)*
- *other myositis* – *infectious eg. cryptococcus*
  - *– postinfectious eg. influenza A, streptococcus*
  - *– inclusion body*
  - *– focal*

JUVENILE ONSET DERMATOMYOSITIS

A multisystem disease involving inflammation of striated muscle and cutaneous lesions.

Associations   HLA-B8, -DR3, DQA1*0501

    Female > male

Clinical features

Muscle   Muscle pain, proximal muscle weakness, dysphagia, dysphonia, palatal regurgitation, respiratory muscle weakness

    Gower sign, waddling gait

Skin   Classic **heliotrope violaceous rash** over eyelids (**pathognomonic**), occlusive vasculitis

    Nail fold dilated capillaries, **Gottron's papules** (red) on DIP, PIP joints and knees, butterfly rash, rash of photosensitive distribution

    Extensor surface skin atrophic and hyperpigmented

    Subcutaneous calcium deposits (20–50%) which may extrude

Joints   Arthralgia, arthritis with contractures

Gastrointestinal   Vasculopathy (ulcerations, bleeding)

Cardiac   Myocarditis (arrhythmias)

Other   Nephritis, CNS involvement, hepatosplenomegaly, interstitial lung disease, pulmonary haemorrhage, retinitis

Investigations

Muscle enzymes	CK ↑, LDH ↑, AST ↑, ALT ↑
Autoantibodies	ANA may be positive, RhF usually negative, more specific antibodies now being defined
EMG	Myopathic
Muscle biopsy	Vasculopathy and consequent muscle fibre necrosis

Management

1. *Physiotherapy and splinting*
2. *Systemic steroids (IV and oral)*
3. *Immunosuppressives (eg. cyclosporin, methotrexate)*
4. *Other eg. IV immunoglobulins, plasmapheresis*

Prognosis

Untreated, the mortality is up to 40%, otherwise 2–5%. 30–40% will remain disabled.

Scleroderma

This is a multisystem disease involving a disturbance of connective tissue, with occlusive vasculitis and fibrosis. It may be localised or diffuse (systemic sclerosis).

Associations Females > males

LOCALISED SCLERODERMA

Clinical features

Skin Discrete plaques (**morphoea**) or linear lesions following **Blashko's lines** (linear scleroderma). Initially erythematous, becoming atrophic and shiny with elevated violaceous borders. Development of hyper/hypopigmentation of lesions. Scarring and fibrosis beneath affected skin may lead to severe contractures and limb shortening
en Coup de Sabre (lesion of half of forehead) may involve underlying vasculitis in the brain and uveitis

Other Tendon nodules, joint stiffness, arthritis

The natural history is usually for the disease to 'burn out' after a number of years.

Adenocarcinoma , Carcinoid tumours .

SYSTEMIC SCLEROSIS

Rare in children, systemic manifestations cause significant morbidity and mortality.

Clinical features

Hands	Raynaud's phenomenon, digital ulcers, sclerodactyly (sausage fingers)
Skin	Diffuse thickening and tightening, beak nose, small mouth, telangiectasia

Musculoskeletal	Synovitis, tenosynovitis, myopathy
Gastrointestinal	Dysphagia (oesophageal involvement), malabsorption
Lungs	Fibrosis, pulmonary hypertension
Cardiac	Pericarditis, cardiac failure
Renal	Obliterative endarteritis, hypertension, chronic renal failure

Adenocarcinoma

Investigations

ESR	Normal
Autoantibodies	ANA (positive), RhF (may be positive), Scl70 (positive in systemic form)
Skin biopsy	Typical features of morphoea
Muscle biopsy	Perivascular infiltration and fibre necrosis may be present

Management

1. *Physiotherapy*
2. *Localised disease – topical and systemic steroids*
3. *Systemic disease – cold protection, systemic steroids, immunosuppressants*

Mixed connective tissue disease (MCTD)

One of the **overlap syndromes**. This may not be a distinct entity and includes features of SLE, rheumatoid arthritis, dermatomyositis and scleroderma. Mostly girls over six are affected. High titres of anti-RNP (ribonucleoprotein) autoantibodies and speckled ANA.

Prognosis is variable; renal involvement may occur and it may progress to classic SLE or scleroderma.

Sjögren syndrome

Very rare in children, this disease involves:

- *dry eyes (keratoconjunctivitis sicca)*
- *dry mouth (xerostomia)*

Dryness of the vagina and skin may also occur. Mothers who are Anti-Ro positive may have infants with congenital heart block.

Associations	HLA-B8, –DR3
	Connective tissue disease (eg. SLE, vasculitis, Raynaud's phenomenon)
	Autoimmune disease (eg. thyroid disease, chronic active hepatitis)
	Renal tubule defects (eg. nephrogenic DI, renal tubular acidosis)

Clinical features

Eyes	Photophobia, burning eyes
Glands	Parotid and salivary gland enlargement
Mouth	Decreased taste, dysphagia, angular cheilitis, fissured tongue
Nose	Decreased sense of smell, epistaxis

Respiratory   Bronchitis, otitis, hoarseness
Malignancy   Lymphoma risk

Investigations

Autoantibodies   Anti-Ro (SSA) (70%), anti-La (SSB)
                    ANA (positive 70%)
Schirmer test   Filter paper placed inside eyelid. Wetting of <10 mm in five minutes
                   indicates decreased tear production
Biopsy   Lip or salivary gland (focal lymphocytic infiltration)

Management

Symptomatic (artificial tears, and lozenges)
Systemic steroids or immunosuppression may be needed

Ehlers–Danlos syndromes

A group of connective tissue disorders of different genetic origin, involving deficiencies of collagen.

Clinical features

Normal at birth
Skin   Hyperelasticity, fragility, easy bruising, atrophic 'cigarette paper scars'
Joints   Hypermobile, tendency to dislocate

There are several different types (10 at present), each possessing specific clinical features which include:

- *premature birth (with PROM)*
- *mitral valve prolapse, dissecting aortic aneurysm*
- *bowel rupture, uterine rupture*

Mutations have been found in collagen III and other genes.

Vasculitis

CLASSIFICATION OF VASCULITIS

Polyarteritis   Macroscopic, eg. PAN
                   Microscopic

Kawasaki disease
Granulomatous vasculitis   Churg Strauss syndrome, Wegener granulomatosis
Leucocytocytoclastic vasculitis   Henoch-Schönlein purpura (HSP) (see p. 228)
                                     Hypersensitivity arteritis
Cutaneous polyarteritis   Post-streptococcal angitis
Secondary to connective tissue disease   SLE, dermatomyositis, scleroderma, juvenile
                                            chronic arthritis, MCTD

Giant cell arteritis	Takayasau disease
Miscellaneous vasculitides	Behçet's, familial Mediterranean fever

(Ref: MJ Dillon, 5:11:8, p. 1402, Oxford textbook of Rheumatology, 2nd edition, PJ Maddison, DA Senberg, P Woo, DA Glass, 1998.)

KAWASAKI DISEASE (MUCOCUTANEOUS LYMPH NODE SYNDROME)

An infantile polyarteritis involving the following diagnostic criteria.

- *Fever >38.5°C for >5 days and four of:*
    1. *Bilateral non-purulent conjunctivitis*
    2. *Oral mucosal changes – 'strawberry tongue', erythema, cracked lips*
    3. *Cervical lymphadenopathy with one node >1.5 cm*
    4. *Extremities (feet and hands) – erythematous, swollen or peeling of palms and soles*
    5. *Rash – polymorphous, no vesicles or crusts*

- *Other features*
    Extremely irritable
    Profuse watery diarrhoea
    Cough, coryzal symptoms

Cardiac complications

1. *20% of untreated children will develop* **coronary artery aneurysms**, *a major cause of morbidity*
2. *Cardiac tamponade*
3. *Cardiac failure*
4. *Myocarditis, myocardial infarction*
5. *Pericarditis*

Investigations

FBC	Marked thrombocythaemia (2nd–3rd week)
	Anaemia, WCC ↑

Acute phase proteins	ESR, CRP ↑
Cardiac	ECG, CXR, two-dimensional echocardiogram

Management

1. *High dose IVIG (2 mg/kg) over 12 hours, within 10 days of disease*
2. *Aspirin for six weeks or until coronary aneurysms gone*
3. *Two-dimensional echocardiogram at presentation and follow-up*

POLYARTERITIS NODOSA (PAN)

A necrotising vasculitis of medium and small arteries. Males > females, uncommon in children.

Clinical features

General	Malaise, fever, weight loss, myalgia
Joints	Migratory arthralgia, arthritis
Renal	Chronic renal failure, hypertension, (major cause of death)
Neurological	Mononeuritis multiplex, seizures, stroke
Cardiac	Aneurysms, myocardial infarction, cardiac failure
Lungs	Microinfarcts, alveolar haemorrhages
Abdominal	Splenic and coeliac vessels affected causing liver pain
Skin	Nodules, ulcer, rashes

Investigations

FBC	Anaemia, WCC $\uparrow$
ESR	$\uparrow$
Autoantibodies	p-ANCA (may be positive)
Biopsy	Tissue may show characteristic features
Angiography	Mesenteric or renal microaneurysms

Management
Steroids and imunosuppressants

TAKAYASAU DISEASE

An arteritis of the aorta and major branches ('pulseless disease'), this is probably an autoimmune disease. Most common in young women. Poor prognosis in children.

Associations	Orientals, blacks

Clinical features

CVS	Claudication in arms and legs, absent peripheral pulses, BP $\uparrow$
General	Fever, malaise, myalgia

Investigations

ESR	$\uparrow$
FBC	Anaemia, neutrophilia
Doppler and angiography	(occlusion, stenosis and aneurysms)

Management

- *Systemic steroids and cytotoxic agents may be considered*
- *Surgery as necessary*

CHURG–STRAUSS SYNDROME

Rare in childhood. A necrotising vasculitis of small vessels associated with eosinophilia, extravasculer granulomas on biopsy, and asthma. Peak age 30–40 years.

Clinical features

Respiratory	Asthma, transient pulmonary infiltrates, paranasal sinus pain
Skin	Subcutaneous nodules, purpura
Peripheral nerves	Neuropathy (mono- or polyneuropathy)
Kidneys	Chronic renal failure

Investigations

Autoantibodies	p-ANCA or c-ANCA
CXR	Transient shadows

Management

Steroids. Cytotoxics (eg. cyclophasphamicle) may be needed.

WEGENER GRANULOMATOSIS

A systemic necrotising vasculitis affecting mainly the respiratory tract with granulomas and glomerulonephritis. Usual age of onset 25–30 years.

Clinical features

Upper respiratory tract	Rhinorrhoea, nasal ulceration, granulomas
Lungs	Cough, pleurisy, haemoptysis, granulomas
Kidneys	Proliferative glomerulonephritis
Other	Malaise, fever, weight loss, arthritis, arthralgia, splenomegaly, rash

Investigations

Autoantibodies	c-ANCA (90%)
CXR	Pulmonary infiltrates
Renal function	Microhaematuria, red cell casts
Biopsy	Granulomatous inflammation (wall of arteriole or artery)

Management

Steroids and cyclophosphamide.

BEHÇET SYNDROME

Very rare in children.

Associations Turkish, Arabic

A vasculitis of small and medium-sized vessels involving:

1. *Oral ulcers*
2. *Genital ulcers*
3. *Eye inflammation (anterior or posterior uveitis, retinal vasculitis may lead to blindness)*

Associated features include:

Skin	Erythema nodosum, erythema multiforme, pustules, acne, ulcers on mucous membranes (with scarring in neonates only)
Joints	Arthritis (asymmetrical, recurrent, knees, wrists, ankles)
Vascular	DVT, arterial aneurysms, pericarditis
CNS	Cranial nerve palsies, psychosis, meningoencephalitis
Other	Fevers, colitis

Diagnosis
Clinical only.

Management
Immunosuppressive therapy (eg. steroids, methotrexate, chlorambucil)

Amyloidosis

This is characterised by deposition of amyloid in the extracellular matrix around blood vessels and in parenchymal organs. It may be primary or secondary.

Type	Amyloid characteristics	Associated disease	Clinical features
Primary	AL (homologous with immunoglobulin K or L light chains)	Myeloma Macroglobulinaemia	Arthritis, macroglossia, carpal tunnel syndrome, neuropathy, cardiac failure, malabsorption, gastrointestinal bleeding
Secondary	AA (unique protein)	Systemic JCA Familial mediterranean fever Inflammatory bowel disease	Nephrotic syndrome Diarrhoea Hepatosplenomegaly Anaemia Hypergammaglobulinaemia

Diagnosis
Biopsy Staining with Congo red dye, green under polarising light

Treatment
Treat underlying disorder; alkylating agents (eg. chlorambucil) may be used in secondary amyloid.

Osteogenesis imperfecta

A syndrome of fragile bones due to a defect in the α-chain of type 1 collagen. The clinical features involve multiple fractures, with impairment of growth and premature death (severity depends on type).
Incidence: 1: 20 000–1: 50 000 live births.

Type	Inheritance	Sclera	Deafness	Other features
I	AD	Blue	Common	Common type Reach adult life
II	AR, sporadic	Blue	None	Lethal *in utero* or neonatal period
III	AR, sporadic	Variable	Uncommon	Severe disease, few reach adult life
IV	AD	Normal	Uncommon	Similar to type I

Clinical features (in general)

Skeletal	Bone fragility, multiple fractures, resulting deformity
	Joint hypermobility, kyphoscoliosis, soft teeth (dentinogenesis imperfecta)
ENT	Conductive deafness
CVS	Aortic regurgitation

Investigations

Blood   Alkaline phosphatase (N or ↑), acid phosphatase (↑)
Urine   24-hour hydroxyproline (↑)
X-rays   Wormian bones (skull), fractures, osteopenia, deformity

Management

Orthopaedic (fracture management and corrective surgery)

Blue sclera – differential diagnosis:

Marfan syndrome, Ehlers–Danlos syndrome, pseudoxanthoma elasticum

Osteopetrosis (marble bone disease)

A disease of increased skeletal density and brittle bones. There are several forms; the type presenting in the newborn period with early death, **osteopetrosis with precocious manifestations**, an autosomal recessive condition, is described.

Clinical features

General	Failure to thrive
Marrow failure	Anaemia, thrombocytopenia, infections, hepatosplenomegaly
Hyperostosis	Optic atrophy, blindness, deafness, cranial nerve palsies, hydrocephalus

Investigations

Blood   Ca ↓, PO$_4$ ↓, alkaline phosphatase ↑
          Hb ↓, platelets ↓, WCC ↓
X-rays Bone density ↑
          'Bone in bone' appearance of vertebral bodies
          Clubbed metaphyses, 'rugby jersey' pattern of spine
          Osteosclerosis

Management

- *Low-calcium diet, phosphate supplements*
- *Drugs – steroids, interferon-α*
- *BMT*
- *Neurosurgery to the orbital roof*

Osteochondrodysplasias

ACHONDROPLASIA

A pure skeletal dysplasia. Incidence: 1: 15 000–27 000. New mutations (mostly), autosomal dominant.

Clinical features

Proportions	Short limbs and trunk, large head
Other skeletal	Exaggerated lumbar lordosis, genu varum, trident hands and brachydactyly, mid-facial hypoplasia, relative prognathism, narrow nasal airways
Neurological	Hydrocephalus (1–2%)
	Obstructive sleep apnoea
	Spinal canal stenosis
	Intelligence normal
	Hypotonia and delayed motor milestones
ENT	Serous otitis media

NB. These patients have their own growth charts devised. Lifespan is normal.

THANATOPHORIC DWARFISM

A 'lethal' dwarfism, though a few survive >1 year.

Clinical features

- *Similar proportions to achondroplasia (large head, small body)*
- *Severe thoracic dysplasia with respiratory distress*
- *Bow limbs, flat nasal bridge, brachydactyly*
- *X-rays – thin vertebral bodies, femoral head banana shaped, metaphyseal flaring and cupping*

ELLIS–VAN CREVELD SYNDROME

Autosomal recessive syndrome featuring:

- *skeletal dysplasia including mild thoracic involvement*
- *four limb postaxial polydactyly*
- *conical teeth, oligodontia, dysplastic nails*
- *CHD (40%)*

STICKLER'S DYSPLASIA

A group of autosomal dominant disorders with a defect in COL2A1 gene for type II collagen on chromosome 12q.

Clinical features

- *Marfanoid habitus, hyperextensible joints, enlargement of large joints*
- *Retinal detachment, myopia, deafness, cleft palate*
- *X-ray – 'Dumbbell'-shaped long bones*

SPONDYLOEPIPHYSEAL DYSPLASIAS

These diseases are characterised by disproportionate short stature (short trunk). They include three main forms.

Type	Inheritance	Clinical features
Congenita	AD COL2A1 gene (type II collagen) Chromosome 12	Cleft palate, hypertelorism, myopia, retinal detachment. Hip and shoulder epiphyseal dysplasia, short limbs, platyspondyly, pectus carinatum, talipes equinovarus
Pseudochondrodysplasia	AD, AR	Progressive scoliosis, normal head, long bone epiphyseal irregularities
Tarda	Variable	***Pseudorheumatoid*** subgroup involves progressive joint deformity, arthritis in some, short stature, platyspondyly, hip and back pain and stiffness

MULTIPLE EPIPHYSEAL DYSPLASIAS

These are similar to spondyloepiphyseal dysplasias, with mild spinal disease, short phalanges and fragmentation of the epiphyses of hips, knees and other joints.

Other musculoskeletal conditions

OSTEOCHONDRITIDES

Boys > girls. Usual age 3–12 years.

A group of disorders in which the primary or secondary ossification centre in the growing child undergoes aseptic necrosis with resorption of the dead bone and replacement by new osseous tissue. They are associated with trauma or avascular necrosis of the affected area.

LEGG–CALVE–PERTHES DISEASE

This is an osteochondrosis caused by avascular necrosis of the femoral head. Males 5: females 1, usually 4–8 years at presentation. 20% have bilateral disease.

Clinical features

1. *Intermittent pain in anterior thigh or knee (referred pain)*
2. *Painless limp*
3. *Decreased range of movement of the hip (internal rotation and abduction)*
4. *Leg length inequality*

Investigations

Hip X-rays	Increase in the medial joint space, fragmented, flattened femoral head, increased density of femoral head, subchondral fracture
MRI hip	This may show the above features earlier
Radionucleide scan	Reduced uptake in affected femoral head, later increased uptake with neovascularisation

Management

If <6 years	Conservative
If >6 years	1. Abduction exercises and bed rest
	2. Abduction casts and femoral osteotomy if necessary

Other osteochondritides

Disease	Osteochondrosis	Clinical features
Osgood–Schlatter disease	Tibial tubercle	Tenderness and swelling over the tibial tubercle
Kohler disease	Tarsal navicular	Foot pain and limp
Freiberg's infraction	Second metatarsal head	Pain on weight bearing, swelling at 2nd metatarsal head
Thiemann disease	Phalangeal epiphyses	Painless enlargement of the PIP joints
Irregularity of the epiphyses of the digits
Scheuermann disease	Midthoracic or lumbar	See below

KYPHOSIS

This may be postural, idiopathic or congenital.

Postural kyphosis
Caused by bad posture. Smooth back contour on examination. Child able to correct the deformity. X-rays normal.

Idiopathic kyphosis (Scheuermann disease)
A common disease presenting as kyphosis in adolescence. Child unable to correct the deformity. May have back pain.

X-rays:

1. *Narrow disc space*
2. *Loss of anterior height of the vertebrae, causing wedging in ≥3 vertebrae*
3. *Schmorl's nodes*
4. *Endplate irregularities*

Management

- *Conservative management usually*
- *Casting or surgical fusion*

Congenital kyphosis
Presentation in infancy. Due to vertebral malformations:

1. *vertebral body anomaly*
2. *failure of anterior segmentation of the spine*

SCOLIOSIS

This may be congenital, neuromuscular or compensatory.

Congenital   This presents in infants. Associated with renal abnormalities in 20% Due to vertebral malformations: 1. Vertebral body anomaly
2. Failure of segmentation

Neuromuscular   Scoliosis secondary to neuromuscular disease eg. muscular dystrophy

Compensatory   This is due to a compensation for differing *leg length* from any cause.

Management
Physiotherapy may help for neuromuscular disease. Surgical fusion used for congenital disease.

SLIPPED UPPER FEMORAL EPIPHYSIS (SUFE)

The epiphysis of the femoral head 'slips' off the neck, a disorder seen in adolescence.

Associations   Hypogonadism
              Hypothyroidism
              Pituitary disfunction

Growth hormone is thought to weaken the growth plate and thus it is weakest at puberty.

Clinical features

1. *Pain on hip movement (acute presentation)*
2. *Antalgic gait (limp), hip externally rotated (chronic presentation)*
3. *Referred knee pain only*

On examination, decreased internal rotation of the hip is present.

X-ray hip ('Frog-leg lateral view')

- *Widening of growth plate*
- *Femoral neck anteriorly rotated*

Management
Surgical pinning of the femoral head.

Complications

1. *Osteonecrosis*
2. *Chondrolysis (articular cartilage degeneration)*

GENU VARUM (BOW LEGS)
Causes:

- *Familial*
- *Rickets*
- *Idiopathic (Blount disease)*
- *Local damage – trauma, tumour, infection*
- *Skeletal dysplasia – achondroplasia, neurofibromatosis*

Blount disease
Idiopathic disorder resulting from abnormal growth of the proximal medial tibial epiphysis. Common in Africans.

If <4 years: females > males, 20% unilateral
If >4 years: males > females, 50% unilateral

Associations   Obesity

Clinical features

- *Leg length discrepancy*
- *Internal tibial torsion*

Investigations
X-ray legs – 'Beaking' of the medial metaphysis of the tibia.

Management
If <4 years: splinting or surgical treatment
If >4 years: surgical osteotomies

SYNDROMES INVOLVING ABSENT RADII

1. *Absent thumbs*
2. *Holt–Oram syndrome*
3. *Fanconi anaemia*
4. *VATER syndrome*
5. *TAR syndrome (thrombocytopenia with absent radii), 100% have cows milk protein sensitivity*

Treatment options include splinting and surgery.

FURTHER READING

Cassidy JT, Petty RE *Textbook of Paediatric Rheumatology*, WB Saunders, Philadelphia, 1997
The Oxford textbook of rheumatology 2nd Ed. Maddison PJ, Senberg DA, Woo P, Glass DN Eds. Oxford University Press, Oxford, 1998

13

Neurological and neuromuscular disorders

- *Physiology and anatomy*
- *Investigations*
- *Development*
- *Structural brain anomalies*
- *Epilepsy*
- *Headaches*
- *Neuroectodermal syndromes*

- *Ataxia*
- *Cerebral palsy*
- *Neurodegenerative disorders*
- *Stroke*
- *Spinal cord disorders*
- *Neuromuscular disorders*
- *Autism*

Physiology and anatomy

The nervous system can be divided into:

1. *central nervous system (CNS) – brain and spinal cord*
2. *peripheral nervous system (PNS) – somatic and autonomic nervous systems conveying information into* (afferent, sensory) *and away from* (efferent, motor) *the CNS*

For a detailed review, anatomy and physiology texts must be consulted.

BRAIN

Some major areas of function within the cerebral cortex are shown in Figure 13.1 and the ventricular system is outlined in Figure 13.2.

The internal carotids and the basilar artery supply the circle of Willis, from which the three cerebral arteries (anterior, middle and posterior) branch. The vertebrobasilar system supplies the cerebellum and brainstem and the cerebral arteries supply the cerebrum (see Figure 13.3).

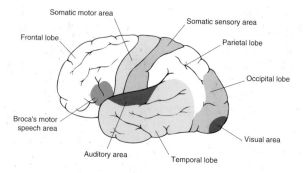

Figure 13.1 Major functional areas of the cortex

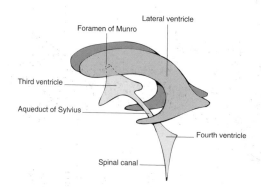

Figure 13.2 The ventricular system

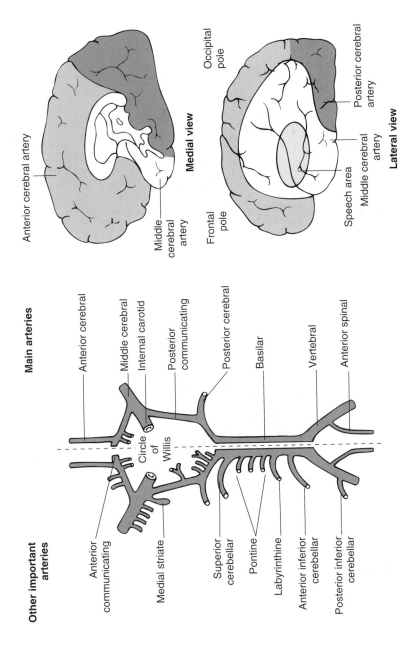

Figure 13.3 Blood supply to the brain

CRANIAL NERVES

For detailed outline see an anatomy text.

Number	Name	Motor component	Sensory component
I	Olfactory	None	Smell
II	Optic	None	Vision
III	Oculomotor	Eye movements (all EOM except lateral rectus and superior oblique)	None
IV	Trochlear	Superior oblique muscle (intorsion)	None
V	Trigeminal	Masseter muscles	Facial, buccal mucosa and anterior 2/3rds tongue via: V1 (ophthalmic branch) V2 (maxillary branch) V3 (mandibular branch)
VI	Abducens	Lateral rectus muscle (outward lateral gaze)	None
VII	Facial	Facial muscles Stapedius muscle Secretomotor to submandibular, sublingual and lacrimal glands	Taste (anterior 2/3rds tongue via chorda tympani)
VIII	Vestibulocochlear	None	Hearing (cochlear nerve) Balance (vestibular nerve)
IX	Glossopharyngeal	Tongue (stylopharyngeus) Secretomotor to parotid gland	Taste (posterior 1/3rd) Gag afferents Sensation from tonsils, pharynx, posterior 1/3rd tongue
X	Vagus	Gag efferent Larynx, bronchial muscles, alimentary tract, epiglottis Secretomotor to alimentary tract, bronchial muscle glands	Dura, external auditory meatus Respiratory tract, alimentary tract, heart
XI	Accessory	Sternomastoid, trapezius	None
XII	Hypoglossal	Tongue muscles	None

MOTOR AND SENSORY SYSTEMS

Motor system

Corticospinal tracts (pyramidal system)
These originate in the cortex (layer V) and terminate on the: motor nuclei (cranial nerves) or anterior horn cells (spinal cord).

The nerve fibres *decussate* (cross over) in the medulla.

Disease of the pyramidal system causes an upper motor neuron (UMN) lesion and disease of the anterior horn cells and peripheral nervous system results in a lower motor neuron (LMN) lesion.

Extrapyramidal system
Basal ganglia, involved in movement. Lesions result in a reduction in movement, involuntary movements and rigidity.

Cerebellum
Involved in posture and balance, lesions producing classic cerebellar signs.

Peripheral nerves run from the anterior horn cell via α motor nerve fibres to the motor endplate (the *LMN pathway*).

UMN lesion	Sign	LMN lesion
↑ (spastic)	Tone	↓ (hypotonia)
Weakness	Strength	Weakness
No wasting	Muscles	Wasting, fasciculation
↑	Reflexes	↓
Upgoing	Plantar response	Downgoing/equivocal

Reflexes	Level
Supinator	C5–6
Biceps	C5–6
Triceps	C7
Knee	L3–4
Ankle	S1

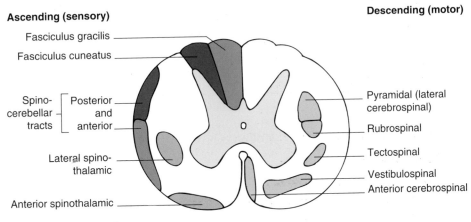

Ascending (sensory)   **Descending (motor)**

Fasciculus gracilis
Fasciculus cuneatus

Spino- [Posterior   Pyramidal (lateral
cerebellar and   cerebrospinal)
tracts [anterior   Rubrospinal

Lateral spino-   Tectospinal
thalamic   Vestibulospinal
                                                      Anterior cerebrospinal
Anterior spinothalamic

Figure 13.4 Motor and sensory tracts

Clinical signs of cerebellar disease
Gait   Ataxic, broad based. Patient falls to the side of the lesion
Movements   Dysmetria (imprecise movements in force and distance)
            Dysdiadokinesis, past-pointing on finger–nose testing

Tremor	Intention tremor
	Titubation (head tremor)
Nystagmus	Towards the affected side
	Coarse, horizontal
Speech	Dysarthria, 'scanning' speech
Reflexes	Pendular

Lesions within a lateral lobe produce symptoms in the same side of the body. Midline lesions produce truncal ataxia.

Sensory system

Peripheral nerves run from free or specialised nerve endings to the dorsal root ganglia and along the spinal cord (see Figure 13.4) via:

- *posterior columns (vibration, proprioception, light touch). Decussate in the medulla*
- *spinothalamic tracts (crude touch, temperature, pain). Cross in the cord at entry*

RAISED INTRACRANIAL PRESSURE

This may be an acute emergency or a chronic disorder.

Causes

Benign intracranial hypertension (BIH)	
CSF disorder	Hydrocephalus
Trauma	Cerebral oedema, intracranial haemorrhage
Intracranial mass	Tumour, haematoma, cysts, abscess
Infection	Meningitis, encephalitis
Other	Bleeding from AV malformation or aneurysm
	CVA with oedema
	Hepatic encephalopathy
	Malignant hypertension

Acute ↑ ICP

Vital signs	Cushing reflex (BP ↑ and pulse ↓ due to medullary ischaemia), pupillary dilatation
False localising signs	III and VI cranial nerve lesions
Coning	(Herniation of brain contents) Bradycardia, hypertension, respiratory depression, bilateral pupillary dilatation, decerebrate posturing, death

Emergency management

1. *Mannitol (0.25 g/kg over 30 min on 2 or 3 occasions)*
2. *Hyperventilation – aim for pCO$_2$ 25–35 mmHg (causes cerebral vasoconstriction)*
3. *Minimise cerebral metabolism – sedation, analgesia, muscle paralysis, antipyretics, moderate hypothermia (35°C), anticonvulsants (if seizures suspected)*
4. *Treat cause – eg. steroids for cerebral oedema, surgery for acute bleed*

Chronic ↑ ICP

- *Headache (early morning, frontal or vertex, worse on lying down and with coughing and crying)*
- *Drowsiness, diplopia, vomiting*
- *Papilloedema*
- *Infant – bulging fontanelle, macrocephaly, failure to thrive*

Management

Drugs   Acetazolamide
        Steroids (may make BIH worse)

Surgery Ventriculoperitoneal shunts

Treat underlying cause.

Benign intracranial hypertension (BIH)

This is a condition of raised intracranial pressure in the absence of an obstruction to CSF flow.

Associations   Obese pubertal girls
               Steroid withdrawal, oral contraceptive pill, isotretinoin, tetracycline, head injury
               Calcium (↑ or ↓)

Clinical features

Those of chronic ↑ ICP.

- *Diplopia*
- *Marked papilloedema*
- *Infarction of the optic nerve may occur with subsequent blindness*

Investigations

- *Lumbar puncture – diagnostic (v. high pressure)*
- *CT brain – normal*

Management

- *Lumbar puncture*
- *Thiazide diuretics, dexamethasone (if prolonged ICP ↑)*
- *Surgical shunting may be necessary*
- *Weight loss*

PAPILLOEDEMA

This is swelling of the papilla (optic disc).

Causes

Intracranial   Space-occupying lesion
                    Chronic cerebral oedema

Subarachnoid haemorrhage

Benign intracranial hypertension

Metabolic $CO_2 \uparrow, O_2 \downarrow, Ca^{2+} \uparrow$ (long-standing)

Accelerated hypertension

Optic Ischaemic optic neuropathy

Infiltration (eg. leukaemia)

Retinal vein obstruction

Clinical features

Symptoms Blurred vision and enlarged blind spot (later in disease)

Disc Blurring, erythema, heaping up of the margins

Retina Loss of retinal vein pulsation and dilatation, obliteration of physiological cup and retinal haemorrhages

OPTIC ATROPHY

This is visible as disc pallor. Causes include:

Optic nerve compression eg. tumour, aneurysm

Ischaemia eg. severe anaemia, arteritis

Optic and retrobulbar neuritis eg. multiple sclerosis

Deficiency eg. vitamin B_{12}.

DIDMOAD

Hereditary optic neuropathy

Infection eg. orbital cellulitis, sinusitis, syphilis

Toxic neuropathy eg. methyl alcohol, quinine, tobacco

Causes of papilloedema

CAUSES OF CATARACT

Familial Aut. Dominant (usually) autosomal recessive

Congenital infection *Any* infection eg. Rubella, CMV, toxoplasmosis

Drugs Corticosteroids

Metabolic Hypocalcaemia

Galactosaemia 'oil droplet' cataract

Diabetic mother, diabetic child (uncommon, snowflake cataracts)

Lowe syndrome, chrondrodysplasia punctata

Chromosomal Down syndrome, Turner syndrome, Trisomy 13, Trisomy 18

Idiopathic

CAUSES OF REDUCED CONSCIOUSNESS AND COMA

Consciousness Is awareness of oneself and surroundings in a state of wakefulness

Coma Is a state of unrousable unresponsiveness

Causes

Diffuse brain dysfunction   Infection, eg. meningoencephalitis, sepsis
                               Epilepsy (after generalised seizure)
                               Traumatic brain injury (accidental or abuse)
                               Toxins, drugs, eg. CO, lead, salicylates, alcohol, glue
                               Metabolic imbalance, eg. glucose, calcium, sodium ($\uparrow$ or $\downarrow$)
                               Inborn error of metabolism
                               Hypothermia
                               Systemic organ failure eg. liver failure, Reye syndrome
                               Hypoxic ischaemic brain injury
                               Subarachnoid haemorrhage
                               Hypertensive encephalopathy
Brainstem dysfunction   Infarction, neoplasm, trauma, coning

Investigations

ELECTROMYOGRAPHY (EMG) AND PERIPHERAL NERVE CONDUCTION

EMG

A needle electrode is inserted into voluntary muscle and an amplified recording is made.

Changes seen   Myopathic, myotonic, myaesthaenic, denervation, reinnervation

Peripheral nerve conduction

Measurements are taken of conduction velocity, distal motor latency, sensory and muscle action potentials.

ELECTROENCEPHALOGRAM (EEG)

Notes on EEG interpretation

1. *Obvious pattern present, eg. hypsarrythmia, 3 per second spike and wave*
2. *No obvious pattern, check:*
   - *Scale (amplitude)*
   - *Montage (map)*
   - *Time marker*
   - *Individual traces. Look for a feature that stands out:*
     Nature of the feature eg. spikes, slow waves
     Whether it is generalised (in all channels)
     Or focal (in certain channels only)

Some basic EEG patterns
1. **Absence seizures**. 3 per second spike and wave activity

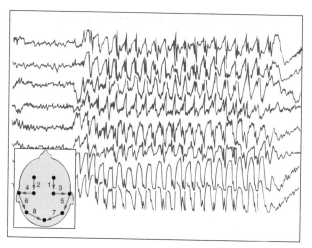

Figure 13.5a Absence seizures

2. **Myoclonic epilepsy**. Bursts of generalised spikes and slow waves

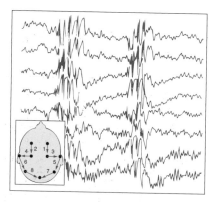

Figure 13.5b Myoclonic epilepsy

3. Focal activity left temporal area (eg. caused by a left temporal infarct). High-amplitude slow activity over the left temporal and posterior temporal areas

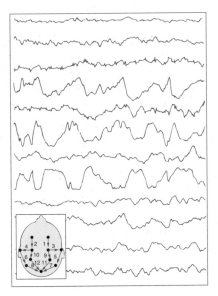

Figure 13.5c Focal activity in left temporal area

4. **Hypsarrhythmia**. A mixture of high-amplitude irregular slow activity and some discharges, following no pattern

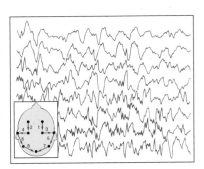

Figure 13.5d Hypsarrhythmia

5. **Acute encephalopathy**. Typical pattern of irregular slow activity caused by encephalopathy of any cause

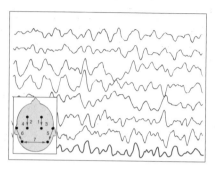

Figure 13.5e Acute encephalopathy

6. **Burst suppression pattern**. Isoelectric EEG with bursts of spikes and other activity. These findings indicate a hopeless prognosis for recovery in a child.

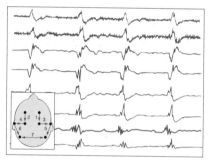

Figure 13.5f Burst suppression pattern

Development

AREAS OF CHILD DEVELOPMENT

- *Gross motor*
- *Fine motor*
- *Language and hearing*
- *Social skills*
- *Vision*

KEY DEVELOPMENTAL MILESTONES

Age	Fine motor	Gross motor	Language	Social
3 months	Fixes and follows Smiles (from 6 weeks) Opens hand	Pushes up with arms Head control	Cries, laughs May babble	Smiles
6 months	Palmar grasp, reaches, transfers	Sits unsupported	Babbles	Solid food in mouth
9 months	Pincer grasp (9–10 months)	Sits well Pulls to stand	Daddy (non-specifically)	Stranger awareness
1 year	Pincer grasp Releases object	Walks or shuffles	Mummy, daddy (specific)	Waves bye-bye Cup drinking
18 months	Scribbles 3-cube tower	Walks upstairs	>5 words	Mimics
2 years	Circular scribbles 6-cube tower	Kicks, runs	2-word sentences	Uses spoon Undresses Symbolic play
3 years	Draws circle Bridge 3 cubes	Jumps	Says first name Colours	Dresses Has friend
4 years	Draws cross	Stands on one leg Hops	Good speech Says surname	Does buttons
5 years	Draws triangle	Bicycle	Good speech	Shoe laces

Hand dominance appears at 18–24 months and development under one year may indicate brain damage.

REFLEXES

Primitive reflexes

These are all present from birth and persistence for longer than usual is seen in cerebral palsy.

Reflex	Disappears	
Palmar grasp	3–4 months	
Plantar grasp	12–18 months	
Stepping reflex	2 months	When held and 'walked' with the feet touching the ground, the feet move in a stepping sequence
Moro reflex	4–5 months	Sudden neck extension causes extension, abduction and adduction of upper extremities and flexion of fingers, wrists and elbows
Asymmetric tonic neck reflex	6 months	In a supine infant, turning the head laterally causes extension of the arm and leg on the side to the turn and flexion of both on the side away from the turn (the fencer position)

Postural responses

Reflex	Appears	Disappears	
Forward parachute	5–6 months	Stays for life	When held prone by the waist and lowered, the arms and legs extend
Landau reflex	3–6 months	1 year	When held prone, the legs, spine and head extend
Lateral propping reflex	7 months	Stays for life	When sitting and pushed sideways, the arms extend to prevent a fall

The *Babinsky reflex* is upgoing initially and downgoing from around one year.

VISION

Visual acuity tests

Normal vision   6/6
Partially sighted   4/60–6/24
Registered blind   3/60
Infants   3/60 vision at three months, achieving adult levels at approximately 2–3 years

Age	Test
Birth	Face fixation, preference for patterned objects
6 weeks	Fixes and follows a face through 90° (not to the midline until 3 months) 90 cm away
	Optokinetic nystagmus on looking at a moving, striped target
3 months	Fixes and follows through 180° 90 cm away
6 months	Reaches for toys
10 months	Picks up a raisin
1 year	Picks up hundreds and thousands
2 years	Identifies pictures of reducing size
3 years	Letter matching using single letter charts eg. Sheridan Gardiner, Stycar
5 years	Identifies letters on Snellen chart by name or matching letters.

STRABISMUS (SQUINT)

A common condition due to misalignment of the visual axes. A squint present after 2–3 months of age should be referred to an ophthalmologist as binocular vision should be developing by this time.

Squints may be:

- *non-paralytic (concomitant) or paralytic*
- *convergent (esotropia), divergent (exotropia) or vertical*
- *constant (manifest), intermittent (latent), or alternating*

Concomitant (non-paralytic, common)

Convergent   (most common concomitant type) eg. infantile strabismus – few months of age, surgery often required

Accommodative strabismus – 2–4 years in hypermetropic children

Divergent   eg. intermittent childhood divergent squint – 2–5 years temporary squint with fatigue

Paralytic (rare)

- *Divergent eg. IIIrd nerve palsy*
- *Convergent eg. VIth nerve palsy*
- *Vertical eg. IVth nerve palsy (head tilt occurs)*

Tests for squint

Corneal light reflection test   Pen torch shone to produce reflections in both cornea. If the reflection is in different places in each cornea, a squint is present

Eye movements   Detect a paralytic squint

Cover test   Eyes covered individually with a card using a toy for fixation. If the fixing eye is covered, the squint eye moves to take up fixation.

On removal of the cover, the eyes move again as the normal fixing eye takes up fixation (manifest). Used to detect a latent squint where the eye squints when covered. An alternating squint is where each eye moves in turn when covered.

HEARING TESTS

Mild hearing loss   25–35 dB
Moderate hearing loss 40–60 dB
Severe hearing loss   60–90 dB
Profound hearing loss >90 dB

Age	Objective test
Birth	Otoaccoustic emission (OAE) Brainstem-evoked potential
9–24 months	Distraction testing/behavioural audiometry
15 months–2 years	Cooperative testing (whisper instructions with hand covering mouth)
2 years–3 years	Performance testing (condition eg. balls into a bucket), (play audiometry)
2 years–4 years	Speech discrimination tests (similar words eg. man, lamb)
>3 years	Pure tone audiometry

Criteria for performing OAEs

- *Family history of deafness*
- *Craniofacial malformations*
- *Birth weight <1500 g*
- *Neonatal meningitis*
- *Severe perinatal asphyxia*
- *Potentially toxic levels of ototoxic drugs*

- *Neonatal jaundice requiring exchange transfusion*
- *Congenital infection (eg. rubella, CMV, toxoplasmosis)*
- *Parental concern at six-week check*

Audiograms

Hearing loss may be conductive (common in children) or sensorineural (uncommon).

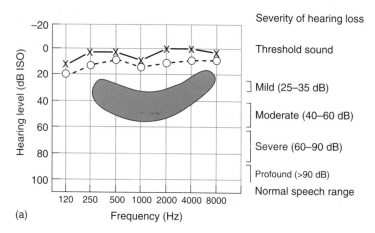

(a) Frequency (Hz)

Figure 13.6 Audiograms. (a) Normal hearing + speech range. (Continued on page 367)

Structural brain anomalies

CRANIOSYNOSTOSES

This is premature closure of the cranial suture.

People with craniosynostosis are at increased risk of:

- *hydrocephalus, ↑ ICP, papilloedema, optic atrophy*
- *deviated nasal septum, choanal atresia, speech disorders and deafness. Craniofacial surgery may be necessary*

Some craniosynostoses have been found to have mutations in the FGFR2 (fibroblast growth factor receptor 2) gene eg. Apert's, Crouzons.

Abnormal head shapes (see Figure 13.7)

Brachycephaly	Flat occiput, eg. Down syndrome
Scaphocephaly (dolichocephaly)	Long, narrow, eg. premature babies, Hurler syndrome
Turricephaly	Tall head
Trigonocephaly	Keel-shaped forehead, hypotelorism
Kleeblattschädel deformity	Cloverleaf shape
Plagiocephaly	Asymmetrical, parallelogram (as if skull pushed one side and pulled the other)

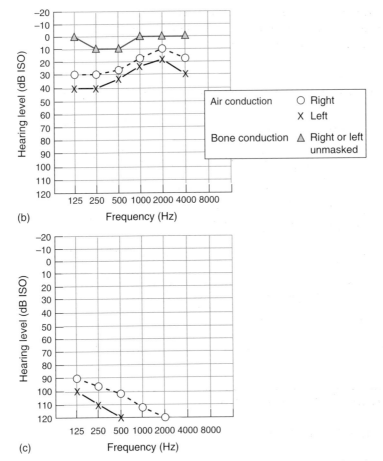

Figure 13.6 (continued) Audiograms. (b) Bilateral conductive hearing loss. (c) Bilateral profound sensorineural hearing loss

Syndrome	Inheritance	Features
Crouzon	AD	Usually causes brachycephaly from coronal suture closure Proptosis Hypertelorism, frontal bossing Small maxilla
Apert	Sporadic, AD	Multiple suture closure, results in asymmetrical head and face Syndactyly of 2nd, 3rd, 4th fingers and toes Mental retardation (66%) Progressive calcification and fusion of cervical spine, hands and foot bones
Carpenter	AR	Multiple sutures affected, brachycephaly, Kleeblattschädel skull Syndactyly and brachydactyly hands and feet Mental retardation CHD, genu valgum, coxa valga, preaxial polydactyly of feet

Chotzen	AD	Asymmetrical fusions, plagiocephaly
		Ptosis, hypertelorism
		Brachydactyly
		Syndactyly 2nd and 3rd fingers
Pfieffer	Sporadic, AD	Turricephaly, brachycephaly
		Prominent eyes, hypertelorism
		Short, broad thumbs
		Syndactyly

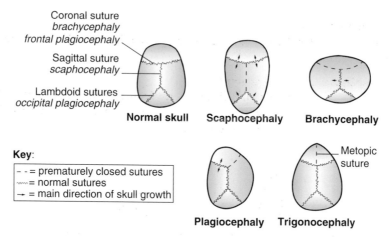

Figure 13.7 Cranial sutures and abnormal head shapes

FONTANELLE CLOSURE

Normally the anterior fontanelle closes between nine and 18 months, and the posterior at 6–8 weeks.

Delayed closure	Premature closure
Rickets	Craniosynostosis
Hypothyroidism	Microcephaly
Malnutrition	Hyperthyroidism
Osteogenesis imperfecta	
Alpert syndrome	
Hydrocephalus	
Chromosomal abnormality,	
eg. Down syndrome,	
Rubinstein-Taybii syndrome, trisomy 13	

NEURAL TUBE DEFECTS (NTD)

These result from failure of the neural tube to close on day 21–26 of intrauterine life and may involve brain or spinal cord.

Associations   Folate deficiency, sodium valproate, previous NTD

Antenatal detection   Raised α-FP in amniotic fluid, direct view on USS

Recurrence risk   1 previous NTD 4%

                        2 previous NTD 10%

Spina bifida occulta

5% population affected. Failure of vertebral arch fusion (L5, S1) (NB. This is normal <10 years).

Clinical manifestations   Mostly asymptomatic

                                Skin lesion (hair tuft, sinus, lipoma, pigmented lesion)

                                Neural tethering may cause bladder and lower limb problems (cauda equina syndrome)

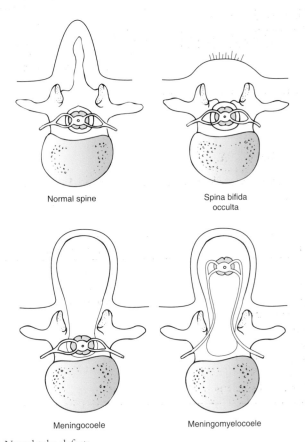

Normal spine

Spina bifida occulta

Meningocoele

Meningomyelocoele

Figure 13.8 Neural tube defects

Meningocoele

Protrusion of meninges through vertebral defect.

Meningomyelocoele

Incidence 1:1000 live births. Herniation of nerves and meninges.

Clinical manifestations   Paralysis (UMN) and sensory loss in legs
Neuropathic bladder and bowel (involvement <S1)
Talipes, hip dislocation, scoliosis
Hydrocephalus

Raschisis (open myelocoele)

Failure of fusion of the neural tube with CSF leakage. Incompatible with survival.

Encephalocoele

Midline defect of the skull with protrusion of brain. Usually occipital, may be frontal or nasofrontal.

Clinical manifestations   Developmental delay, visual defects, hydrocephalus, seizures, microcephaly

Meckel–Gruber syndrome

- *Autosomal recessive*
- *Occipital encephalocoele*
- *Cleft palate*
- *Microphthalmus, microcephaly*
- *Abnormal genitalia, polycystic kidneys*
- *Polydactyly*

Anencephaly

Incidence 1:1000 live births. Failure of closure of the rostral neuropore results in rudimentary brain and a large defect of the meninges and skull. Other anomalies in 10–20%. Incompatible with life.

HYDROCEPHALUS

This is dilatation of the CSF spaces.

Causes

↑ *CSF production*
Choroid plexus papilloma (rare).

Obstruction to CSF pathways

Intraventricular block   1. Congenital aqueductal stenosis (aqueduct of Sylvius)
                                     2. Dandy–Walker syndrome:
                                            Occlusion of the exit of the fourth ventricle
                                            Enlarged fourth ventricle and cerebellar hypoplasia
                                     3. Arnold–Chiari malformation:
                                            Elongated medulla, downward displacement of cerebellar tonsils and brainstem
                                            ± spina bifida, syringomyelia
                                     4. Neoplasm or vascular malformation
                                     5. Meningitis

Extraventricular block   Posthaemorrhagic (premature infants SAH)
                                     Infection eg. TB meningitis
                                     Leukaemic infiltrates

Decreased CSF reabsorption

Venous hypertension   Dural venous sinus thrombosis (severe dehydration)

Hydrocephalus can be classified into non-communicating and communicating types but these terms have been used with different meanings and are therefore misleading.

Clinical manifestations

These are variable depending on the duration and rate of increase of the CSF pressure and age of onset.

Infant	Head circumference crossing centiles
	Bulging fontanelle, distended scalp veins
	'Setting-sun' eye sign
	Developmental delay, ataxia
Older child	Signs of raised intracranial pressure

Investigations

Neuroimaging (USS/CT/MRI) Dilated ventricles, structural malformations

Management

Treat the cause.

Surgery	Ventriculoperitoneal (VP) shunt
Shunt complications	Blockage, infection

NEURONAL MIGRATION DISORDERS

These occur during foetal development and may be very minor or have major sequelae. They are diagnosed on MRI brain scans. Important types include the following.

Lissencephaly (smooth brain)

- *Absent cerebral convolutions and rudimentary Sylvian fissure*
- *Large lateral ventricles, microcephaly, microphthalmia*
- *Manifest as severe developmental delay, failure to thrive and seizures*

Miller-Deiker syndrome

- *Lissencephaly, characteristic facial dysmorphism*
- *Chromosome deletions of 17p 13.3*

Schizencephaly

- *Clefts in the cerebral hemispheres from the cortex to the ventricles, the entire cleft being coated with cortex*
- *Presents with epilepsy and/or focal neurology*

Porencephaly

- *Cysts within the brain*
- *Presents with focal neurology*

AGENESIS OF THE CORPUS CALLOSUM

X-linked recessive, autosomal dominant, sporadic. This may be completely asymptomatic (if isolated) or produce severe intellectual impairment when associated with other defects.

Associations Cell migration defects (eg. pachygyria, microgyria), Trisomy 18

Aicardi syndrome

- *Agenesis of the corpus callosum*
- *Retinal abnormalities (eg. coloboma, pits)*
- *Seizures refractive to treatment*
- *Severe mental retardation*
- *Vertebral abnormalities*

Epilepsy

A *seizure (convulsion)* is an abnormal burst of electrical activity in the brain, which may manifest in various ways. *Epilepsy* is recurrent seizures unrelated to fever or acute cerebral insult.

Generalised seizures Whole cortex involved diffusely
Partial seizures One area of the cortex involved; may become generalised

---

INTERNATIONAL CLASSIFICATION OF EPILEPTIC SEIZURES

Generalised seizures

Absence:
   Typical
   Complex
Myoclonic eg. Juvenile myoclonic epilepsy, infantile spasms
Tonic
Tonic-clonic
Atonic

Partial seizures

Simple partial (remain conscious):
   Motor
   Sensory
   Autonomic
   Psychic
Complex partial (impaired consciousness):
   Simple partial extended
   Initial complex partial eg. temporal lobe epilepsy
Partial with secondary generalisation

INVESTIGATING EPILEPSY

Full history and clinical examination including developmental check. For first convulsion, investigate only if <6 months old or unwell child or findings on examination.

Investigations

EEG

Lumbar puncture   In an unwell child. Low threshold in febrile convulsion if child <18 months. NB. Not if raised intracranial pressure signs

Blood   Glucose (when fitting)
         Electrolytes, metabolic screen, congenital infection screen

Neuroimaging   USS (infants)
         Skull X-ray (calcification, trauma)
         CT scan (urgent if unwell)
         MRI scan

COMMON SEIZURE TYPES

Absence seizures

Typical   Sudden loss of awareness, no motor activity, eyelid fluttering
         No postictal phase
         Last <30 seconds

Complex	Motor component (myotonic movements, loss of body tone)
EEG	Typical 3/sec generalised spike and wave
Treatment	Ethosuximide
	Sodium valproate (NB. Potential for precipitating fulminant liver failure)
	Lamotrigine

Generalised tonic-clonic seizures

These may follow a partial seizure. May be idiopathic or induced by infections, stress or drugs. An 'aura' suggests a focal origin.

Features

Tonic phase	Sudden loss of consciousness, tonic contraction, apnoea, cyanosis, eyes roll backwards
Clonic phase	Rhythmic contractions of all muscle groups
	Tongue biting, sphincter control lost
Postictal	Semiconscious for 30 minutes – 2 hours
Treatment	Sodium valproate, carbamazepine
	Lamotrigine
	Clobazam

Simple partial seizures

These are usually motor, involving asynchronous tonic or clonic movements. Aura may occur. May be confused with tics (which can be suppressed temporarily).

Complex partial seizures

These involve altered consciousness and may follow on from a simple partial seizure. Temporal lobe epilepsy (a form of complex partial seizure) may produce outbursts of emotions. Automatisms are a common feature (lip smacking, chewing, drooling).

EEG	Focal spikes or sharp waves
	Brought on by sleep deprivation
MRI scan	Looking for structural brain abnormalities

EPILEPSY SYNDROMES

Childhood absence epilepsy

Usually age 3–10 years, girls > boys, family history in 40%.

Seizure types	Typical or atypical absence seizures
Induced by	Hyperventilation, emotion, hunger
Treatment	As for absence seizures

Juvenile myoclonic epilepsy

5% of all epilepsy. Onset 12–16 years.

Associations	25% family history
	90% develop generalised tonic-clonic seizures
	25% develop absences

Features	Myoclonic jerks, worse in the morning (cannot brush their teeth, spill their tea)
	No impairment of consciousness
EEG	Normal background, 4–6/sec irregular polyspike and wave discharge pattern
	Photosensitivity
Treatment	Sodium valproate
	Lamotrigine (may help)

Infantile spasms

Incidence 1:3000. Onset age 4–6 months, boys > girls. Associated with arrested development.

Features	Symmetrical contractions, occur in bursts
	May be extensor, flexor (Salaam spasms, jack-knife) or mixed
EEG	Hypsarrhythmia (chaotic EEG with high-amplitude activity)

Cause

Cryptogenic (20%)	Normal prior development, examination and CT scan
Symptomatic (80%)	Structural, eg. tuberose sclerosis, lissencephaly
	Metabolic disease
	Birth injury, eg. hypoxic ischaemic encephalopathy, IVH
	Postnatal injury, eg. trauma, infection

Investigations of cause

- *MRI brain*
- *Metabolic screen (see p. 286)*
- *Chromosome analysis*
- *If tuberous sclerosis (TS) is suspected, renal USS, echocardiogram*

Treatment options

- *Vigabatrin* –
- *ACTH or prednisolone (second line)*

West syndrome

A triad of:

1. *infantile spasms*
2. *hypsarrhythmia*
3. *mental retardation*

Temporal lobe epilepsy

Complex partial seizures originating in the temporal lobe area. They may manifest as outbursts of emotions.

EEG	Anterior temporal lobe focal spikes or sharp waves
MRI	To look for temporal lobe abnormalities

Benign rolandic epilepsy (benign partial epilepsy with centrotemporal spikes)

Common partial epilepsy with good prognosis. Onset 2–14 years (peak 9–10 years).

Features	Drooling, abnormal sensations in mouth
	Secondary generalisation
	75% occur in sleep, 25% occur on waking
EEG	Repetitive spike focus in the Rolandic area (centrotemporal)
Treatment	Carbamazepine
	Spontaneous resolution usually occurs in early to mid teenage years

Landau–Kleffner syndrome (LKS)

- *Onset five years, male > female*
- *Loss of language skills associated with seizures of several types in 70%*
- *EEG abnormalities more common during sleep*

Rasmussen encephalitis

- *Subacute inflammatory encephalitis with frequent focal seizures*
- *Associated with progressive hemiplegia*

Pyridoxine deficiency

- *Neonatal, infancy or adult onset generalised tonic-clonic seizures*
- *Autosomal recessive*
- *Treat with pyridoxine supplements*

Lennox–Gastaut syndrome

This is an electroclinical syndrome comprising:

1. *multiple seizure types (myoclonic, atypical absences, atonic 'drop' attacks, tonic nocturnal seizures, generalised tonic-clinic seizures)*
2. *EEG shows slow spike and wave (2–3/sec)*

Onset mostly 4–5 years. Pre-existing severe seizures in 60%. Mental handicap initially 75% and regression. Epilepsy often intractable.

FEBRILE CONVULSIONS

These are convulsions associated with fever or a rapid temperature rise from an infection (not directly involving the CNS), often due to an URTI. Incidence 2–5% children under five years. Males > females. Family history in 30%.

Typical	Complex
6 months to 5 years	<6 months or >5 years
Generalised tonic or tonic-clonic	Focal
<15 minutes	>15 minutes

Investigations

These depend on the clinical examination looking for a source of infection. Urine specimen for infection should be done. Further investigations depend on clinical evaluation.

Management

- *Admit if first fit*
- *Fever control with paracetamol, tepid sponging*
- *Parental advice on fever control and management of a fit*
- *Rectal diazepam if seizure > 5 minutes*

Risk of later development of epilepsy

General population 0.5%

Febrile convulsions 1% if typical

5–10% if risk factors (atypical, family history epilepsy, febrile seizure <9 months, delayed milestones)

NON-EPILEPTIC 'FUNNY TURNS'

Breath holding attacks

6 months–3 years. Precipitated by fear, anger and pain. A cry, then breath holding. Either: cyanosis, or pallor (vasovagal asystole). This may be accompanied by unconscious, stiffens with clonic movements, then limp with a rapid recovery.

Benign paroxysmal vertigo

1–3 years. Sudden onset, unsteadiness, horizontal nystagmus, vomiting, pallor, remains conscious. This may last <5 min. Ear infection associated.

Night terrors

18 months–7 years. Wake from sleep screaming, thrashing, tachycardia, normal sleep afterwards.

Syncope

Postural (adolescents). Sensitive vago-cardiac reflex (toddlers – trauma) causing bradycardia, collapse, pallor. Cardiac arrhythmia eg. prolonged QT syndrome.

Hysterical fits

Narcolepsy

EMERGENCY MANAGEMENT OF STATUS EPILEPTICUS

NB. Status epilepticus is said to occur when a seizure lasts for >30 minutes.

- *Stabilise the child (airway, breathing, circulation) and give oxygen*
- *IV access*
- *Bloods   BMStix (give IV glucose if low)*
  Glucose, U&E, Ca, Mg, FBC, cultures, ABG, drug screen
- *Drug therapy (protocols vary, see latest APLS guidelines):*
  If no IV access give diazepam 0.4 mg/kg PR, then paraldehyde 0.4 ml/kg (1 ml/year of age if <4 yrs) PR (in olive oil) after 5 mins if still no IV access
  If IV access is obtained rapidly, lorazepam 0.1 mg/kg IV may be given and repeated after 10 mins if necessary
  If the child continues fitting at 10–20 mins give phenytoin infusion 18 mg/kg over 20–30 mins with ECG attached (not if already on phenytoin)
  If fitting continues paralyse and ventilate (IPPV), thiopentone infusion (by anaesthetist)

ANTIEPILEPTIC DRUGS

Drug	Mode of action	Use	Side-effects
Sodium valproate (Epilim)	Unknown	Generalised seizures Atypical absences Partial seizures	Hyperphagia (weight gain) Sedation, tremor, excitation Hepatotoxicity (irreversible) GIT disturbance Thrombocytopenia Alopecia (reversible)
Carbamazepine (Tegretol)	Sodium channel blocker	Partial seizures Generalised tonic-clonic	Enzyme inducer Ataxia, dizziness, drowsiness Blurred vision, diplopia Allergic skin rashes Transient lymphopenia
Phenytoin	Sodium channel blocker	Status Partial seizures	Enzyme inducer Hirsutism, acne Gum hyperplasia Rickets Aplastic anaemia Toxicity: ataxia, tremor, nystagmus, dysarthria

(NB. Phenytoin displays zero-order kinetics and therefore there is a rapid serum rise when the hepatic enzymes are saturated, causing toxicity with no therapeutic benefit. Serum levels must be monitored at some point.)

Phenobarbitone	GABA inhibition	Neonatal seizures	Enzyme inducer Concentration impairment Memory loss, rickets Hyperactivity in children Learning difficulties Dependence
Vigabatrin	GABA transaminase inhibitor	Infantile spasms Intractable epilepsy Partial seizures	Drowsiness, agitation Excitation in children Peripheral retinal atrophy (visual field testing may be necessary), psychosis

Lamotrigine	Presynaptic sodium channel blocker	Generalised seizures	Severe allergic reactions Arousing effect
Gabapentin	Unknown	Partial seizures	Drowsiness, headache Tremor, ataxia, weight gain
Topiramate	Unknown	Severe epilepsy	Cognitive and psychological changes, weight loss

Headaches

These are a common problem and rarely due to a severe underlying organic disorder. A full history and neurological examination should be performed and further investigations only if worrying findings on history (eg. increase in frequency or severity of headaches, developmental deterioration, behavioural change) or examination.

Examination should include:

- *full neurological, especially visual fields (intracranial mass?)*
- *fundoscopy (BP↑?), cranial bruits (AV malformation?)*
- *head size (crossing centiles?), blood pressure (↑?)*
- *teeth (dental caries?), face (sinus pain? rhinorrhoea?)*

TENSION HEADACHE

A common headache.

Clinical features	Dull ache, sharp pain, generalised, at the vertex or unclear location May occur daily for weeks or be continuous; medication often ineffective
Associations	Difficulty sleeping, dizziness, family or school problems No aura, no precipitants, no neurological signs

MIGRAINE

These are recurrent headaches of uncertain pathology, thought to be either neurogenic in origin or secondary to vasoconstriction then vasodilatation

Clinical features	Throbbing, bifrontal, unilateral, photophobia, better in a dark room May wake from sleep, transient hemiplegia or ataxia

Must be accompanied by at least two of: nausea, vomiting, abdominal pain, visual aura, family history.

Management

Avoid stimuli	eg. stress, certain foods (chocolate, cheese, colourings), sun, bright lights
Acute episode	Analgesics (paracetamol), antiemetic if nausea Selective 5-HT agonist if severe (>12 yrs)

HEADACHES OF OTHER UNDERLYING PATHOLOGY

Features

Those of underlying local pathology (eg. sinusitis, toothache, fever). Those of ↑ICP – diffuse, frontal, worse on coughing, sneezing or lying down and in the mornings

Causes

Neurological	Brain tumour, hydrocephalus, meningitis, encephalitis
	Hypertension, post-traumatic, lead poisoning
Other	Sinusitis, dental caries

Neuroectodermal syndromes

These involve a defect in the differentiation of the primitive ectoderm and include:

- *neurofibromatosis*
- *tuberose sclerosis*
- *Sturge–Weber syndrome (see p. 315)*
- *Von Hippel–Lindau disease*
- *ataxia telangiectasia (see p. 37)*
- *hypomelanosis of Ito and incontinentia pigmenti (see p. 319–320)*

NEUROFIBROMATOSIS (NF, VON RECKLINGHAUSEN DISEASE)

Autosomal dominant, 50% new mutation rate. Incidence 1:4000.

NF1 (90%)

Gene on chromosome 17q. Diagnosis if *two or more* of the following occur.

1. *Café-au-lait patches (prepubertal ≥6 × >5 mm, postpubertal ≥6 × >15 mm)*
2. *Axillary freckles*
3. *≥2 neurofibromas or one plexiform neurofibroma*
4. *≥2 Lisch nodules (hamartomas) in iris*
5. *Bone lesion (kyphoscoliosis, sphenoid dysplasia (pulsating exophthalmos), tibial pseudoarthroses)*
6. *Optic glioma*
7. *First-degree relative with NF*

Other features

CNS	Macrocephaly, seizures, learning difficulties, speech defects, attention deficit disorder, aqueduct stenosis
Endocrine	Precocious puberty
Tumours	CNS tumours, Wilms tumour, phaeochromocytoma, leukaemia, sarcomas
Other	Renal artery stenosis, cardiomyopathy, lung fibrosis

NF2 (10%)

Gene on chromosome 22q. Diagnosis if one of the following present.

1. *Bilateral VIII nerve acoustic neuromas*
2. *Unilateral VIII nerve mass in association with any two of: meningioma, neurofibroma, schwannoma, juvenile posterior subcapsular cataracts, glioma*
3. *Unilateral VIII nerve acoustic neuroma or other brain or spinal tumour as above and first-degree relative with NF2*

Clinical features include: cerebellar ataxia, hearing loss, facial nerve palsy, headache. Skin lesions are less common than in NF1.

Management

- *Genetic counselling*
- *Baseline investigations (CT/MRI brain and optic nerves, skeletal survey, EEG, audiogram, brainstem auditory and visual evoked potentials, psychometric testing)*
- *Yearly assessment including: BP, neurological examination, auditory and visual screening*

TUBEROUS SCLEROSIS

Autosomal dominant, 80% new mutations. Gene on chromosome 9q and 16p. Wide variation in severity.

Clinical features

Skin   *Adenoma sebaceum* (angiofibroma) over cheeks and nose >3 years
        Ash leaf patches (pale macules, fluoresce in Woods light)
        Shagreen patches (orange peel skin over lumbar spine)
        Periungual fibromas (>20 years)
        Gingival fibroma
        Fibrous plaque on forehead or scalp
CNS   Epilepsy (infantile spasms, partial)
        Autism
        Cortical tuber (hard nodules with bizarre giant cells); may calcify
        Subependymal glial nodules, project into ventricles, calcify, 'candle-dripping' appearance on CT scan, >3 years
        Gliomas
Eye   *Retinal phakoma* (optic nerve astrocytoma), Mulberry tumour
CVS   Cardiac rhabdomyoma (40–50%)
Renal   *Multiple angiomyolipomas*, hamartomas, polycystic kidneys ·
Lung   Lymphangiomyomatosis

- *Those in italics are pathognomonic features.*

Management

This includes baseline investigations to look for associated features, seizure control, genetic counselling and regular follow-up (renal USS, BP, echocardiogram, CT/MRI brain scan, CXR and eye examination).

VON HIPPEL–LINDAU DISEASE

Autosomal dominant. Gene locus on chromosome 3p25.

Features
Retinal angiomata
Cerebellar haemangioblastomas
Cystic lesions   Renal, pancreas, liver, epididymis, spinal cord
Tumours   Phaeochromocytoma, renal carcinoma (most common
                        cause of death)

Ataxia

This may be due to cerebellar disease or to sensory loss, the former being more common in children.

Causes

Acute	Chronic
Infections	Congenital anomalies:
Acute cerebellar ataxia	Agenesis cerebellar vermis
During infection (coxsackie, echovirus, EBV)	Joubert disease
Postinfectious (varicella)	Dandy-Walker malformation
Toxic Phenytoin, alcohol, piperazine	Cerebral palsy (ataxic)
Acute intermittent	**Progressive**
Seizures	Cerebellar tumour
Migraine	Abetalipoproteinaemia
Hartnup disease	Friedreich ataxia
	Batten disease
	Cerebellar abscess
	Subdural haematoma
	Ataxia telangiectasia

LATE INFANTILE BATTEN DISEASE (CEROID LIPOFUSCINOSIS)

Autosomal recessive.

Clinical features Normal early development, then developmental regression from 2–5
                  years
                  Ataxia, choreoathetosis
                  Seizures
                  Retinitis pigmentosa
Diagnosis   Eye examination
                  EEG
                  Rectal biopsy (typical neurological features)

FRIEDREICH'S ATAXIA

Autosomal recessive. Gene on chromosome 9q13–21.1. A progressive degeneration involving cerebellar tracts and dorsal columns. Presentation usually around 10–12 years (always <20 years) with difficulty walking, with progression of disease and death around 40 years.

Clinical features

- *Progressive ataxia, dysarthria*
- *Loss of deep tendon reflexes with* upgoing plantars
- *Loss of position and vibration sense*
- *Lower limb weakness and amyotrophy*
- *Pes cavus, scoliosis*
- *Optic atrophy, nystagmus*
- *Dilated or restrictive cardiomyopathy, diabetes mellitus*

Investigations

- *Sensory (± motor) conduction velocities slightly decreased*
- *Sensory evoked potential absent or reduced*
- *Visual evoked potential diminished*

Cerebral palsy

Prevalence 2:1000 population. This is a disorder of movement and posture due to a non-progressive lesion in the motor pathways of the developing brain. It is a static encephalopathy.

Associated features

- *Learning impairment*
- *Visual impairment, strabismus*
- *Hearing loss*
- *Speech and language difficulties*
- *Behavioural problems*
- *Epilepsy*

Causes

Antenatal (80%)	Cerebral dysgenesis, cerebral malformation, congenital infection
Intrapartum (10%)	Hypoxic ischaemic encephalopathy
Postnatal (10%)	Cerebral ischaemia, IVH, hydrocephalus, trauma, non-accidental injury (NAI), hyperbilirubinaemia

Types

Spastic
Initial hypotonia, progressing to spasticity with UMN signs. It may be:

- *hemiplegia – unilateral involvement (arm > leg usually), eg. IVH, meningitis*
- *diplegia – legs > arms (arms may be normal), eg. PVL*
- *whole body (quadriplegia) – all limbs involved (arms > legs), eg. birth asphyxia*

Ataxic hypotonic
Hypotonia, poor balance, tremor, incoordinate movements, eg. hydrocephalus.

Dyskinetic

- *Involuntary movements (athetosis, dystonia), eg. hyperbilirubinaemia*
- *Fluctuating muscle tone (dyskinesia)*
- *Poor postural tone*

Presentation may be with the following

- *Delayed motor milestones*
- *Abnormal tone in infancy*
- *Abnormal gait (eg. toe walking, wide based)*
- *Feeding difficulties*
- *Developmental delay (language, social)*
- *Persistence of primitive reflexes*

Investigations

- *Brain imaging – USS in neonates, CT scan*
- *Metabolic screen*

Management

This involves an interdisciplinary approach, to optimise the development of the child. Specialities involved include occupational therapist, physiotherapist, speech therapist, social worker, teacher and developmental psychologist. Physicians involved include the paediatrician, orthopaedic surgeon, neurologist, ophthalmologist and audiologist.

Neurodegenerative disorders

Neurodegenerative disorders involve a progressive deterioration of neurological function with loss of speech, vision, hearing or locomotion and often with associated seizures, feeding difficulties and intellectual impairment. They are a heterogeneous group and classification is variable.

Causes

Lysosomal storage disorders (see p. 298)	GM1 gangliosidosis, Tay–Sachs disease, Sandhoff disease, Niemann–Pick disease Krabbe disease, metachromatic leucodystrophy Gaucher disease

Peroxisomal disorders	Adrenoleukodystrophy (see p. 297)
Ceroid lipofuscinoses	Late infantile Batten disease
Mitochondrial disorders	MERRF, MELAS (see p. 298)
Mucopolysaccharidoses	Hurler, Hunter, etc. (see p. 299)
Cerebellar disorders	Friedreich ataxia
	Ataxia telangiectasia (see p. 37)
	Abetaliproteinaemia (see p. 160)
	Olivopontocerebellar atrophy
Copper metabolism disorders	Wilson disease (see p. 197)
	Menkes kinky hair disease
Infective disorders	SSPE, HIV
Other	Multiple sclerosis, Huntington disease (presents in adulthood)
	Rett syndrome

Investigations

Blood	White cell enzymes (lysosomal storage disorders), very long chain fatty acids, lactate, copper, caeruloplasmin, HIV status
Bone marrow aspirate	Abnormal cells (Gaucher, Niemann–Pick)
CSF	Measles antibody, lactate
Urine	Glycosoaminoglycans (mucopolysaccharidoses)
Hair analysis	Menke's kinky hair disease
Liver biopsy	Wilson disease, glycogen storage disorder
Fibroblast culture	Metabolic disorder eg. peroxisomal disorder, lysosomal storage disorder
MRI brain	Demyelination
EEG	May be characteristic
VER	Batten disease, multiple sclerosis
Chromosome analysis	

RETT SYNDROME

Rare disease of unknown aetiology, a clinical diagnosis. Occurrence in females only (possibly X-linked dominant, lethal to males). The gene ($McCP_2$) has been found at Xq28.

Clinical features

Presentation after one year with:

- *developmental regression (language and motor milestones)*
- *characteristic 'hand-wringing' repetitious movements and loss of hand function*
- *acquired microcephaly*
- *autistic features, ataxic gait, sighing respirations and apnoeas*
- *seizures (generalised tonic-clonic)*
- *death between 10–30 years (often from cardiac arrhythmias)*

SUBACUTE SCLEROSING PANENCEPHALITIS (SSPE)

A chronic encephalitis with high levels of measles antibody in the CSF. Occurs several years after measles infection (or more rarely, measles immunisation).

Clinical features
Presentation often in adolescence with cognitive regression, personality change progressing to severe regression with seizures, choreoathetosis and eventually decerebrate positioning. Death within 1–2 years.

Diagnostic investigations
CSF   Measles antibody (IgG and IgM)
EEG   Characteristic *periodic complexes*: normal background with high-voltage slow wave bursts

No effective treatment.

MENKE'S KINKY HAIR DISEASE

X-linked recessive, gene on chromosome Xq13. Underlying defect in copper transport.

Clinical features
Presentation in early months of life with:

- *progressive neurodegeneration, severe mental retardation*
- *seizures, hypotonia, feeding difficulties, optic atrophy*
- *hair colourless, kinky and fragile*
- *chubby red cheeks*
- *death <3 years*

Investigations
Hair shaft   Trichorrhexis nodosa (fractures along hair shaft)
                Pili torti (twisted hair)
                Monilethrix (brittle hair)
Serum   Copper (↓), caeruloplasmin (↓)

Management
Copper-histidine subcutaneously slows deterioration in some patients.

MULTIPLE SCLEROSIS

A disease of multiple central demyelinating lesions with plaque formation, separated by space and time. Characteristic remissions and relapses occur. It is mostly slowly progressive, though may have a rapid course.

Usual onset 20–35 years, though can occur in children (0.2–2% of cases).

Associations

- *Female > male, lower incidence closer to the equator*
- *First-degree relative with multiple sclerosis, HLA-A3, B7 and DR2*

Clinical features

Neurological symptoms depending on where the demyelination occurs. Some common symptoms are:

- *ataxia, weakness, headache, parasthaesias*
- *optic neuropathy (blurred vision), optic neuritis (swelling of optic disc), optic atrophy*

Unusual features include epilepsy, trigeminal neuralgia.

Investigations

MRI brain	Plaques
CSF	Cells ↑ ($5-60/mm^3$, mononuclear)
	Protein ↑ (0.4–1 g/l) (in 60%)
	IgG ↑ (in 60%)
	Oligoclonal bands (in 80%)
VER	Delay (if optic nerve involvement)

Management

- *Mostly supportive*
- *Steroids may help in acute attacks*

Stroke

A focal neurological deficit with an underlying vascular pathology is defined as:

- *stroke – lasting >24 h*
- *transient ischaemic attack (TIA) – lasting <24 h*
- *reversible ischaemic neurological deficit (RIND) – lasting >24 h but with full recovery*

'Stroke-like episode' – focal neurological deficit lasting >24 h with no obvious vascular pathology, eg. brain tumour, brain abscess

Causes of stroke

Stroke may be due to haemorrhage or to ischaemia. Ischaemia may be caused by vessel spasm, stenosis or dissection or vessel occlusion by thrombosis or embolism.

Ischaemia

Embolism	Cyanotic CHD, endocarditis
Large vessel stenosis	Sickle cell disease
	Varicella, AIDS, homocystinuria
Vessel spasm	Meningitis

Thrombosis	Sickle cell disease
	Severe dehydration (venous sinus thrombosis)
	Homocystinuria, leukaemia, thrombocytosis
	Meningitis
	Clotting disorder eg. protein S or C deficiency, antithrombin III deficiency, lupus antibodies, factor V Leiden
Vessel dissection	Trauma (eg. fall on a pencil in child's mouth)
	Congenital heart disease
Moya moya disease	Moya moya (basal artery occlusion with telangiectasia)
	Also seen in Williams syndrome, Down syndrome

Haemorrhage

Low platelets	ITP
Bleeding disorder	Haemophilia
Vessel disorder	A–V malformation, cerebral aneurysm
Trauma	

Clinical features

- *Hemiparesis, hemisensory signs, visual field defects*
- *Seizures (common in neonates)*
- *Deterioration in level of consciousness (seen in progression of bleed)*

Investigations

These will be led by any underlying disease and history and examination are essential to help elucidate the cause.

MRI brain scan	Outline area affected (thrombosis, bleed, abscess, tumour, etc.)
CT scan	If MRI unavailable (to exclude haemorrhage)
Magnetic resonance angiography (MRA scan)	Vascular outline
Transcranial doppler USS	Large vessel disease
Cerebral angiogram	For more detailed outline, if MRA normal in ischaemia
	Later, after haemorrhage for eg. AV malformation, aneurysm
ECG and echocardiogram	Cardiac anomaly or arrhythmia
Infection screen	
Haematological screen	Including sickle screen, FBC and clotting defects (eg. protein S and C deficiencies, antithrombin III deficiency, see p. 431)
Metabolic screen	If metabolic disease suspected

Management

This is dependent on the cause eg. exchange transfusion acutely in sickle cell disease, anticoagulants may be required in prothrombotic coagulopathy and surgery in AV malformation and cerebral aneurysm.

Spinal cord disorders

SPINAL CORD COMPRESSION

Causes

- *Tumour – spinal cord intradural or extradural tumour, secondary deposit*
- *Trauma*
- *Infection – epidural abscess, TB*
- *Disc protrusion*
- *Vascular malformation*

Clinical features

These depend on whether the transection is partial or involves the whole cord. Basic features are:

1. *pain – back pain and pain at the level of compression (radicular pain)*
2. *paralysis – spastic para- or tetraparesis from the level of compression*
3. *sensory loss – loss to the level of compression*

Complete transection

Paralysis   Initial flaccid muscle paralysis (spinal shock), then spastic paralysis from the level of compression

Loss of voluntary sphincter control (reflex emptying returns)

Sensory loss Total loss of sensation in the regions supplied below the level of injury

NB. Fatal if above 4th cervical cord segment due to paralysis of the diaphragm.

Hemisection (Brown–Séquard syndrome)

Paralysis   Paralysis of muscles on the same side as injury below the level of transection

Sensory loss Same side (paralysed limb) – loss of position sense, proprioception and tactile discrimination in the same side (dorsal columns)

Opposite, unparalysed limb – loss of pain and temperature sensation (spinothalamic)

Investigations

X-ray spine (Bony destruction?)
MRI spine Outline of lesion
Myelogram (May be considered)

SYRINGOMYELIA AND SYRINGOBULBIA

A cystic degeneration of the centre of the cord (myelia) or brainstem (bulbia).

Clinical features

Destruction of spinothalamic tracts Bilateral loss of temperature and pain in a bizzare distribution

Destruction of corticospinal tracts	Spastic paraparesis, absent tendon reflexes upper limbs, wasting of the small muscles of the hand
Brainstem (syringobulbia)	Nystagmus, hearing loss, Horner's syndrome, loss of facial sensation, tongue atrophy and fasiculation

Investigations

- *MRI*
- *Myelogram*

Management

Surgical aspiration may be attempted.

TRANSVERSE MYELITIS

This is acute inflammation of the cord and paraplegia.

Causes

- *Viral infection – EBV, HSV, mumps, rubella, influenza*
- *Multiple sclerosis, radiotherapy, anterior spiral artery occlusion*

Clinical features

Abrupt onset of:

1. *weakness – initially flaccid, becoming spastic, legs*
2. *sensory loss – pain, temperature and light touch, legs*
3. *back pain*
4. *sphincter disturbance*
5. *fever and nuchal rigidity*

Investigations

LP   CSF shows lymphocytes ↑, (protein ↑, N)
MRI *spine* Lesion outlined

Management

Supportive, complete spontaneous recovery may occur.

Differential diagnosis

Guillain–Barré syndrome, acute poliomyelitis, cord compression.

Neuromuscular disorders

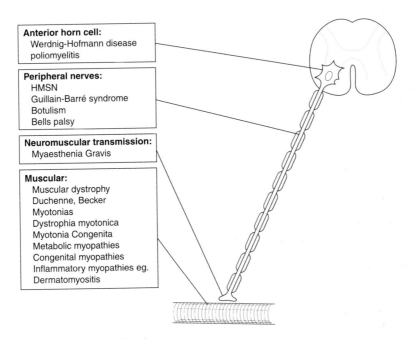

Anterior horn cell:
Werdnig-Hofmann disease
poliomyelitis

Peripheral nerves:
HMSN
Guillain-Barré syndrome
Botulism
Bells palsy

Neuromuscular transmission:
Myaesthenia Gravis

Muscular:
Muscular dystrophy
Duchenne, Becker
Myotonias
Dystrophia myotonica
Myotonia Congenita
Metabolic myopathies
Congenital myopathies
Inflammatory myopathies eg.
Dermatomyositis

Figure 13.9 Neuromuscular disorders

FLOPPY BABY

There are many causes of floppy infants, including:

Central causes Syndrome eg. Prader–Willi syndrome, Down syndrome
Hypoxic ischaemic encephalopathy
Evolving cerebral palsy
Neonatal sepsis
Metabolic disease eg. peroxisomal disorders, MSUD
Hypothyroidism
Hypocalcaemia
Drug therapy

Peripheral causes Spinal muscular atrophy (Werdnig-Hoffmann)
Myopathy
Congenital myotonic dystrophy
Myasthenia gravis (transient neonatal or congenital)

Clinical features

- *Frog-like position*
- *Head lag on pulling up*
- *Flop in ventral suspension*

Paralytic   No antigravity movement eg. spinal muscular atrophy, neuromuscular disorders (ie. reduced power as well as being floppy)

Non-paralytic   Antigravity movement eg. encephalopathy, cerebral palsy

SPINAL MUSCULAR ATROPHY TYPE 1 (WERDNIG–HOFFMANN DISEASE)

Autosomal recessive. Genetic locus on chromosome 5q11–13. This is a degeneration of the anterior horn cells due to failure of arrest of apoptosis.

Clinical features

In utero   Decreased fetal movements, arthrogryphosis

Postnatal Floppy baby, frog-like position, no antigravity movement, respiratory distress
Progressive weakness of skeletal muscles, absent reflexes
Tongue fasciculation
Extraocular muscles not affected

Death <2 years.

Investigations

Muscle biopsy	Characteristic perinatal denervation pattern
EMG	Less definitive changes
Sural nerve biopsy	Mild sensory neuropathic changes
Nerve conduction tests	Slowed sensory conduction

NB. CK normal.

Management

Supportive only (physiotherapy, orthopaedic, occupational therapy).

POLIOMYELITIS

Due to infection with poliovirus type 1,2 or 3. Transmission faecal-oral route.

Clinical features

Incubation 7–14 days. Subclinical infection (95%).

Abortive poliomyelitis (5%)	Fever, sore throat, myalgia
Non-paralytic poliomyelitis (2%)	Above plus meningeal irritation
Paralytic poliomyelitis (0.1%)	Initial fever, sore throat, myalgia, then meningeal irritation, muscle pain (neck and lumbar region). Then asymmetrical paralysis:

Spinal poliomyelitis – limbs, thorax, diaphragm, trunk
Bulbar poliomyelitis (5–30%) motor cranial nerve
paralysis
NB. No sensory involvement

Predisposing factors for paralytic poliomyelitis:

- *exercise early in illness*
- *male*
- *trauma, surgery, IM injection*
- *tonsillitis (bulbar polio)*

Investigations

- *Clinical diagnosis*
- *Viral PCR and culture*

Management
Supportive therapy, early bed rest.

Prevention

- *Trivalent oral poliovaccine (live, Sabin)*
- *Intramuscular killed vaccine available (Salk)*

HEREDITARY MOTOR-SENSORY NEUROPATHIES (HMSN)

Progressive diseases of the peripheral nerves, of which there are several types.

HMSN type I (peroneal muscular atrophy, Charcot–Marie–Tooth disease)
Autosomal dominant. Many loci including 17p and 1q.

Clinical features
Asymptomatic until late childhood.

Peroneal muscular atrophy   Weakness of dorsiflexion, foot drop, reflexes ↓
Pes cavus, gait disturbance
Inverted champagne bottle-shaped legs
Hand involvement milder
Sensory involvement (loss of proprioception and vibration, paraesthesias)

Investigations
Nerve conduction   Reduced motor and sensory velocities
Sural nerve biopsy   'Onion bulb' formations of Schwann cell cytoplasm
CSF   Protein ↑

Management
Supportive only – foot splints, ankle fusion, pillows under legs at night.

HMSN type II (axonal type)

Autosomal dominant. Chromosome 1p35–36. Due to axonal degeneration. Disease similar to type I but milder.

HMSN type III (Dejerine–Sottas disease)

Autosomal dominant. Gene locus chromosome 17p11.2. Phenotypic variant of type I (similar but more severe). Argyll–Robertson pupils common.

GUILLAIN–BARRÉ DISEASE

A postinfectious demyelinating neuropathy.

Clinical features

Trivial viral infection, then 1–3 weeks later:

- *distal limb weakness, ascending, areflexic*
- *muscle pain, paraesthesia*
- *respiratory muscle and facial weakness (20%)*
- *urinary retention or incontinence*
- *autonomic features rare (BP and heart rate lability)*

Investigations

Clinical diagnosis.

Nerve conduction	Delay in motor and sensory conduction
LP	CSF Protein $\uparrow$ ($\times 2$ normal)
	Oligoclonal bands
	WCC normal, glucose normal
Respiratory function tests	Spirometry

Management

Supportive therapy, with spontaneous recovery usual in 2–3 weeks.

γ-Globulin (IV)	Reduces duration and severity
Other options	Steroids, plasmapheresis

Prognosis

Recovery over many months, with relapses sometimes; *may* be incomplete.

Miller–Fischer syndrome

A rare, severe form involving:

- *ataxia*
- *proximal muscle weakness*
- *external ophthalmoplegia*

MYASTHENIA GRAVIS

A disease of immunological neuromuscular blockade. Mostly acquired, may be hereditary. Decreased acetylcholine (ACh) receptors, due to IgG receptor antibodies. Female: male = 2:1. Average age of onset 30 years.

Associations
Drugs (D-penicillamine, lithium, propranolol)
HLA-B8, DR3
Hashimoto thyroiditis
Collagen vascular disease
Thymomas and oat cell carcinoma of lung (Eaton–Lambert syndrome) in adults only

Clinical features
Eyes	External ocular muscle weakness, diplopia and ptosis
Bulbar	Dysphagia
Face	Weakness of facial muscles
Limbs	Proximal weakness, reflexes fatiguable, distal hand weakness
Fatiguability	A cardinal feature

Investigations
Tensilon test	An anticholinesterase (eg. edrophonium), given IV, causes transient relief. NB. Cannot use edrophonium in neonates (causes arrhythmias)
Serum	ACh receptor antibodies (90%)
	Autoimmune tests
	Thyroid profile
Nerve stimulation	Fibrillation and decreased muscle response with repetition

Management
Anticholinesterase drugs	4–6 hourly (eg. pyridostigmine, neostigmine)
Other options	Thymectomy, steroids, plasmapheresis

Care during anaesthetics.

Transient neonatal myasthenia gravis
Due to maternal antibodies crossing the placenta; lasts 2–3 weeks.

Congenital myasthenia gravis
This is a condition of *different aetiology* (due to congenital abnormality of ACh receptor channels and not autoimmune disease) which has similar features to myasthenia gravis but is non-progressive.

MUSCULAR DYSTROPHIES

Genetic myopathies involving progressive disease and death of muscle fibres.

Duchenne muscular dystrophy

X-linked recessive, incidence 1: 3600 live male infants. Due to absence of dystrophin (a muscle protein). Dystrophin gene on chromosome Xp21.3.

Clinical features

Normal early motor development	
Proximal limb weakness	Evident from three years
	Gowers' sign: evident at 3–6 years. A manoeuvre to stand from the supine position, involving rolling over, then using hands to 'climb up' the knees. Waddling (Trendelenberg) gait
Calf muscle pseudohypertrophy	
Progressive deterioration	Eventually wheelchair bound, scoliosis, pharyngeal weakness, respiratory failure
Cardiac	Cardiomyopathy, Q waves in left chest leads
Learning disability (33%)	

Investigations

Genetic testing	Xp21.3 mutation looked for
Creatinine phosphokinase	($\uparrow \times 10$ normal)
Muscle biopsy	Fibre necrosis, fat infiltration, no dystrophin on staining
EMG	Myopathic pattern
Cardiac	ECG, CXR

Management

Supportive (physiotherapy, nutritional support, etc.).

Prognosis

Death by 18 years usually.

Detection

- Female carriers – CK $\uparrow$ in 70%
- Antenatal diagnosis possible with DNA probes

Other muscular dystrophies

	Inheritance	Features
Becker MD	X-linked R Dystrophin gene *abnormal*	Similar but less severe than Duchenne muscular dystrophy
Emery–Dreifuss MD	X-linked R	Scapulohumeral weakness Cardiac involvement causes sudden death
Facioscapulohumeral MD	AD *Anticipation* occurs	A group of disorders Face, shoulder and pelvic girdle Normal life expectancy
Limb girdle MD	AR, AD	A group of disorders Shoulder and pelvic girdles involved. Calf hypertrophy may occur. Rate of progression varies but often wheelchair bound by 30 years

MYOTONIC DYSTROPHY

Autosomal dominant. Chromosome 19q13 expansion with numerous CTG repeats. *Anticipation* occurs (successive generations more severe). A progressive distal muscle weakness with failure of muscle relaxation. Affected mother has difficulty letting go when shaking hands. Worse if inherited from the mother.

Clinical features

Face	Inverted V-shaped upper lip, facial weakness, decreased muscle mass in temporal fossa, high-arched palate
Eyes	Ptosis, cataracts
Cardiac	Cardiomyopathy, conduction defects
Mental	Learning disability (50%)
Hair	Frontal baldness in males
Endocrine	Hypogonadism, small pituitary fossa, glucose intolerance
Immune	IgG ↓
Gastrointestinal	Constipation

Investigations

Clinical diagnosis.

Muscle biopsy	Prognostic value in neonates
EMG	Classic findings after infancy
Serum CK	Mild elevation
Other	Endocrine and immunoglobulin assessment necessary

Management

- *Phenytoin or carbamazepine may help with myotonia (increase depolarisation threshold)*
- *Care with anaesthesia*

MYOTONIA CONGENITA (THOMSEN DISEASE)

- Autosomal dominant (chromosome 7q35) or recessive
- Myotonia with generalised muscle hypertrophy. Appearance of a body builder.

CONGENITAL MYOPATHIES

Congenital myopathies include the following.

Myotubular myopathy

X-linked recessive, autosomal dominant and recessive forms.

Clinical features

In utero	Decreased foetal movements, polyhydramnios
Neonatal	Hypotonia, reduced muscle bulk, feeding difficulties, respiratory distress, ptosis

Diagnosis

Muscle biopsy diagnostic.

Congenital muscle fibre-type disproportion (CMFTD)

Sporadic, autosomal recessive. Features as in myotubular myopathy but less severe with a high degree of clinical variability. Diagnosis on muscle biopsy.

Nemaline rod myopathy

Autosomal dominant or recessive. Variable penetrance of dominant form, with mildly affected individuals having only poorly developed muscles. A severe neonatal form exists, with early death in most infants, and a milder form with motor delay, feeding difficulties and recurrent respiratory infections.

Diagnosis on muscle biopsy (nemaline rods are abnormal structures within the muscle fibres).

POTASSIUM-RELATED PERIODIC PARALYSES

Autosomal dominant. These involve periodic attacks of paralysis with transient alterations in serum potassium:

- $K \downarrow$ *Hypokalaemic periodic paralysis*
- $K \uparrow$ *Hyperkalaemic periodic paralysis*

Normal between attacks in childhood.

Episodes of paralysis (eg. on awakening) lasting minutes or hours. Liquorice may precipitate attacks. Progressive disease with weakness in adulthood. Diaphragmatic muscles unaffected, ECG changes occur during attacks.

Care must be taken during anaesthesia.

HEREDITARY SENSORY NEUROPATHY, FAMILIAL DYSAUTONOMIA: (RILEY-DAY SYNDROME)

Autosomal recessive. Gene at chromosome 9q31–33. Disease of peripheral nervous system involving reduced numbers of small nerve fibres (pain, temperature, taste, autonomic functions).

Associations	Eastern European Jews

Clinical features

Autonomic features	Excessive sweating, blotchy erythema, abnormal tearing. 'Crises' (labile BP, heart rate, vomiting, irritability, sweating, poor temperature control)
Peripheral neuropathy	Insensitivity to pain, feeding difficulties and aspirations, clumsy gait, scoliosis, corneal ulcers, slurred speech
CNS	Breath-holding seizures, mental retardation

Investigations

Diagnosis	Intradermal histamine produces no flare.
	Metacholine infusion causes exaggerated hypotensive response
	Metacholine eye drops produce miosis (no reaction normally)

Plasma	Dopamine-β-hydroxylase enzyme ↓
Urine	VMA ↓, HVA ↑
Sural nerve biopsy	Decreased unmyelinated fibres
CXR	Chronic changes from aspirations
ECG	Prolonged QT

Management

- *Eye drops, protection from injury*
- *Autonomic crises: anxiolytics, antiemetics, electrolyte control*

Prognosis

Death in childhood from chronic pulmonary failure.

Autism (classical or regressive)

Incidence 2:10 000 (rising). Siblings 2–3% prevalence (50–100 × greater than average). Autism is a developmental disorder primarily of social interaction. Features are variable and thought to be part of a spectrum. Most have a low IQ. Usual age of onset 15–21 months.

Clinical features

Social interactions impaired	No eye contact, relates to parts of a person's body (not the whole person), plays alone
Abnormal speech and language development	Delay, echolalia
Narrow range of interests with repetitive behaviour	Repetitive play, fascination with movement, interest in detail, early development of numbers
	Poor concentration span

Asperger's syndrome

Controversy over defining the disorder. Thought to be on the autistic spectrum. These are children who have severe impairment in reciprocal social interaction. They have variable fine and gross motor delay, walking later than they speak, with clumsiness. They have no delay in language, though have unusual language development (eg. have one-sided conversations and interpret literally). There is difficulty understanding non-verbal communication. They generally have a higher level of intelligence. They develop all-absorbing special interests and can memorise large amounts of information, though not necessarily fully comprehend it.

FURTHER READING

Aicardi J *Diseases of the nervous system in childhood*, 2nd Ed MacKeith Press with Blackwell Science Publications, London 1992

14

Haematology

- *Physiology*
- *Anaemia*
- *Genetic haemoglobin disorders*

- *Polycythaemias and thrombocythaemia*
- *Haemostasis*
- *The spleen*

Physiology

HAEMOGLOBIN

A red blood cell contains about 640 million molecules of haemoglobin (Hb). Haemoglobin is composed of four polypeptide chains (normal adult Hb has two α and two β chains, $\alpha_2\beta_2$), each with a haem group.

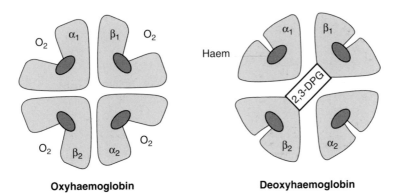

Figure 14.1 Oxyhaemoglobin and deoxyhaemoglobin

HAEMOGLOBIN FUNCTION

Haemoglobin carries oxygen from the lungs to the tissues. Each Hb molecule combines with four O_2 molecules to form oxyhaemoglobin. Deoxyhaemoglobin contains no oxygen molecules and has the metabolite 2,3-DPG in the centre, which acts to decrease its affinity to oxygen.

HAEM SYNTHESIS

This occurs in the mitochondria via a series of biochemical reactions:

$$\text{Glycine + succinyl coenzyme A} \xrightarrow{\hspace{3cm}} \left.\begin{array}{c} \text{Protoporphyrin} \\ + \\ \text{Iron (Fe}^{2+}\text{, ferrous)} \end{array}\right\} \rightarrow \text{Haem}$$

ALA (rate-limiting enzyme)
Vitamin B_6 (coenzyme)

CONTROL OF ERYTHROPOIESIS

Substances necessary for erythropoeisis include:

1. *hormones – erythropoietin, IL-3, stem cell factor, thyroxine and androgens*
2. *metals – iron, manganese, cobalt*
3. *vitamins – B_{12}, folate, C, E, B_6 (pyridoxine), thiamine, riboflavin, pantothenic acid*
4. *amino acids*

ERYTHROPOIETIN

This is a hormone that regulates Hb synthesis. It is a glycosylated polypeptide made mostly in the peritubular complex of the kidney. A low O_2 tension in the kidneys stimulates erythropoietin synthesis.

Recombinant erythropoietin

This is given subcutaneously (or intravenously) three times per week. Indications include endstage renal failure, inherited haemoglobinopathies (eg. thalassaemia) and anaemia of chronic disease. Side–effects include hypertension, high blood viscosity and rarely encephalopathy.

OXYGEN-HAEMOGLOBIN DISSOCIATION CURVE

The oxyhaemoglobin dissociation curve describes the relationship between the affinity of Hb for oxygen and the surrounding partial pressure of oxygen.

METHAEMOGLOBINAEMIA

This is a clinical state where Hb contains iron in the oxidised form (Fe^{3+}, ferric). This can be an inherited condition or result from a drug toxicity reaction oxidising the iron (see p. 104).

RED CELL METABOLISM

Red blood cells generate:

- *energy as ATP via the anaerobic Embden–Meyerhof pathway*
- *reducing power as NADH via this pathway, or NADPH via the hexose-monophosphate pathway*

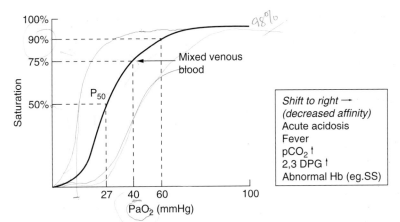

Shift to left ⟵
(increased affinity)
Acute alkalosis
Decreased temperature
pCO_2 ↓
2,3 DPG ↓
Carboxyhaemoglobin
Methaemoglobin
Abnormal haemoglobin (e.g. fetal
haemoglobin)
Cyanotic congenital heart disease

Mixed venous blood

P_{50}

Shift to right ⟶
(decreased affinity)
Acute acidosis
Fever
pCO_2 ↑
2,3 DPG ↑
Abnormal Hb (eg.SS)

Figure 14.2 Oxyhaemoglobin dissociation curve

Embden–Meyerhof (EM) pathway

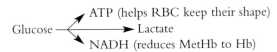

Glucose
→ ATP (helps RBC keep their shape)
→ Lactate
→ NADH (reduces MetHb to Hb)

Hexose monophosphate (HM) pathway

Glucose-6-phosphate ──G6PD──→ 6-phosphogluconate ──→ ribulose-5-phosphate
↘ NADPH (maintains Fe in ferrous state)

Haemopoiesis sites		
Fetus	0–2 months	Yolk sac
	2–7 months	Liver, spleen
	5–9 months	Bone marrow
Infant		Bone marrow (all bones)
Adult		Bone marrow (vertebrae, ribs, pelvis, skull, sternum, proximal end femur)

Extramedullary haemopoiesis is when Hb is synthesised in the liver and spleen outside fetal life.

Haemoglobin types

Adult blood: HbA $\alpha_2\beta_2$ (96–98%)   Fetal blood: HbF $\alpha_2\gamma_2$ (age dependent)

HbA2 $\alpha_2\delta_2$ (1.5–3.2%)   HbA2 $\alpha_2\delta_2$ (age dependent)

HbF $\alpha_2\gamma_2$ (0.5–0.8%)

The switch from fetal haemoglobin (HbF) to adult haemoglobin occurs by 3–6 months of age.

RED BLOOD CELLS (Fig. 14.3)

Cell	Condition
Target cells	Iron deficiency anaemia
	Abnormal Hb (eg. thalassaemia, HbSC disease)
	ELCAT deficiency
	Lipid abnormalities eg. abetalipoproteinaemia, liver disease
Pencil cells	Iron deficiency anaemia
Acanthocytes	Lipid abnormality eg. abetalipoproteinaemia, liver disease
Burr cells	Chronic renal failure
Heinz bodies★	G6PD deficiency
Basophilic stippling	Lead poisoning, thalassaemia, B_{12} deficiency
Ring sideroblasts (in bone marrow)	Sideroblastic anaemia
Howell–Jolly bodies	Postsplenectomy, hyposplenism
Prickle cells	Pyruvate kinase (PK) deficiency
Red cell fragments	Microangiopathic anaemia
Bite cells	G6PD deficiency
Blister cells	G6PD deficiency
Dimorphic film	Post-transfusion
	B_{12}/folate + iron deficiency (eg. coeliac disease)
	Partially treated iron deficiency anaemia
	Sideroblastic anaemia
	Chronic haemolysis with no folic acid
★ = special stain needed	

Anaemia

This can be defined as an inadequate level of haemoglobin.

Normal Hb ranges in childhood

Age	Hb (g/dl)
Birth	14.9–23.7
2 weeks	13.4–19.8

---

2 months	9.4–13.0
6 months	11.1–14.1
1 year	11.3–14.1
2–6 years	11.5–13.5
6–18 years	11.5–16.0

Clinical manifestations

Fatigue, headaches, fainting

Breathlessness, palpitations

General signs – pallor, tachycardia, flow murmur, cardiac failure, retinal haemorrhages (if severe)

Specific signs – eg. koilonychia (iron deficiency), jaundice (haemolysis)

Investigations

Red cell indices   Size: MCV (normocytic, microcytic, macrocytic)

Haemoglobin content: MCH, MCHC (normochromic, hypochromic)

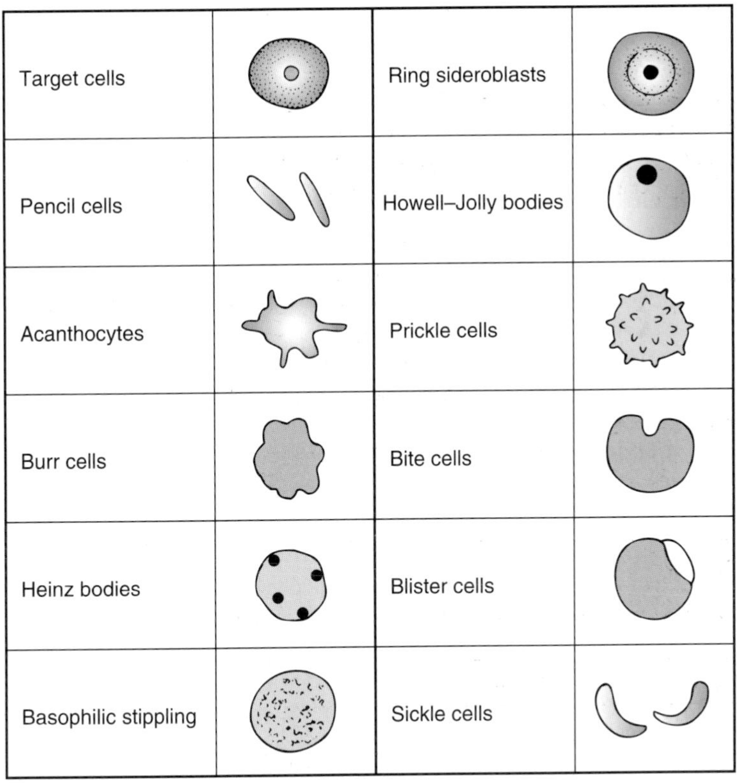

Target cells		Ring sideroblasts	
Pencil cells		Howell–Jolly bodies	
Acanthocytes		Prickle cells	
Burr cells		Bite cells	
Heinz bodies		Blister cells	
Basophilic stippling		Sickle cells	

Figure 14.3 Red blood cells

Reticulocyte count	This rises within 2–3 days of a bleed. Low count suggests marrow failure. High in haemolysis. Normal = 1.5–2%
Platelet and WCC	Low in pancytopenia Rise in haemolysis, haemorrhage or infection
Blood film	Red cell morphology Dimorphic blood film is when features of both microcytosis and macrocytosis are present
Bone marrow	**Aspiration** – smear of bone marrow to view developing cells **Trephine** – core of bone and marrow, useful to view overall marrow architecture, cellularity and abnormal infiltrates

MICROCYTIC HYPOCHROMIC ANAEMIA

Causes

- *iron deficiency*
- *anaemia of chronic disease*
- *sideroblastic anaemia (congenital)*
- *thalassaemia*

Iron deficiency anaemia

Iron metabolism

Iron absorption (maximum 3–4 mg/day) occurs in the duodenum and jejunum (as Fe^{2+}) mainly derived from cereals. Absorbed iron is transported as transferrin (a β-globulin, with Fe^{2+}) in the plasma.

Body iron is present as two-thirds incorporated into Hb molecule, one-third in stores as ferritin (two-thirds) or haemosiderin (one-third) or other iron proteins. These are found in the RE cells of the liver, spleen and bone marrow and in parenchymal liver cells.

A small fraction of ferritin circulates in the serum. The amount of serum ferritin is related to tissue iron stores.

Iron is lost mainly in the stool (in iron-laden macrophages). Loss occurs with nail, hair and skin cell turnover. High requirements are present in rapid growth periods and in pregnancy. In females menstruation accounts for significant losses.

As iron can only be absorbed in the ferrous soluble form, much iron in the diet is unavailable and as there is no physiological mechanism for excretion of iron, the control of iron balance is through absorption. Thus iron deficiency is the commonest cause of anaemia worldwide and iron overload may occur in certain situations. In iron overload, excess iron is transferred to parenchymal cells (eg. those in the heart, pancreas, liver, endocrine organs).

Specific clinical features

Mouth	Painless glossitis, angular stomatitis
Nails	Koilonychia (spoon shaped), brittle, ridged
GIT	Pharyngeal web (Paterson-Kelly, Plummer-Vinson syndrome), pica, atrophic gastritis

Specific investigations

Anaemia

1. RBC indices and film	Hypochromic, microcytic
	Anisocytosis
	Target cells, pencil-shaped poikilocytes
	Moderately raised platelets
2. Serum iron	↓
3. Total iron-binding capacity (TIBC)	↑
4. Serum ferritin	↓
5. Free erythrocyte porphyrin (FEP)	↑
6. Bone marrow	No iron stores in macrophages and no siderotic granules in erythroblasts. Small erythroblasts.

Underlying causes

This should include dietery and absorption history and investigations and a search for blood loss (endoscopy, colonoscopy, Meckel's scan, hookworm ova, haematuria, etc.).

Management

- Treat cause
- Oral iron (tablet, elixir)   Ferrous sulphate (67 mg iron in 200 mg tablet)
       Ferrous gluconate (37 mg iron per 300 mg tablet)
- Parenteral iron (rarely needed)   Intravenous or intramuscular. NB. Anaphylactic reactions can occur

Sideroblastic anaemia

This is an anaemia with hypochromic peripheral cells and increased marrow iron and **ring sideroblasts**. There is disordered haem synthesis.

Causes

1. Inherited	X-linked disease, mitochoncrial (Pearson syndrome)	
2. Acquired	Primary	Myelodysplasia (RARS – refractory anaemia with ring sideroblasts)
	Secondary	Malignant disease of marrow
		Drugs eg. isoniazid, alcohol
		Lead poisoning. NB. Basophilic stippling occurs
		Other conditions eg. malabsorption, haemolytic anaemia

Investigations

1. Blood film. Microcytic, hypochromic, often dimorphic
2. Bone marrow. Erythroblasts with a ring of iron granules on staining with Perls' reaction

Management

- *Withdraw cause*
- *Pyridoxine therapy (especially inherited disease) and folate therapy if deficient*
- *Repeated blood transfusions*

Laboratory tests in hypochromic anaemias

	Iron deficiency	Chronic disease	Sideroblastic	Thalassaemia
MCV, MCH, MCHC	↓	↓ or N	↓ (congenital) ↑ (acquired)	↓↓
Serum iron	↓	↓	↑	N
TIBC	↑	↓	N	N
Serum ferritin	↓	N or ↑	↑	N or ↑
Marrow iron stores	Absent	Present	Present	Present

MACROCYTIC ANAEMIA

This is divided into macrocytic and megaloblastic.

Causes

Megaloblastic anaemia	Macrocytosis
Vitamin B_{12} deficiency	Newborn
Folate deficiency	Pregnancy
DNA synthesis defects eg. orotic aciduria	Liver disease
	Reticulocytosis
	Hypothyroidism

Megaloblastic anaemia

In megaloblastic anaemia there are erythroblasts with delayed maturation of the nucleus present in the bone marrow. Defective DNA synthesis is the underlying cause. There may also be platelet and WCC deficiencies.

Vitamin B_{12} metabolism

Found in animal produce only (liver, fish, dairy produce). Body stores of 2–3 years present.

Diet ⟶ IF-B_{12} complex ⟶ Absorbed in ⟶ Plasma bound to ⟶ Bone marrow
(stomach)   terminal ileum   TC I and TC II   (TC II necessary)
IF = intrinsic factor (made by parietal cells)
TC = transcobalamin (I and II)

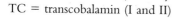

Causes of B$_{12}$ deficiency

- Low intake   Vegans
- Impaired absorption   Gastrectomy, ileal resection
                       Pernicious anaemia
                       Bacterial overgrowth
- Abnormal metabolism   Transcobalamin II deficiency
                       Nitrous oxide

Pernicious anaemia

This is caused by a deficiency or absence of intrinsic factor (IF). It may be congenital (aut. recessible).

- Associations   Older people, Northern European, blue eyes, blood group A
                 Vitiligo, autoimmune thyroid disease, Addison's disease, hypoparathyroidism
                 atrophic gastritis
- Findings   Parietal cell antibodies 90%. Non-specific
                 IF antibody 50% (inhibits B$_{12}$ binding). Specific for PA
                 NB. No antibodies in congenital PA

Folate

Found in green vegetables, liver and kidney. Stores of 3–4 months present. Absorbed in the small intestine.

Causes of folate deficiency

- Inadequate intake   Special diets, coeliac disease, Crohns disease
- Increased utilisation   Physiological: Prematurity, pregnancy
                      Pathological: Haemolysis
                                  Malignant disease
                                  Inflammatory disease
- Increased urine loss   Acute liver disease
- Antifolate drugs   Phenytoin, methotrexate, trimethoprim

Specific clinical features of megaloblastic anaemia

Mouth   Glossitis (sore, beefy red tongue), angular stomatitis

Skin   Lemon yellow (mild jaundice), purpura, melanin pigmentation (unknown mechanism)

Neuropathy   NB. This is in B$_{12}$ deficiency only. (Often associated with a polyneuropathy)

Subacute combined degeneration of the cord:

- a progressive neuropathy of posterior and lateral columns (vibration, proprioception) of the spinal cord
- difficulty walking, ataxia, tingling hands and feet
- absent ankle jerks (peripheral), increased knee jerks (cord)
  Optic atrophy, retinal haemorrhage, dementia may also occur

Investigations

Blood film	Macrocytic
	WCC and platelets may be low
	Neutrophils have hypersegmented nuclei (five or more lobes)
Bone marrow	Hypercellular, megaloblastic changes
Chemistry	Unconjugated bilirubin ↑, hydroxybutyrate ↑, LDH ↑ (due to marrow cell breakdown from ineffective erythropoiesis)
Iron and ferritin	N or ↑

B_{12} and folate tests

Test	B_{12} deficiency	Folate deficiency
Serum B_{12}	↓	N
Serum folate	N, ↑	↓
Red cell folate	N, ↓	↓

Underlying cause

- B_{12} Dietary history, B_{12} absorption (Schilling test), endoscopy, gastric function (IF, gastric acid)
- Folate Dietary history, intestinal malabsorption tests, jejunal biopsy, antendomysial abs

Schilling test

This is used to differentiate inadequate intake from malabsorption and pernicious anaemia.

Oral radioactive-labelled cyanocobalamin is given. Absorption is measured by detecting the amount in a 24-hour urine after 'flushing' it into the urine by giving a large unlabelled IM dose simultaneously, or by whole-body counting of labelled cyanocobalamin. The test is repeated with an IF preparation to see if this allows absorption to occur.

Management

- B_{12} (hydroxycobalamin) Intramuscular, 6 × 1000 μg over three weeks, then three-monthly injections
- Folate Oral supplements daily (1–5 mg)

HAEMOLYTIC ANAEMIAS

These result from an increased rate of red cell destruction. Normal RBC lifespan is 120 days.

Causes

Hereditary	Membrane	Spherocytosis, elliptocytosis
	Metabolism	G6PD deficiency,★ PK deficiency
	Haemoglobin	HbS, HbC, thalassaemias
Acquired	Immune	Autoimmune★ Warm Ab
		Cold Ab

Alloimmune Transfusion reactions★
Haemolytic disease of the newborn
Transplant eg. BMT, cardiac transplant

Drugs induced antibodies★ eg. quinine

Red cell fragmentation syndromes★

Prostheses, ECMO eg. cardiac valves
Microangiopathic HUS, TTP, DIC
Meningococcal septicaemia
Kassabach–Merritt syndrome

Systemic disease eg. renal, liver
Infections★ eg. malaria
Toxins eg. burns, drugs (diapsone, sulphasalazine)
Membrane defect eg. paroxysmal nocturnal haemoglobinuria (PNH)★

★*Denotes that intravascular haemolysis may occur*

Clinical features

- *Pallor*
- *Fluctuating mild jaundice (acholuric, urobilinogen in the urine)*
- *Splenomegaly*
- *Pigment gallstones*
- *Ulcers*
- *Aplastic crises precipitated by parvovirus (eg. SS disease)*
- *Folate deficiency (due to rapid Hb turnover)*

Investigations

Increased RBC production	Reticulocytosis
	Erythroid hyperplasia of bone marrow
Increased RBC breakdown	Unconjugated hyperbilirubinaemia (albumin bound)
	Urine urobilinogen ↑
	Faecal stercobilinogen ↑
	No serum haptoglobins (become saturated with Hb and removed)
Damaged RBC	Microspherocytes, elliptocytes, fragments
	Osmotic fragility ↑
	Autohaemolysis
	Shortened RBC survival (using chromium labelling)
Autoimmune tests	Coombs' test, other Abs

Intravascular haemolysis

This is destruction of the RBC within the circulation. The particular features are:

1. *haemoglobinaemia, haemoglobinuria*
2. *haemosiderinuria (from breakdown of Hb in renal tubules)*
3. *methaemoglobinaemia*
4. *red cell fragments.*

Hereditary spherocytosis (HS)

Autosomal dominant, variable expression. Spherical RBCs (ie. not biconcave discs), due to a defect in spectrin (a membrane protein). Their shape results in the cells being unable to pass through the splenic microcirculation, so they die prematurely.

Associations: Northern Europeans (incidence 1:5000)

Clinical manifestations

Neonatal jaundice
May be asymptomatic
Haemolytic anaemia symptoms as above, particularly:

- *splenomegaly*
- *pigment gall stones, leg ulcers*
- *aplastic or anaemic crises especially with parvovirus*

Investigations

Blood	Anaemia (may not be present)
Film	Reticulocyte counts of 5–20%
	Microspherocytes
Others	Osmotic fragility ↑
	Autohaemolysis ↑

Management

Splenectomy after childhood if severe anaemia, requiring transfusion or impaired growth. Folic acid supplements.

Hereditary elliptocytosis

Autosomal dominant.
  This is similar to spherocytosis.
  The cells are elliptical and the clinical features are milder.

Glucose-6-phosphate dehydrogenase deficiency (G6PD)

X-linked. Females may be mildly affected. NB. Carrier state protects against falciparum malaria. Millions affected worldwide.

  G6PD is an enzyme involved in the hexose-monophosphate pathway (see p. 403), and is the only source of NADPH for a red blood cell. Defective activity of the enzyme results in a susceptibility of the RBC to acute haemolysis with oxidant stress.

There are several types, the commonest being:

- *type A, African type – milder, young RBCs have normal enzyme activity*
- *type B, Mediterranean type – severe, all RBCs affected*

Clinical features

- Neonatal jaundice
- *Haemolytic crises (rapidly developing intravascular haemolysis) induced by oxidant stress, including:*

  1. *sepsis*
  2. *drugs, eg. antimalarials (primaquine, chloroquine, fansidar, maloprim), sulphonamides (co-trimoxazole), chloramphenicol, naphthalene (moth balls), aspirin*
  3. *fava beans (type B only).*

Investigations

Blood   Hb normal between attacks
Enzyme   G6PD levels in RBC. NB. These may be normal in a crisis
During a crisis Bite cells, blister cells, Heinz bodies, reticulocytes, intravascular haemolysis
               NB. No spherocytes.

Management of a crisis

- *Stop causative drug*
- *High fluid input (IV)* → analgesia
- *Transfusions as required*

Pyruvate kinase deficiency

Autosomal recessive   Prevalence: thousands worldwide EM plw.
  Pyruvate kinase is an enzyme involved in the Embden–Meyerhof pathway, deficiency resulting in a reduction in ATP formation and rigid RBCs

Clinical features

Anaemia (Hb 4–10 g/dl) with relatively mild symptoms due to compensatory increased 2,3 DPG levels
  Splenomegaly, jaundice, gallstones, frontal bossing.

Investigations

Blood film   Prickle cells, poikilocytes, reticulocytes
Haemolysis   Autohaemolysis increased
Enzyme   Direct assay of PK

Management

- *Repeated transfusions*
- *Splenectomy*

Autoimmune haemolytic anaemias (AIHA)

These occur as a result of autoantibody production. They are divided into 'warm' and 'cold' types, depending on the temperature at which the antibody reacts better with the red cells. They all have a positive direct antiglobulin test (DAT, Coombs' test).

	Warm AIHA	Cold AIHA
Type of Ab	IgG	IgM
Best temperature for attachment of Ab to RBC	37°C	4°C
Causes	Idiopathic Autoimmune: SLE, RhA Lymphomas CLL Methyldopa	Idiopathic Infections: EBV, CMV, Mycoplasma Lymphomas Paroxysmal cold haemoglobin-uria (NB. IgG Ab)
Clinical features	Haemolytic anaemia Splenomegaly **Evans syndrome =** warm AIHA and ITP, ± neutropenia	Haemolytic anaemia Splenomegaly Acrocyanosis (blue peripheries)
Investigations	Those of haemolytic anaemia Spherocytosis in peripheral blood Positive Coombs' test	Those of haemolytic anaemia Less spherocytosis Positive Coombs' test
Management options	Remove cause Steroids (high dose initially) Splenectomy (if poor response to steroids) Immunosuppression, eg. azathioprine, cyclophosphamide Folic acid and blood transfusions as necessary High-dose immunoglobulin	Remove cause Keep warm Alkylating agents may help

Red cell fragmentation syndromes

These result from physical damage to red cells from:

1. *abnormal surfaces eg. artificial heart valves or grafts*
2. *microangiopathic anaemia when red cells pass through:*

   - fibrin strands in small vessels during DIC
   - damaged vessels in HUS, TTP, meningococcal sepsis or preeclampsia.

Investigations as listed above (intravascular haemolysis).

Paroxysmal nocturnal haemoglobinaemia (PNH)

Acquired defect of red cells making them susceptible to be destroyed by complement. Platelets and WBCs may also be affected.

Clinical features

- Haemolysis
- Dark urine (haemosiderinuria, haemoglobinuria)
- Thrombosis

Specific investigations

Ham's test – red cell lysis occurs at low pH (due to complement activation at low pH).

Management

- Supportive only
- Consider anticoagulation
- Development into leukaemia or aplastic anaemia may occur

APLASTIC ANAEMIAS

This is a pancytopenia (anaemia, leucopenia and thrombocytopenia) due to bone marrow aplasia.

Causes

Primary	Congenital	Fanconi anaemia
		Dyskeratosis congenita
	Idiopathic (50%)	
Secondary	Drugs	1. Regular effect eg. cytotoxics
		2. Sporadic effect eg. chloramphenicol, azathioprine, penicillamine
	Infection	Viral hepatitis, measles, EBV, parvovirus, TB
	Radiation	
	Pregnancy	

Clinical features

Those of bone marrow suppression.

Investigations

Blood film	Anaemia (normocytic, normochromic or macrocytic)
	Leucopenia (particularly neutrophils)
	Thrombocytopenia
Bone marrow	Trephine biopsy (hypoplasia with replacement with fat cells)

Management

- *Remove any cause*
- *Initial supportive therapy*
- *Specific therapy options:*

  1. *bone marrow transplant may be indicated*
  2. *drugs eg. cyclosporin, methylprednisolone, androgens, haemopoietic growth factors, antilymphocyte globulin*

Fanconi anaemia

Autosomal recessive
Presentation at 5–10 years.

Features

Growth retardation

Skeletal	Absent radii or thumbs, microcephaly
Renal	Pelvic or horseshoe kidney
CNS	Mental retardation
Skin	Café-au-lait patches, hypopigmented areas

Increased chromosomal breakages, with AML often developing

Management

BMT (androgen therapy delays progression of disease).

Prognosis

Without BMT, most die from bone marrow failure or AML <30 years.

RED CELL APLASIA

This is an isolated anaemia due to reduced or absent erythroblasts in the bone marrow. It may be a chronic problem or an acute, transient disease lasting 2–3 months.

Causes

Chronic disease

Congenital→Diamond-Blackfan syndrome
Acquired   Idiopathic
                Thymoma, SLE, leukaemia

Acute disease

Infections Parvovirus infection in patients with shortened red cell survival (eg. SS, spherocytosis)
               Infants following viral infection
Drugs   eg. azathioprine, co-trimoxazole

Management

- *Supportive therapy with regular transfusions and iron chelation*
- *Specific treatments include steroid therapy and growth factors*
- *BMT rarely needed*

Diamond–Blackfan syndrome

Autosomal recessive. A pure red cell aplasia, presenting with profound anaemia by 2–6 months of age. Other congenital anomalies (eg. dysmorphic facies, triphalangeal thumbs) in 30%.

Blood film shows a macrocytic anaemia, young red cell population and reduced reticulocytes.

Thrombocytosis and neutropenia may be present initially. Bone marrow shows reduced erythrocyte precursors.

Treatment is with steroids and transfusions as necessary. If steroid unresponsive, immunosuppression, androgens and BMT may be tried.

Genetic haemoglobin disorders

SICKLE CELL HAEMOGLOBINOPATHIES

These involve synthesis of an abnormal haemoglobin. Sickle haemoglobin (HbS) = Hb $\alpha_2\beta_2^S$ (in the β chain, valine is substituted for glutamic acid in position 6).

In low O_2 tensions HbS is insoluble and polymerises as long fibres which result in the red cells becoming sickle shaped. The cells block areas of the microcirculation and result in microinfarcts.

HbS also releases O_2 in the tissues more readily than HbA (ie. the Oxy-Hb dissociation curve shifted to the right).

- *Sickle cell anaemia = HbSS (homozygous disease) 85–95% HbS, 5–15% HbF, no HbA*
- *Sickle cell trait = HbSA (heterozygous disease) 40% HbS, 60% HbA*

Sickle cell anaemia

HbSS disease, seen in Africans, Mediterraneans and Indians.

Clinical features

- *Anaemia – severe haemolytic*
- *Crises*
  1. Painful crises *(vascular-occlusive)*
     Precipitated by cold, hypoxia, infection or dehydration.
     These occur in: bone (commonest)
     dactylitis (hand-foot syndrome) (digital infarcts in small children, resulting in fingers of differing lengths)

chest (sickle chest syndrome)
cerebral (strokes)
kidney, liver, heart
spleen (autosplenectomy)

2. Aplastic crises *(sudden fall in Hb and reticulocytes)*
   Occur with parvovirus infection
3. Acute sequestration *(sickling within organs with blood pooling)*
   Splenic, chest, liver
4. Haemolytic crises *(haemolysis, usually accompanying a painful crisis)*

- *Other – leg ulcers, pigment gall stones, salmonella osteomyelitis, priapism (pooling of blood in the corpora cavernosa), proliferative retinopathy. Splenomegaly in infancy with autosplenectomy later.*

Investigations

Blood film	Hb 6–8 g/dl
	Sickle cells, target cells, Howell–Jolly bodies
Sickledex test	Blood sickles when deoxygenated with dithionate and Na_2HPO_4
Hb electrophoresis	To detect quantities of HbS, HbF and HbA

Management

General	Folic acid 5 mg daily
	Oral penicillin daily
	Triple vaccination (pneumococcal, Hib and meningovax)
	Avoid crisis precipitants
Crisis	Analgesia (strong, usually opiates intravenously)
	Fluids (oral or intravenous)
	Rest
	Antibiotics if infection present
	Transfusion if necessary
	Consider exchange transfusion (severe painful crises, neurological damage, sequestration, sickle chest)
Surgery	Preoperatively for major surgery, transfusions are performed to reduce HbS fraction to <30%
	Anaesthetic care is taken to keep patient warm, well oxygenated and hydrated, and avoid acidosis
New therapies	1. BMT (if unaffected HLA-identical sibling and severe disease)
	2. Hydroxyurea (may increase HbF and decrease frequency of crises)

Sickle trait

Heterozygous expression of the sickle Hb gene. This is HbSA. HbS is 25–45% of the haemoglobin. This blood type appears to protect against *Falciparum malariae*.

Clinical course is usually benign with no anaemia. In severe hypoxia sickling can occur, with resulting ischaemic consequences. Haematuria is the commonest symptom. Care is needed with general anaesthetics and pregnancy.

Diagnosis by Hb electrophoresis and sickle testing.

HAEMOGLOBIN C

In HbC, lysine replaces glutamic acid at position 6 on the β chain.

• *Heterozygous state (HbAC)*	*No anaemia, target cells*
• *Homozygous state (HbCC)*	*Haemolytic anaemia, splenomegaly, target cells*
• **HbSC disease** *(HbS and HbC genes)*	*Hb 9–10 g/dl, target cells*
	Less severe than HbSS
	Thrombosis, pulmonary embolism and retinal vascular changes
	Large spleen

THALASSAEMIAS

These are a heterogeneous group of disorders where there are total or partial deletions of globin chain genes, resulting in a reduced rate of synthesis of normal α- or β-chains and precipitation of the excess chains in the red cells which causes haemolysis. In α-thalassaemias whole α-globin genes are deleted, whereas in β-thalassaemia mainly point mutations within the β-globin genes occur (over 100 mutations have been identified)

Thalassaemia comes from the Greek 'thalassa' for 'sea', as the disease was found in people on the shores of the Mediterranean. It is found in tropical and subtropical areas (Asia, N. Africa and Mediterranean).

- • *β-thalassaemia*   *Due to reduced or absent β-globin chains (excess α-chains precipitate)*
- • *α-thalassaemia*   *Due to reduced or absent α-globin chains (excess β-chains precipitate)*

Chromosome 16 codes for α-globin.
Chromosome 11 codes for β, δ and γ-globins.

Clinical types

- • *α-Thalassaemias*
- • *β-Thalassaemia major*
- • *Thalassaemia intermedia*
- • *Thalassaemia minor*

Haemoglobin types involved

HbA	$\alpha_2 \beta_2$
HbA2	$\alpha_2 \delta_2$
HbF	$\alpha_2 \gamma_2$
HbH	β_4
HbBarts	γ_4 (no oxygen carrying ability)

β-Thalassaemia major

Homozygous disease. Either β° (no β-chains) or β^+ (small amounts).

Haemoglobin electrophoresis:	HbF	70–90%
	HbA2	2%
	± HbA	0–20%

Clinical features

Severe anaemia from 3–6 months	When switch from γ to β-chain production normally occurs
Hepatosplenomegaly	Due to haemolysis and haemopoiesis
Extramedullary and medullary haemopoiesis	Thalassaemic facies, frontal bossing, maxillary hyperplasia
	'Hair on end' skull X-ray appearance
	Cortical thinning with fractures
Iron overload	See below. Due to multiple transfusions
Infections	Hepatitis B and C (multiple blood transfusions)
	Yersinia enterocolytica (seen with desferrioxamine therapy)
	Encapsulated organisms (autosplenectomy)

Investigations

Blood film	Microcytic hypochromic anaemia, target cells, basophilic stippling, nucleated red cells
Hb electrophoresis	As above
DNA analysis	May be used to identify the genetic defect

Management

Transfusions	4–6 weekly (transfuse when Hb >10 g/dl; this is 'hypertransfusion')
Folic acid	5 mg daily
Iron chelation	Subcutaneous desferrioxamine for 8–12 hours, five days per week. NB. Need auditory and ophthalmological assessments, while on desferrioxamine
	Chelated iron is excreted in the urine and stools
Vitamin C	200 mg/day. Increases iron excretion
Splenectomy	May be needed to decrease blood requirements (done >6 years)
Endocrine therapy	As necessary (pituitary, insulin, thyroid, parathyroid)
BMT	Recommended in childhood (if unaffected HLA-identical sibling)

Iron overload

Damage caused:

1. *Liver – cirrhosis, hepatoma*
2. *Heart – Cardiomyopathy (arrhythmias, cardiac failure)*
3. *Endocrine – IDDM, growth failure, delayed puberty, hypothyroidism, hypoparathyroidism, osteoporosis*
4. *Skin – 'Slate-grey' appearance*

Investigation and management (see p. 198).

β-Thalassaemia minor (trait)

Heterozygous disease with reduced β-chains.

Clinical features	Asymptomatic
Blood film	Mild or no anaemia (Hb 10–15 g/dl)
	Microcytic, hypochromic picture, target cells
Hb electrophoresis	HbA
	HbA2 >3.5%
	HbF ↑

Thalassaemia intermedia

This is a clinical syndrome, resulting from several different gene defects:

- *homozygous β-thalassaemia with persisting HbF*
- *homozygous β-thalassaemia with coexisting α-thalassaemia*
- *heterozygous β-thalassaemia (trait) with coexisting extra α-chains*

Clinical features

Variable.

- *Symptomatic anaemia (Hb 7–10 mg/dl)*
- *Splenomegaly, hepatomegaly, extramedullary haemopoiesis, leg ulcers, gall stones, infections*

Management

Transfusions may be required
Hydroxyurea
Splenectomy if necessary

α-Thalassaemias

These all involve decreased synthesis of α-chains. There are **four** genes for α-globin because the gene is duplicated on chromosome 16. Deletion of one α-globin gene results in a silent carrier with only a mild microcytosis.

Hydrops foetalis (Hb Barts)

No α-chains (4 genes deleted).

Hb electrophoresis	Hb Barts (γ 4)
	No HbF

Death occurs *in utero* due to lack of HbF unless there is early prenatal diagnosis and intrauterine transfusions.

HbH disease

Three α-globin genes are deleted.

Hb electrophoresis	HbH, HbA, Hb Barts (in fetus)
Blood film	Microcytic, hypochromic anaemia (Hb 7–10 g/dl)
	'Golf ball' cells (aggregates of β-globin chains)
Splenomegaly	Thalassaemia intermedia syndrome.

No treatment required.

α-Thalassaemia trait

One or two α-globin genes are deleted.
Asymptomatic.

Investigations:

Hb electrophoresis	Normal ± HbH
Blood film	No/mild anaemia, hypochromic, microcytic cells
Globin chain synthesis studies	α:β-chain synthesis ratio is reduced
DNA studies	

Antenatal and neonatal diagnosis of sickle cell and thalassaemia

Antenatal diagnosis

This can be done with:

Fetal blood sampling (electrophoresis)	Umbilical cord blood in second trimester (18–20 weeks), to check normal chain manufacture
DNA analysis	Amniotic fluid (second trimester)
	Chorionic villous sampling in first trimester (8–10 weeks)

Neonatal diagnosis

Hb electrophoresis can be done at birth but the switch from γ-chains (HbF) to β-chains occurs at 3–6 months, making testing at six months accurate. DNA analysis can be used to identify the defect on each allele.

Polycythaemia and thrombocythaemia

POLYCYTHAEMIA

These are blood changes involving increased Hb levels to above the upper limit of normal and increased haematocrit. They may be 'relative', due to decreased circulating volume.

Causes

Primary	Polycythaemia rubra vera (PV)	
Secondary	Appropriate	Cyanotic heart disease
		Lung disease
		High altitude
		Central hypoventilation
	Inappropriate	Renal disease (eg. hydronephrosis, cysts, tumour)
		Adrenal disease (eg. CAH, Cushing syndrome)
		Tumour (eg. cerebellar haemangioblastoma, hepatocellular carcinoma)

Relative   Neonatal (eg. infant of diabetic mother, IUGR, twin-twin transfusion)

Dehydration (eg. gastrointestinal losses, burns, etc.)

Stress polycythaemia

Clinical features

- *Haemorrhage or thrombosis*
- *Headaches*

Management

- *Treat cause*
- *Venesection if necessary*
- *Chemotherapy (for PV)*

THROMBOCYTHAEMIA

Causes

Endogenous   Essential thrombocythaemia

CML, PV

Reactive   Haemorrhage

Postoperative

Kawasaki disease

Chronic infections

Connective tissue disease

Postsplenectomy

Iron deficiency and haemolytic anaemia, malignancies

Clinical features

Usually asymptomatic; risk of thrombosis is rare.

Management

Often no treatment is required. To reduce the risk of thrombosis, platelet pheresis, low-dose aspirin or anagrelide (antiplatelet drug) may be used.

Cytotoxics or α-interferon are used in essential thrombocythaemia.

Haemostasis

Haemostasis involves:

- *normal vasculature*
- *platelets*
- *coagulation factors*

PLATELETS

Produced from megakaryocytes in the bone marrow, lifespan 7–10 days.

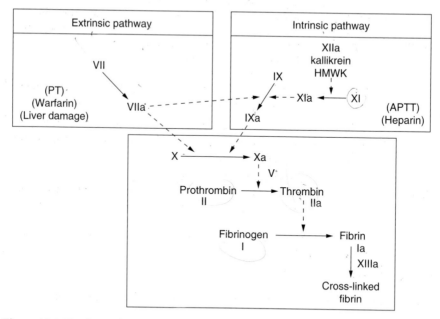

Figure 14.4 Blood coagulation cascade: HMWK = High molecular weight kininogen

Functions

Mechanical plug formation in vascular trauma. This involves adhesion (VWF involved), secretion of granule contents (including arachidonic acid), aggregation and procoagulant activity (involving PF3 and coagulation factors).

BLOOD COAGULATION CASCADE

This involves activation of the blood coagulation factors, resulting in production of thrombin and a fibrin clot. Fibrin stabilises the initial platelet plug.

INVESTIGATIONS OF COAGULATION

Blood count and film	Platelets (morphology, count), other abnormalities
Bleeding time	Measures platelet plug formation *in vivo*
	Prolonged in thrombocytopenia and platelet function disorders
Prothrombin time (PT)	Measures factors VII, X, V, prothrombin, fibrinogen (extrinsic and common pathways). Tissue thromboplastin and calcium added to sample
	Normal = 10–14 seconds (INR = 1)
	May be expressed as international normalised ratio (INR)

	Prolonged in liver disease, vitamin K-dependent clotting factors
	Used to monitor warfarin therapy
Activated partial thromboplastin time (APTT)	Measures factors V, VIII, IX, X, XI, XII, prothrombin, fibrinogen (intrinsic and common pathways). Surface activator, phospholipid and calcium added
	Normal = 30–40 seconds
	Used to monitor heparin therapy
Thrombin clotting time (TT)	Abnormal in fibrinogen deficiency or thrombin inhibition. Thrombin added to sample. Normal = 14–16 seconds

NB. Prolonged PT or APTT due to factor deficiency are corrected when normal plasma is added. If correction is incomplete with normal plasma, then an **inhibitor of coagulation** may be present (eg. lupus anticoagulant).

Coagulation factors	Specific assays of individual clotting factors
Fibrinolysis tests	Detection of fibrinogen or fibrin degradation products (FDPs) Plasminogen ($\downarrow$ in enhanced fibrinolyis), plasminogen activator ($\uparrow$)

VASCULAR DISORDERS

These involve abnormalities in the vessels or the perivascular connective tissues.

Causes
Inherited Hereditary haemorrhagic telangiectasia
Acquired Easy bruising
 HSP (Henoch-Schönlein purpura)
 Infections eg. meningitis
 Scurvy
 Drugs eg. steroids
 Connective tissue disorders eg. Ehlers-Danlos

Clinical features
Not usually severe. Skin and mucous membrane bleeding (easy bruising, petechaiae, ecchymoses).

Investigations
Screening tests normal (including the bleeding time).

Hereditary haemorrhagic telangiectasia
Autosomal dominant. Telangiectasia in the skin, mucous membranes and internal organs, becoming more numerous throughout life. Recurrent GI bleeding occurs.

PLATELET DISORDERS

These include thrombocytopenia and platelet function disorders.

Thrombocytopenia

Causes of thrombocytopenia
Decreased production
  Isolated megakaryocyte depression Infections
                                      TAR syndrome
                                      Drugs
  Abnormal megakaryocytes   Wiskott–Aldrich syndrome
  Bone marrow failure   Aplastic anaemias
Increased consumption
  Immune disease   ITP
                                      Drug induced eg. quinine, trimethoprin
                                      Postinfectious eg. malaria
                                      Neonatal isoimmune (maternal antiplatelet
                                      antibodies)
                                      SLE, heparin
                                      Post-transfusional (Pl^{A1} antibodies)
  DIC
  TTP, HUS
Abnormal distribution
  Splenomegaly

Idiopathic thrombocytopenic purpura (immune thrombocytopenia, ITP)
Common in children
Mechanism not established, immune complex suspected.
Associations: Following infection eg. VZV, measles, EBV or vaccination

Clinical features
1–4 weeks postinfection: bleeding, bruising, petechiae, mucosal bleeding, intracranial bleeds (very rare).

Investigations
Blood film   Platelets $\downarrow$ (<10–20×10^9/l)
                  Hb and WCC normal
Bone marrow   Megakaryocytes $\uparrow$ or N
Antibodies   Antiplatelet IgG, antiplatelet IgM

Management options

- *Monitoring only*
- *Steroids*
- *Intravenous immunoglobulin (IVIG)*
- *Platelet transfusions (in emergency, they are quickly destroyed)*
- *Immunosuppression and/or splenectomy only if no response to treatment and chronic disease*

Prognosis

Spontaneous remission   Most cases
Chronic disease   5–10% in childhood (commoner in adults)

Thrombotic thrombocytopenic purpura (TTP)

This is a serious disease involving thrombocytopenia with arteriolar thrombi. Features are similar to HUS, with more widespread involvement.

Clinical features

A classic pentad of:

1. *fevers*
2. *haemolytic anaemia*
3. *thrombocytopenia – purpura*
4. *CNS – fluctuating neurological signs*
5. *Renal – ischaemic damage*

Investigations

Blood film   Platelets ↓
              Microangiopathic anaemia
Serum   LDH ↑

Management options

- *Plasmapheresis, FFP*
- *Steroids, cytotoxics, antiplatelet drugs*

Thrombocytopenia absent radius (TAR) syndrome

This involves:

1. *thrombocytopenia, megakaryocytes ↓, anaemia, eosinophilia*
2. *bilateral absent radii and thumbs, abnormal humerus and ulnar*
3. *leg involvement (50%) – CDH, patella and knee dislocations, small feet, tibial torsion*
4. *other associations – CHD, renal abnormalities, mental retardation, spina bifida, 100% have cows milk protein intolerance*

Platelet function disorders

Causes

Hereditary   Bernard-Soulier syndrome
              Glanzmann disease
              Grey platelet syndrome
              Hermansky–Pudlak syndrome (platelet function + albinism)
Acquired   Drugs: aspirin (cyclo-oxygenase inhibition)
                     heparin (inhibits segregation and secretion)
              Myeloproliferative disorders
              Uraemia

Investigations

Blood film   Normal platelet count

Bleeding time Prolonged
Specific tests Platelet aggregation studies with ADP, adrenaline, collagen, ristocetin
Other tests eg. adhesion studies, nucleotide pool measurement
von Willebrand factor assay
Factor VIII assay

Bernard–Soulier syndrome

- *Autosomal recessive, deficiency of membrane glycoprotein Ib*
- *Platelet adhesion defects (no aggregation with ristocetin)*
- *Large platelets with some thrombocytopenia*

Glanzmann disease

Autosomal recessive, failure of platelet aggregation due to deficiency of membrane glycoproteins IIb and IIIa.

CLOTTING FACTOR DISORDERS

Haemophilia A

- *Incidence 30–100: 1 000 000*
- *X-linked recessive, 30% spontaneous mutation rate*
- *Gene located at Xq2.8*
- *Disease of absent or low factor VIII*

Clinical features

Spontaneous bleeding Joints (haemarthroses), painful, swollen, resulting in deformity
Muscle haematomas
'Pseudotumours' in bones due to repeated subperiosteal bleeds
Haematuria
Intracerebral bleeds (rare)
Excessive traumatic bleeding Surgery eg. postcircumcision, dental extractions
Infection (transfusion related) HIV, hepatitis B and C (subclinical liver disease)

Severity depends on the amount of factor VIII (% of normal) present:
<1% severe disease with frequent spontaneous bleeds
1–5% severe bleeds with injury, occasional spontaneous bleeds
>5% mild disease

Investigations

1. *Factor VIIIc activity*
2. *APTT ($\uparrow$)*

Management

This can involve:

1. *Recombinant factor VIII infusions as prophylaxis.*
2. *Recombinant factor VIII infusions after injury or prior to surgery:*

Injury	Factor VIII levels aimed for (% of normal)
Minor bleed	>30%
Severe bleed	>50%
Pre major surgery	100%

3. *DDAVP (desmopressin)*   *Use in mild disease, intravenous or inhaled (causes a rise in the patient's own factor VIII levels)*
4. *Fibrinolytic inhibitor*   *eg. tranexamic acid, may be given with DDAVP*
5. *Advice*   *Avoid contact sports, good oral hygiene*

Factor VIII antibodies

These occur in 10% of haemophiliacs. Management options include:

- *give very large doses of factor VIII*
- *immunosuppression*
- *give factor IX concentrate which bypasses the factor VIII, recombinant factor VIII or porcine factor VIII*

Antenatal and carrier detection

Carrier female   Plasma factor VIII activity (usually < half normal)
DNA probes (more accurate)
Antenatal   Foetal DNA using chorionic villous biopsy at 8–10 weeks
Foetal factor VIII activity using foetal blood sampling at 18–20 weeks

Haemophilia B (Christmas disease)

- *Incidence 1: 30 000 males*
- *X-linked recessive, gene at Xq2.6*
- *Deficiency of factor IX*
- *Clinical features identical to haemophilia A*
- *Management is with factor IX concentrate*

von Willebrand disease

- *Incidence 30–100: 1 000 000*
- *Autosomal dominant, variable expression, worse in females*
- *Disorder of: Low vWF (causing low factor VIII activity)*
  Platelet adhesion abnormalities
- ***von Willebrand factor (vWF)***   *Is the carrier protein for factor VIII*
  Promotes platelet adhesion

Clinical features

Variable.
Excessive bleeding   Cuts, operative, mucous membranes (menorrhagia, epistaxis)
Spontaneous bleeds   Haemarthroses and muscles (rare except in homozygotes)

Investigations

Bleeding time	Prolonged
Factor VIIIc activity	↓
VWF levels	↓
Platelet aggregation with ristocetin	↓

Management

Acute bleeds treated with factor VIII concentrate containing vWF, DDAVP or fibrinolytic inhibitors.

Vitamin K deficiency

This affects the Vitamin K-dependent clotting factors **II, VII, IX and X**. Vitamin K is a fat-soluble vitamin, present in green vegetables and synthesised in the gut.

Causes of vitamin K-dependent clotting factor deficiency

Low vitamin K stores	Haemorrhagic disease of the newborn
	Inadequate diet
Malabsorption of fat-soluble vitamins	Hepatic obstruction
	Small bowel disease
Vitamin K antagonists	eg. warfarin

Investigations

PT   ↑↑
APTT   ↑ or N

Management

Vitamin K	IV takes six hours to work
	IM or oral (as prophylaxis)
FFP	Immediate effect
Prothrombin concentrates	Immediate effect

Disseminated intravascular coagulation (DIC)

This is a consumption of platelets and clotting factors with widespread intravascular fibrin deposition. It may be acute or more chronic.

Causes

Sepsis	eg. meningococcal, Gram-negative, viral (purpura fulminans)
Widespread tissue damage	Trauma, burns, surgery
Obstetric	Eclampsia, amniotic fluid embolism
Malignancy	Acute promyelocytic leukaemia
Hypersensitivity reactions	Anaphylaxis
Other	Hypoxia, hypothermia, snake venom, Kasabach-Merritt syndrome

Clinical features

Severely unwell patient with generalised bleeding (acute disease).

Investigations

Blood count and film	Platelets ($\downarrow$), microangiopathic anaemia
TT	$\uparrow$
APTT	$\uparrow$
PT	$\uparrow$
FDPs	$\uparrow$, fibrinogen $\downarrow$
Factors	V and VIII ($\downarrow$)

NB. Chronic disease may have normal screening results, due to production of new factors.

Management

1. *Underlying cause*
2. *Supportive therapy (blood, FFP, fibrinogen, platelets)*
3. *Heparin and antiplatelet drugs controversial*

Haemostasis tests

	BT	Plts	PT	APTT	TT	FVIIIc	FIX	vWFAg
Haemophilia A	N	N	N	$\uparrow$	N	$\downarrow$	N	N
Haemophilia B	N	N	N	$\uparrow$	N	N	$\downarrow$	N
VW disease	$\uparrow$	N	N	$\uparrow$ or N	N	$\downarrow$	N	$\downarrow$
Liver disease	N,$\uparrow$	$\downarrow$	$\uparrow$	$\uparrow$	N,$\uparrow$	N	$\downarrow$	N
DIC	N,$\uparrow$	$\downarrow$	$\uparrow$	$\uparrow$	$\uparrow\uparrow$	$\downarrow$	$\downarrow$	$\downarrow$

THROMBOSIS

Pathogenesis of thrombosis is related to Virchow's triad of:

1. *hypercoagulability*
2. *intravascular stasis*
3. *vessel wall damage*

- *Arterial thrombosis occurs mainly as a result of vessel wall damage eg. arteriosclerosis.*
- *Venous thrombosis occurs mainly as a result of hypercoagulability and venous stasis.*

Causes of venous thrombosis

Hypercoagulability

Congenital	Antithrombin III deficiency
	Protein S or C deficiency
	Increased fibrinogen or factor VIII levels
	Factor V Leiden
	Abnormal plasminogen or fibrinogen
Acquired	Trauma
	Lupus anticoagulant
	Pregnancy and OCP
	Malignancy
	Thrombocytosis

Stasis   Immobilisation
            Venous obstruction
            Dehydration
            Pump failure

Investigations

These may include:

Blood count and film Platelets (↑), haematocrit (↑), malignancy

PT, APTT May be shortened. NB. If prolonged and does not correct with normal plasma, suggests lupus anticoagulant

TT, reptilase time Prolonged if fibrinogen abnormal

Fibrinogen assay
Protein S and C assay
Antithrombin III assay
Factor V Leiden (PCR)

The Spleen

SPLENECTOMY

This may occur naturally (autosplenectomy) or as a result of therapeutic surgical removal of the spleen, eg. sickle cell anaemia (autosplenectomy), ITP (therapy).

The consequences are:

Immediate Marked thrombocytosis (platelets > $1000 \times 10^9/l$), usually for 2–3 weeks, then moderate increase

Long term Susceptibility to encapsulated organisms (eg. pneumococcus), and malaria Young infants at particular risk of pneumococcal infections, *Haemophilus influenzae* and *Niesseria meningitidis*

Blood count and film findings in hyposplenism

- *Platelets may be high*
- *Monocytosis, lymphocytosis*
- *Howell–Jolly bodies, Pappenheimer granules, target cells, irregular contracted red cells*

Management

- *Try to avoid splenectomy in children <6 years (increased susceptibility to infections)*
- *Prophylactic penicillin (for life)*
- *Triple vaccination >2 weeks prior to splenectomy (pneumovax, Hib and meningovax)*
- *Malaria prophylaxis when travelling to endemic areas*

SPLENOMEGALY

This can result in abdominal discomfort and a pancytopenia (hypersplenism), as the spleen sequesters and destroys cells.

Causes of splenomegaly

Massive splenomegaly	Malaria, Kalar–Azar, CML, myelofibrosis
Infections	Acute: EBV, SBE, septicaemia
	Chronic: TB, brucellosis, schistosomiasis
Extra-medullary	
haemopoeisis	Haemolytic anaemias, haemoglobinopathies, osteopetrosis
Neoplasms	Leukaemia, lymphoma, haemangioma
Portal hypertension	
Storage diseases	Gaucher disease, Niemann–Pick, Langerhans cell histiocytosis, muccopolysaccharoidoses
Systemic disease	SLE, RhA (Felty's), amyloidosis

FURTHER READING

Hann IM, Lake BD, Lilleyman J, Pritchard J, Weatherall DJ *Colour Atlas of Paediatric Haematology*, Oxford University Press, Oxford, 1996

Lilleyman JS, Hann IM, Blanchette VS *Paediatric Haematology* 2nd Ed, Churchill Livingstone, Edinburgh, 1999

Nathan DG, Orkin SH *Hematology of Infancy and Childhood*. 5th Ed Vol 1 and 2 Ed: Nathan SH, Orkin SH, WB Saunders, Philadelphia, 1997

15

Oncology

- *General*
- *Specific cancers*

General

CHILDHOOD CANCER

Incidence: 1 : 650 children develop cancer by age 16 years.

Relative frequencies		
	Leukaemia	34%
	Brain tumours	23%
	Lymphomas	11%
	Neuroblastoma	6%
	Wilms tumour	6%
	Bone tumours	5%
	Rhabdomyosarcoma	4%
	Retinoblastoma	3%

Aetiology
Factors that influence the development of cancer, involve inherited cancer genes and altered somatic genes.

Genetic factors
Oncogene expression	eg. activation of C-myc oncogene – All
Loss of tumour suppression genes	eg. retinoblastoma *RB1* gene
DNA Repair gene defects	eg. Ataxia relangiectasia, xeroderma pigmentosum

Environmental factors
Ionising radiation	eg. leukaemia, thyroid carcinoma, breast cancer
Ultraviolet radiation	eg. skin cancers
Viruses	eg. retrovirus – T cell leukaemia
	EB virus – Burkitt lymphoma and Hodgkin disease, nasopharyngeal carcinoma
Drugs	eg. diethylstilboestrol in pregnancy – vaginal adenocarcinoma in the daughter
	the immunosuppressive drugs – generalised risk
	anabolic steroids – liver tumours

Management is complex, involving many specialists and therapies, including chemotherapy, radiotherapy, surgery and bone marrow transplant.

CHEMOTHERAPEUTIC AGENTS

Drug	Action	Toxicity
Antimetabolites		
Methotrexate	Folic acid antagonist Inhibits dihydrofolate reductase	Cirrhosis Severe perforating enteritis Myelosuppression Dermatitis, stomatitis Renal impairment
6-Mercaptopurine (6-MP)	Purine analogue Inhibits purine synthesis	Myelosuppression Hepatic necrosis
Alkylating agents		
Cyclophosphamide	Inhibits DNA synthesis	Myelosuppression Secondary malignancy Sterility Lung fibrosis SIADH Haemorrhagic cystitis (give Mesna)
Vinca alkaloids		
Vincristine	Inhibits microtubule formation	Peripheral neuropathy Seizures, ptosis Constipation, SIADH Local cellulitis (extravasation injuries) Minimal myelosuppression Jaw pain
Vinblastine	Inhibits microtubule formation	Leucopaenia, local, cellulitis
Antibiotics		
Doxorubicin and daunorubicin	Bind to DNA	Cardiotoxicity Red urine Nausea and vomiting Hair loss Myelosuppression Necrosis on extravasation
Bleomycin	Binds to DNA	Lung fibrosis Dermatitis, stomatitis
Enzymes		
L-Asparaginase	L-asparagine depletion	Pancreatitis, hyperglycaemia Allergies Coagulopathy Encephalopathy
Others		
Cisplatin	Inhibits DNA synthesis	Nephrotoxic

Etoposide	Topoisomerase inhibitor	Neurotoxic, ototoxic Myelosuppression Myelosuppression Secondary AML

BONE MARROW TRANSPLANT (BMT)

A bone marrow transplant replaces the marrow with normal stem cells. The initial marrow is ablated with high-dose chemotherapy and radiotherapy and then the patient rescued with the BMT. Used for therapy after relapse of leukaemia and now also in initial consolidation therapy.

Autologous BMT
The patient acts as their own donor. Marrow is harvested (may be purged of malignant cells) and cryopreserved and then reinfused. Peripheral blood stem cells may be harvested with granulocyte colony-stimulating factor (GCSF).

Complications

- *Residual cancer cells cause relapse*
- *Conditioning toxicity (including infertility and secondary malignancy)*
- *Infections in cytopaenic phase (two weeks for peripheral blood stem cell transplant, four weeks for BMT)*

Allogeneic BMT
Marrow from a matched donor (HLA screened). Best donor is an HLA–identical sibling (matched related donor). The conditioning with chemotherapy and radiotherapy here is also used to destroy the patient's immune system to prevent rejection.

Complications

- *Marrow rejection*
- *GVHD (acute or chronic)*
- *Infections*
- *Acute regimen-related toxicity (initial ablative therapy causes venoocclusive disease, pneumonitis, haemorrhagic cystitis)*

GRAFT-VERSUS-HOST DISEASE (GVHD)

This is due to donor T lymphocytes mounting an immune response to host MHC antigens. There is a beneficial graft-versus-leukaemia (GVL) effect of the process.

Acute GVHD (<100 days of BMT)
This is characterised by:

Rash	Pruritic maculopapular on ears, palms, soles, then trunk May progress to bullae or exfoliation, usually occurs in the third week.

Cholestatic hepatitis

Enteritis	Bloody diarrhoea
Other features	Fever, protein-losing enteropathy, marrow aplasia, infections
Predisposing factors	HLA differences between donor and host, sex mismatch, active malignancy at time of BMT
Prevention	T cell depletion of donor marrow

Chronic GVHD (>100 days post–BMT)

This is characterised by:

Rash	Hyperpigmented nodules, lichenoid, erythema, hypopigmented, then scleroderma-like
Other	Arthritis, hepatitis, malabsorption
Autoimmune features	SLE, scleroderma, Sjögren syndrome, primary biliary cirrhosis
Infections	Bacterial, fungal, viral
Predisposing factors	Acute GVHD, increasing age, buffy coat transfusions

Management

This is with further immunosuppression eg. cyclosporin A, steroids.

TUMOUR LYSIS SYNDROME

This results from a high rate of cellular breakdown and occurs in fast-growing tumours (especially with high WCC ALL and bulky NHL) and when chemotherapy is given. It is potentially life threatening and dialysis may be necessary.

Features

1. *Firstly K $\uparrow$ within hours*
2. *Then $PO_4 \uparrow$ with simultaneous Ca $\downarrow$ (within 1–2 days)*
3. *Then urate $\uparrow$.*

Preventive measures

1. *Intravenous fluids (with no added K) and alkalinisation prior to chemotherapy*
2. *Regular monitoring of biochemistry*
3. *Allopurinol*
4. *Dialysis or haemofiltration (used prophylactically in bulky tumours)*

NAUSEA AND VOMITING

These are common side-effects of chemotherapy.

Centres involved

- *Visceral afferents*
- *Chemoreceptor trigger zone (CTZ)*
- *Vomiting centre (in the medulla)*

- *Higher centres (emotional)*
- *Vestibular apparatus*

Common antiemetics

Drug	Action	Adverse effects
Ondansetron	5-HT3 antagonist	Elevated transaminases
Metoclopramide	CTZ + peripheral gut	Acute dystonic reactions (oculogyrate crises, spasms)
Cyclizine	Antihistamine	Those of antihistamines (drowsiness, dry mouth, blurred vision)

Specific cancers

NEUROBLASTOMA

A tumour arising from *neural crest cells* of the sympathetic nervous system developing in:

- *adrenal medulla − 50%*
- *sympathetic chain − anywhere from the posterior cranial fossa to the coccyx*

Tumours of neural crest cells may be benign ganglioneuromas, ganglioneuroblastomas or malignant neuroblastomas and may spontaneously regress in infants.

Cytogenetic abnormalities
Carry a poor prognosis if these are present.

- *Chromosome 1p partial deletion*
- *Chromosome 17 abnormalities*
- *Amplification of N-myc oncogene*

Clinical features
Usually <5 years
Abdominal mass
Metastatic disease (70%) Weight loss, pallor, malaise
Hepatomegaly, lymphadenopathy
Bone pain, limp
Proptosis, periorbital bruising
Cord compression (paraplegia)
Skin nodules
Horner syndrome

Investigations
CT or MRI scan
MIBG scan Meta-iodobenzylguanidine (a catecholamine precursor, outlines metastases)
Urine catecholamines Homovanillic acid (HVA) and vanillylmandelic acid (VMA) (↑)
Tissue biopsy Necessary to confirm diagnosis

Blood tests	FBC (anaemia, thrombocytopaenia), coagulation (abnormal) LDH, ferritin, creatinine (all ↑)
Bone scan	Metastases?

Staging

A   Grossly resectable tumour

B   Localised unresectable tumour

C   Lymph node metastases

D   Further metastases

Ds   Neonates with small adrenal tumour and metastases in skin, liver or bone marrow only (Ds can undergo spontaneous remission)

Management

Options involve:

Surgical resection	
Chemotherapy	Before and/or after surgery
Radiotherapy	With chemotherapy or palliative

Prognosis

30% five-year survival with metastatic disease.

Screening

Attempted in Japanese infants using urine catecholamine screen. Results controversial as pick-up rate for aggressive tumours is low.

NEPHROBLASTOMA (WILMS TUMOUR)

Incidence 7.8:million. 5% have bilateral disease at presentation.

Associations	Genitourinary anomalies	4.4%
	Hemihypertrophy	2.9%
	Aniridia	1.1%
	Neurofibromatosis	
	Beckwith–Weidemann syndrome	
	Chromosome 11 loci deletions	

Clinical manifestations

- *Mean age three years*
- *Abdominal mass (most common presentation)*
- *Abdominal pain, vomiting*
- *Hypertension*
- *Haematuria*

Staging

I   Kidney only

II   Beyond the kidney, but completely excisable

III   Unresectable local tumour

IV   Haematogenous metastases (usually lung)

V   Bilateral

Investigations

Imaging Abdominal USS
           CT
           CXR (lung metastases?)

Urine   Haematuria (micro- or macroscopic)

Management options

- *Primary nephrectomy then chemotherapy*
- *Initial chemotherapy and delayed nephrectomy (if large tumour)*
- *Radiotherapy only for advanced disease*

Prognosis

80% overall survival

60% survival if metastatic

Poor survival if relapse

SOFT TISSUE SARCOMAS

Incidence 1.4:million per year. More common in caucasians.

They comprise:

1. *rhabdomyosarcoma >50%*
2. *non-rhabdomyosarcoma soft tissue tumours (NRSTS) – eg. liposarcoma, angiosarcoma, leiomyosarcoma, neurofibrosarcoma and fibrosarcoma.*

Rhabdomyosarcoma

Tumour of primitive mesenchymal tissue (tissue that striated skeletal muscle arises from).

Associations Neurofibromatosis
               Li-Fraumeni syndrome

They may occur anywhere, but the most common sites are:

- *head and neck*   *40%*
- *genitourinary (GU) tract* *20%*
- *trunk*   *10%*

Clinical features

Head and neck tumour Proptosis
                       Nasal obstruction, blood-stained nasal discharge, facial swelling, cranial nerve palsies

GU tract tumour   Obstruction, dysuria, blood-stained vaginal discharge

Metastatic disease is present in 15% at diagnosis (liver, lung, bone).

Staging

I   Completely resectable

II   Microscopic residual tumour
III   Macroscopic residual tumour
IV   Metastatic

Investigations

Imaging of relevant area	CT, USS, MRI scan
Metastases search	Bone scan, CXR and CT, bone marrow
Tumour tissue	Histology

Management options

This depends on tumour stage and location.

- *Initial surgical resection then chemotherapy (and radiotherapy if residual disease or metastatic)*
- *Preoperative chemotherapy (if large primary)*

Prognosis

80% survival if resectable (some sites have a better prognosis than others)
66% survival if incompletely resected
<50% survival if metastatic

BONE TUMOURS

Incidence 5.6: million in white children and adolescents. Commonest age=second decade. Male > female.

The most common bone tumours are osteosarcoma and Ewing sarcoma; rarer ones are chondrosarcoma and fibrosarcoma.

	Osteosarcoma	Ewing sarcoma
Associations	More common Retinoblastoma Li-Fraumeni syndrome Pagets Osteogenesis imperfecta	Less common 11 : 22 translocation
Site	Metaphysis (proximal end) of long bones Distal femur, proximal tibia	Flat bones (ribs, pelvis, vertebrae) Diaphysis of long bones
Presentation	Bone pain and mass	Bone pain and mass Soft tissue component, fever
X-ray findings	Skip lesions, sclerotic	Lytic lesions 'Onion skinning' periosteal reaction
Cells	Spindle cell neoplasm	Small round cells*
Metastases	Lung, bones	Lung, bones
Management	Surgery and chemotherapy	Surgery or radiotherapy to primary Chemotherapy
Prognosis	66% survival non-metastatic <20% survival metastatic	60% survival non-metastatic 20–30% survival metastatic

* Other similar small round cell undifferentiated neoplasms include primitive neuroectodermal tumours (PNET), also known as peripheral neuroepithelioma (PN).

RETINOBLASTOMA

This usually develops in the posterior portion of the retina. Incidence 1: 16 000 live births.

Mean age at diagnosis   11 months (bilateral)
23 months (unilateral)

Both hereditary and sporadic forms exist.

Hereditary form

- *Retinoblastoma (RB1) gene on chromosome 13q*
- *Autosomal dominant, incomplete penetrance*
- *Risk of osteosarcoma <10 years = 1%*
- *Risk of secondary malignancy <40 years = 30%*

Hereditary tumour (40%)   All the bilateral tumours
20% of unilateral tumours

Sporadic tumour (60%)   Unilateral tumours

Clinical features

- *Leucocoria (white pupillary reflex)*
- *Strabismus*
- *Decreased vision*
- *More advanced disease – pupillary irregularity, hyphaema, orbital pain, proptosis, raised ICP*

Investigations

- *Fundoscopy*
- *Orbital imaging – CT or MRI of orbits, USS orbits*

Management options

- *Radiotherapy, photocoagulation or cryotherapy*
- *Enucleation if unavoidable*
- *Chemotherapy if metastatic or residual orbital disease*

Prognosis
Overall survival 90%
Poor survival if extensive, metastatic disease

GONADAL AND GERM CELL TUMOURS

These are tumours arising from primitive pluripotent germ cells, which migrate from the foetal yolk sac to form the gonads. They are mostly benign, though may be malignant. Extra-gonadal tumours occur due to abherrant germ cell migration.

Associations   Cryptorchidism, gonadal dysgenesis

Classification is based on the differentiation pathway:

✳ *Embryonic differentiation*	Teratoma (usually benign), eg. sacrococcygeal teratoma
	Embryonal carcinoma
✳ *Extraembryonic differentiation* ◦	Choriocarcinoma Highly malignant
	Gonadal or extragonadal
	β-HCG ↑
	Yolk sac carcinoma AFP ↑
Suppressed differentiation	Germinoma
	Seminoma
	Dysgerminoma (ovarian tumours)

Investigation of germ cell tumour

- *CXR*
- *CT scan or MRI affected area*
- *Bone scan*
- *Biological markers – AFP and βHCG*
- *Histology of lesion (biopsy or surgical excision)*

Management

This involves surgical excision wherever possible and chemotherapy if malignant.

Sacrococcygeal teratoma

- *Most common tumour in newborns*
- *Rectum and urinary tract may be involved, 90% have external component*
- *10% malignant at birth*
- *70% malignant at two months*

✳ Testicular germ cell tumours ✳

Present as	Testicular swelling (painless or painful)
	Gynaecomastia (if secretes HCG)
	Metastases (retroperitoneal, LN, lung)
Seminoma (1/3rd)	No biological markers (radiosensitive)
	Dysgerminoma is the ovarian counterpart
Teratoma (2/3rds)	

Ovarian germ cell tumours

Present as	Abdominal pain (acute or chronic) and swelling
	Abdominal mass

LIVER NEOPLASMS

Incidence 1.6:million children.

Primary	Benign 50%	Haemangioma, liver cell adenoma
		Haemangioendothelioma
		Hamartoma, focal nodular hyperplasia

Malignant 50%   Hepatoblastoma 65%

Hepatocellular carcinoma 35%

Metastatic   Neuroblastoma, Wilms tumour

	Hepatoblastoma	Hepatocellular carcinoma (HCC)
Age	<3 years	12–15 years
Associations	Hemihypertrophy	Preexisting cirrhosis (33%)
	Beckwith–Wiedemann syndrome	
	Meckel's diverticulum	
	Hernia (umbilical, diaphragmatic)	
	Renal anomalies	
Cells	Immature hepatic epithelial tissue	Abnormal hepatocytes
Clinical features	Abdominal mass	Abdominal mass (RUQ)
	Systemic signs rare	Systemic signs more common
Markers	AFP ↑ 60%	AFP ↑ 50%
Metastases	Lung, lymph nodes	Lung, lymph nodes
Prognosis	Three-year survival:	Very poor
	90% (resectable)	75% recurrence in resected tumours
	65% (initially unresectable)	
	10–20% (metastatic)	

Investigations

These include CT or MRI scans to search for extent of tumour and metastases. It can be difficult to differentiate between the two tumours.

Management

- *Primary surgical excision (possible in 50% of hepatoblastomas and 33% of HCC)*
- *Chemotherapy (preoperatively if initially unresectable or for metastases)*
- *Transplantation is a possibility in a minority*

BRAIN TUMOURS

These are almost always primary in children.

<2 years   Equal frequencies of posterior fossa and supratentorial tumours

2–12 years   66% are infratentorial (posterior fossa)

Clinical features

Signs of raised intracranial pressure (ICP):

- *Headache (morning), vomiting*
- *Diplopia, papilloedema (late sign in young children), strabismus*
- *Bulging fontanelle, loss of pulsation, macrocephaly*
- *Head tilting and nuchal rigidity*
- *Nystagmus Horizontal in unilateral cerebellar tumours, worse on looking to the side of the lesion*
  All directions in cerebellar vermis or fourth ventricle tumours
  Horizontal, vertical and rotatory in brainstem tumours

- Cranial nerve palsy (IV and VI)   4   6
- Vital sign abnormalities (bradycardia, BP ↑, hyperventilation, respiratory arrest)

Focal neurological signs:

Long-tract signs	Hemiparesis
Seizures	Complex partial
Ataxia	Truncal (cerebellar vermis)
	Ipsilateral (cerebellar hemisphere)

Behavioural changes

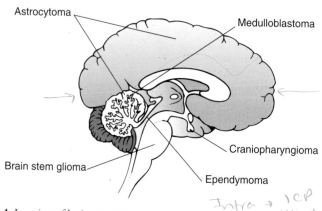

Figure 15.1 Location of brain tumours

Infratentorial tumours

Astrocytoma 20%

- Usually cystic, slow growing
- May be in a cerebellar hemisphere or midline
- Cause ICP ↑ by blocking the fourth ventricle or aqueduct of Sylvius
- Treatment is surgical resection (irradiation also, rarely)
- Five-year survival >90%

Medulloblastoma 20%

- Usually midline
- Cause ataxia and ICP ↑
- 20% have spinal metastases at diagnosis
- Treatment is surgical resection (irradiation and chemotherapy if necessary)
- Five-year survival 50%

Brain stem glioma 10%

- May be 1. diffusely infiltrating the brain stem (poor outlook)
          2. low-grade focal midbrain or medulla tumour (good outlook if resectable)
- Causes cranial nerve palsies, ataxia, long-tract signs

- *Treatment is mostly radiotherapy, unless low-grade focal tumour is resectable*
- *Five-year survival 20%*

Ependymoma 10%

- *Behaves as a medulloblastoma*
- *Causes ICP ↑*
- *Treatment is with surgery and radiotherapy*
- *Five-year survival 50%*

Supratentorial tumours

— Germ cell tumour.
— meningioma,

Craniopharyngioma (see Chapter 10)

- *Develops from a squamous remnant of Rathke's pouch in the sella turcica*
- *Solid and cystic areas; 90% have calcification on skull X-ray*
- *Causes endocrine abnormalities, ICP ↑, bitemporal hemianopia*
- *Treatment is surgical with radiotherapy only if necessary*

Optic nerve glioma
No treatment until progression is observed as the natural history is variable. 30% associated with neurofibromatosis.
Cause:

- *Decreased acuity and disc pallor*
- *Diencephalic syndrome – anorexia, or increased appetite, emaciation, hyperalert, euphoric (occurs if hypothalamus invaded)*

Treatment options involve surgery, radiotherapy and/or chemotherapy.

Astrocytoma
These have a much less favourable prognosis when supratentorial.

Choroid plexus papilloma → intra
These secrete CSF and cause slowly progressive hydrocephalus. Prognosis is excellent after resection.

Pineal tumours
A variety of tumour types can occur in the pineal gland in children. Therapy and prognosis are dependent on the aetiology.

LEUKAEMIAS

These are the most common childhood cancers. They include:

- *ALL 75% – peak incidence four years*
- *AML 20% – stable incidence <10 years, higher incidence during adolescence and older*
- *CML 3%*
- *juvenile CML/myelodysplastic syndromes 2–3%*

The leukaemias are classified according to morphology and cytochemistry, immunophenotyping, chromosome analysis and gene rearrangements.

Acute lymphoblastic leukaemia (ALL)

These arise from early cells in the lymphoid series.

Genetic associations

Chromosomal mutations	eg. trisomy 21, hyperdiploidy (good prognosis) hypodiploidy (poor prognosis)
Chromosomal rearrangements	eg. translocations − t (9:22) Philadelphia chromosome and t (4:11) infant ALL
	These are poor risk leukaemias, with allogeneic BMT indicated in first remission
	t (12:21) probably associated with good prognosis

Classifications

French-American-British (FAB) system (morphological)
L1   Small lymphoblasts, little cytoplasm (good prognosis)
L2   Larger and pleomorphic, more cytoplasm
L3   Cytoplasmic vacuoles, finely stippled nuclear chromatin

Immunophenotypes classification
Precursor B-ALL 75% (includes c-ALL (common), null-ALL and pre-B-ALL)
T-ALL 20% − m > f
B-ALL 5% − mediastinal mass, 'Burkitt', t (8:14), t (2:8) and t (22:8)

Clinical features

Bone marrow failure	1. Hb (↓) – pallor, lethargy
	2. WCC (↓ or N) – infections, fever
	3. Platelets (↓) – bruises, gum bleeding, menorrhagia
Infiltration	Hepatosplenomegaly, lymphadenopathy, testicular swelling
	Limp (bone pain), acute renal failure
	Meningeal syndrome (features of ICP ↑, papilloedema, retinal haemorrhage)
	Anterior mediastinal mass (T-ALL)

Prognostic indicators

Good	Bad
Low initial WCC	High initial WCC (>50)
Female	Male
2–10 years	Age <2 years or >10 years
<4 weeks to remission	>4 weeks to remission
t (12:21)	t (9:22), t (4:11) *MLL gene rearrangement*
Hyperdiploidy	Tumour bulk
c-ALL	CNS involvement
	T cell ALL
	B cell leukaemia

Investigations

Peripheral blood count and film	Anaemia (normochromic, normocytic)
	WCC $\downarrow$, N or $\uparrow$
	Platelets $\downarrow$
	Blasts present
Bone marrow	Aspirate or biopsy. Shows >30% leukaemic blast cells
CXR	?Mediastinal mass
CSF	(Blasts seen in cytospin if CNS involvement)
Renal function + uric acid	
Special classification tests	Chromosomal analysis, immunophenotyping, cytochemistry
	Immunoglobulin and T cell receptor (TCR) gene rearrangements

Treatment

1. *Induction of remission*
2. *Consolidation of remission:*

   - *Intensive multiagent chemotherapy*
   - *CNS prophylaxis – treatment that crosses the blood–brain barrier eg. high-dose IV methotrexate, CNS radiotherapy, intrathecal chemotherapy*

3. *Intensification (2–3 blocks of therapy). Aim to clear submicroscopic or minimal residual disease (intensive, multiagent chemotherapy)*
4. *Maintenance or continuing chemotherapy (two years). An outpatient treatment usually with oral 6-MP, methotrexate, vincristine and prednisolone*

Consider allogeneic BMT if very poor features such as initial WCC >100, Philadelphia positive or t (4 : 11).

Relapse

Common sites are the bone marrow, CNS and testes. Give intensive chemotherapy as treatment, with cranial irradiation and intrathecal chemotherapy in CNS relapse. BMT may offer the best chance of cure.

Prognosis

Dependent on type; overall approximately >80% five-year survival in c-ALL.

Acute myeloid leukaemia (AML)

The predominant form of congenital leukaemia that probably arises from a pluripotent cell or myeloid progenitor committed to erythroid, granulocytic-monocytic or megakaryocytic lines.

Associations	Trisomy 21
	Fanconi anaemia
	Bloom syndrome
	Previous chemotherapy (secondary AML)
	Myelodysplasia, aplastic anaemia

Classification

French-American-British (FAB) system	
M0 Undifferentiated	No Auer rods
M1 Myeloblastic, no maturation	No Auer rods
M2 Myeloblastic, some maturation	t (8:21), good prognosis, chloroma common, few Auer rods
M3 Acute promyelocytic	t (15:17), DIC common, retinoic acid as initial therapy, good prognosis, many Auer rods
M4 Myelomonocytic	Chromosome 16 material inversion, eosinophilia, good prognosis
M5 Monocytic	Renal damage common, meningeal involvement, gum swelling
M6 Erythroleukaemia	Poor prognosis
M7 Megakaryoblastic	Marrow fibrosis

Clinical features

Non-specific	As in ALL
Bone marrow failure	As in ALL (WCC may be ↓, N or ↑)
Other	Gum hypertrophy (M4 and M5 especially)
	DIC (M3)
	Chloroma (a localised mass of leukaemoid cells; common sites are retro-orbital, skin and epidural)
	Bone pain less common than in ALL

Diagnosis

As for ALL. Bone marrow must contain at least 30% blast cells; blasts may contain Auer rods.

Management

1. *Induction of remission:*

   - *chemotherapy eg. daunorubicin, cytosine arabinoside, thioguanine or etoposide*
   - *80% achieve remission (if not achieved, BMT is necessary)*

2. *Consolidation:*

   - *eg. daunorubicin, cytosine arabinoside, thioguanine or etoposide*
   - *intrathecal chemotherapy (± cranial irradiation) if CNS leukaemia at diagnosis or CNS relapse*

3. *Further consolidation:*

   - *total of 4–5 courses of multiagent chemotherapy, eg. etoposide, cytosine arabinoside, m-amascrine*
   - *BMT is usually only considered after relapse of AML in children*

Other treatments
All-trans-retinoic acid (ATRA) in M3.

Prognosis
60–70% overall cure rate in children. Cure rate decreases with increasing age.

Myelodysplastic syndromes

Juvenile myelomonocytic (JMML)
This is unlike adult CML, generally occurring at a young age and having features of AML. Philadelphia chromosome *not* present.

Predominant findings	Abnormal monocytes on the blood film
	Hb F elevated
	Platelets ↓
	Leucocytosis
	Hepatosplenomegaly, bleeding tendency, lymphadenopathy, eczema
	Chronic desquamative maculopapular rash

Due to resistance to treatment, allogeneic BMT is recommended.

Myelodysplasia (including monosomy 7)
Children initially develop only anaemia, thrombocytopenia or leucopenia. The bone marrow has characteristic dysplastic features and blast cells. Underlying chromosomal changes associated include trisomy 8 and complete or partial deletion of chromosome 5 or 7. Monosomy 7 is the most common abnormality in infants with myelodysplasia and AML. The condition usually evolves into AML and so patients are treated as for AML. BMT is considered more often as this condition is more resistant to chemotherapy.

Chronic myelogenous leukaemia (CML, adult type)
This is a malignancy of a haematopoietic stem cell capable of entering both myeloid and lymphoid lineages and containing the Philadelphia chromosome. The Philadelphia (Ph) chromosome has the translocation: t (9:22). This produces a fusion gene (bcr-abl) which encodes the bcr-abl protein (ie. activates the abl oncogene).

Phases in CML

Chronic phase	3–4 years. Cell counts easily controlled with chemotherapy
Accelerated phase	More difficult to control
Blast crisis	ALL or AML

Clinical features

Hypermetabolism	Fever, weight loss, anorexia, night sweats
Massive splenomegaly	
Anaemia, bleeding, bruising	

| *Leucostasis* | Visual disturbance, priapism |
| *Renal failure, gout* | |

Investigations

Peripheral blood film	Hb N or ↓, platelets ↑, N or ↓, WCC ↑↑, immature myeloid cells but few blasts on film
Bone marrow	Hypercellular, myeloid hyperplasia
Others	Neutrophil alkaline phosphatase score ↓, uric acid ↑, B_{12} ↑
Cytogenetic studies	Philadelphia chromosome (>95%)

Management

| *Chemotherapy* | eg. busulphan, hydroxyurea, α-interferon (suppresses the Ph chromosome) signal transduction inhibitors (STI) are in trial with encouraging results |
| *BMT in chronic phase* | only known cure |

Prognosis

- *If BMT during chronic phase, survival is 80% (matched sibling), 50–60% (partially matched or unrelated)*
- *If BMT during accelerated phase, survival is 20–30%*
- *If BMT during blast crisis, survival is 0–10%*

LYMPHOMA

Incidence 13: million children per year. In the lymphomas there is replacement of normal lymphoid tissue with collections of abnormal cells.

Hodgkin disease

This is a malignancy of lymphoid tissue with the histological feature of the presence of Reed–Sternberg (RS) cells. The origin of the malignant cells is unclear. Bimodal age distribution: peak in mid-20s and >50 years. Male 2: female 1.

Histological classification

Nodular sclerosing 50%	Good prognosis, females > males, mediastinal mass common
Mixed cellularity 40%	Present with more advanced disease, HIV associated
Lymphocyte predominant 10%	Best prognosis, males > females
Lymphocyte depleted (v. rare)	Present with disseminated disease, poor prognosis, seen in HIV

Clinical features

| *Lymphadenopathy* | Painless, firm Cervical, supraclavicular, axillary, inguinal Mediastinal (cough, airway compression), retroperitoneal |
| *'B' symptoms* | Fever (Pel–Ebstein), night sweats, weight loss |

Other constitutional symptoms	Fatigue, pruritis, anorexia
Extranodal involvement	Hepatosplenomegaly, SVC obstruction, lungs, bone, skin
	Bone marrow failure (rare)

Investigations

Routine   Clinical examination

FBC   Normocytic normochromic anaemia, platelets (initially high, low in advanced disease), neutrophils ↑, eosinophils ↑

ESR   ↑ (used to monitor disease progress)

LFTs   LDH ↑ (poor prognosis)

Biopsy (lymph node) Diagnosis and histological classification

CT chest/abdomen/pelvis

Other   MRI

Biopsy (liver) (may need to be radiologically guided).

Bone marrow aspirate (stage II–IV disease)

Bone scan

Lymphangiography

Stages of disease

I	Single lymph node region (LNR)
II	≥ 2 LNR same side diaphragm
III	LNR both sides diaphragm
	± spleen
IV	Disseminated involvement of extralymphatic organs (e.g. B.M, liver)
The stage is also A	absence of 'B' symptoms
or B	presence of 'B' symptoms

Management

Stages IA and IIA	Radiotherapy only
Advanced disease	Chemotherapy, eg. ABVD (adriamycin (doxorubicin), bleomycin, vinblastine, dacarbazine) usually
	± Radiotherapy
Relapse	Alternative combination chemotherapy (eg. MOPP) and autologous BMT may be used

Prognosis

Stage I and II	>90% five-year survival
Stage IIIA	>70% five-year survival
Stage IIIB, IV	>50% five-year survival

Non-Hodgkin lymphoma

These are characterised by collections of abnormal T or B lymphocytes or histiocytes.

Associations   Congenital immunodeficiency disorders, HIV

Autoimmune disorders

Children have high-grade, diffuse disease. There are several classifications.

National Cancer Institute histological classification of high-grade lymphomas

1. *Small non-cleaved cell (SNCC)*   *B cell tumours (like B-ALL)*
   (Burkitt)   *All have either: t (8 : 14), t (2 : 8), t (8 : 22), which*
        contain: c-myc oncogene and an immunoglobulin gene
        (μ, κ or λ)
2. *Lymphoblastic*   *T cell tumours (like T-ALL)*
3. *Large cell*   *T cell, B cell, non-B or non-T cell phenotypes*

Clinical features

These are dependent on the site of the primary.

Abdomen (31%)	Abdominal distension, nausea, vomiting, bowel habit change, acute abdomen, hepatosplenomegaly
Mediastinum (26%)	Dyspnoea, pleural effusions, superior vena cava obstruction
Oropharyngeal	Sore throat, stridor
Lymph nodes	Painless masses. Cervical LN most commonly affected
Bone marrow	Bone marrow failure symptoms and signs
CNS	Headache, raised intracranial pressure, cranial nerve palsies
Other organ	Skin, testes
Systemic symptoms	Fever, night sweats, weight loss

Investigations

Excision biopsy or fine-needle aspirate	
Bloods	Anaemia, platelets ↓, neutropenia, lymphoma cells
	U&E, creatinine, uric acid, bone profile
	LDH ↑ (prognostic marker)
Bone marrow	Involvement (20%)
CSF	? CNS involvement
Imaging studies	CT scan (chest, abdomen, pelvis), bone scan
Special tests	Chromosome analysis, immunological markers

Staging

This is as for Hodgkin disease, though is less clearly related to prognosis than is the histological type.

Management

This depends on the grade of malignancy. High-grade malignancy seen in children is usually treated with multiagent chemotherapy like ALL protocols. Relapses are treated with intensive chemotherapy, radiotherapy and autologous or allogeneic BMT.

Prognosis

- *Limited-stage disease – >90% cure*
- *Stage III and IV – 70% cure*

Burkitt lymphoma

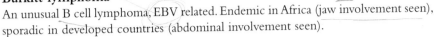

An unusual B cell lymphoma, EBV related. Endemic in Africa (jaw involvement seen), sporadic in developed countries (abdominal involvement seen).

Clinical features

- Massive jaw lesions
- Abdominal extranodal involvement
- Ovarian involvement

Specific investigations

Lymph node biopsy   'Starry sky' appearance (a few histiocytes amongst masses of lymphocytes)

Cell culture   EB virus

Chromosome analysis   t (8 : 14) usual

Management

Intensive sequential chemotherapy, with BMT in relapse. Traditionally it has been associated with a poor prognosis but recently very good results have been obtained (70% cure).

CHILDHOOD HISTIOCYTOSIS SYNDROMES

These diseases involve a proliferation of cells in the bone marrow of the monocyte-macrophage system. They are classified histologically and mostly not considered true malignancies.

Class I – Langerhans cell histiocytosis

This includes the old classification of:

Eosinophilic granuloma   Bone lesions, lung involvement

Hand–Schüller–Christian disease   Hypothalamic findings (eg. diabetes insipidus), proptosis

Letterer–Siwe disease   Infants, severely unwell, hepatosplenomegaly

Histology

Cells of monocyte lineage containing the EM findings of a Langerhans cell (ie. the Birbeck granule).

Clinical features

Very variable presentation, including:

Skeleton (80%)   Lytic lesions   Skull (punch out lesions)
Pathological fractures of spine and long bones
'Free floating teeth'

Skin (50%)   Refractive seborrhoeic dermatitis of the scalp and nappy area (and elsewhere)
Petechiae, papular rash

Lymphadenopathy (33%)	Localised or disseminated
Hepatosplenomegaly (20%)	
Others	Exophthalmos, pulmonary infiltration
	Pituitary dysfunction (diabetes insipidus, growth retardation)

Investigations

Tissue biopsy	Skin or bone lesions
Blood tests	FBC, clotting, U&E, creatinine, LFTs
Skeletal survey	
Urine	Osmolality

Management

Single-system disease	Radiotherapy
Multisystem disease	Chemotherapy

Class II histiocytoses

These include: Haemophagocytic lymphohistiocytosis (HLH), which may be familial associated, viral associated, leukaemia, or others.

Histology

Antigen-processing cells (macrophages). Allogeneic BMT is the only chance of cure.

Class III histiocytoses

These include:

Acute monocytic leukaemia

Histology

Malignancies of cells of monocyte–macrophage lineage.

FURTHER READING

Pizzo PA, Poplack DG *Principles and Practice of Paediatric Oncology* 3rd Ed. Lippincott-Raven, New York, 1997

16

Neonates

- Neonatal definitions
- Antenatal diagnostic techniques
- Delivery
- Normal neonate
- Birth injuries
- Twins
- Congenital infections

- Intrapartum infections
- Postnatal infections
- Small for gestational age (SGA)
- Large for gestational age (LGA)
- Prematurity
- Neonatal intensive care
- Neonatal systems

Neonatal definitions

Embryo	<9 weeks gestation
Fetus	9 weeks gestation – delivery
Neonate	Infant below 28 days old
Small for gestational age (SGA)	Birth weight <10th centile
Large for gestational age (LGA)	Birth weight >90th centile
Appropriate for gestational age (AGA)	Birth weight between 10th–90th centile
Low birth weight (LBW)	Infants = ≤2500 g at birth
Very low birth weight (VLBW)	Infants = ≤1500 g at birth
Extremely low birth weight (ELBW)	Infants = ≤1000 g at birth
Stillbirth	Fetal death and expulsion from the uterus after 24 weeks gestation
Abortion	Fetal death and expulsion from the uterus before 24 weeks gestation
Stillbirth rate	Number of stillbirths per 1000 of all births (live and still)
Neonatal mortality rate	Number of deaths of liveborn infants within 28 days of birth per 1000 live births
Perinatal mortality rate	Number of stillbirths plus deaths within the first seven days per 1000 births (live and still)
Postneonatal mortality rate	Number of deaths between 28 days and one year per 1000 live births
Infant mortality rate	Number of deaths between birth and one year per 1000 live births

Antenatal diagnosis techniques

Maternal blood tests	Blood group and antibodies (rhesus and other red cell antigens)

Rubella, syphilis, hepatitis B

HIV status (with maternal consent)

Toxoplasmosis (if specifically indicated only in UK)

Down syndrome (12–16 weeks):

Triple test:	Serum AFP ($\downarrow$)
	Serum HCG ($\uparrow$)
	Serum unconjugated oestriol (uE3)($\downarrow$)
Neural tube defects:	Serum AFP raised in 80–90% of NTDs
	(NB. Nuchal fold thickness now done instead)

Ultrasound screening   Gestational age estimate at 8–12 weeks (reliable if <20 weeks)

Congenital structural malformations scan at 18–20 weeks

Amniotic fluid volume

Fetal growth measurements (serial monitoring of head circumference, abdominal circumference and femur length)

34 week anomaly scan if concerns

Nuchal fold thickness (thick in Down syndrome) at 11–14 weeks

Amniocentesis   Around 16 weeks, 1 : 100–200 risk of miscarriage

Chromosomal analysis (amniocytes used)

Enzyme analysis: (inborn error of metabolism)

Bilirubin level: (rhesus disease)

Chorionic villus sampling   Around 12 weeks, 1 : 100 risk of miscarriage

More rapid and earlier analysis than amniocentesis achieved

Chromosomal analysis

Enzyme analysis: (inborn error of metabolism)

DNA analysis using PCR (eg. haemoglobinopathies, cystic fibrosis)

Congenital infection: viral particles using PCR

Foetal blood sampling   Severe rhesus or platelet isoimmunisation (estimation of severity)

Congenital infection: viral serology

Delivery

RESUSCITATION

Infants who do not establish normal respiration quickly (a small minority of infants) will require assessment and resuscitation (done on a Resuscitaire). Apgar scores are performed at one, five and 10 minutes (and further if necessary).

Basic resuscitation	Advanced resuscitation
Start the clock	Endotracheal intubation and ventilation
Dry and stimulate baby	Drug therapy
Nasopharyngeal suctioning (if excess fluid)	Blood/fluid therapy via umbilical venous catheter
Mask ventilation	Transfer to SCBU
External cardiac massage	
Naloxone IM or IV (if opiates likely to be present) (NB. Contraindicated in maternal drug abuse)	

NB. If meconium aspiration is suspected the pharynx can be suctioned after delivery of the head. If the infant is not vigorous on delivery pharyngeal suctioning (and beyond the cords if meconium seen at the larynx) is performed *prior* to IPPV in order to prevent further meconium damage.

Drugs used

Adrenaline IV or ETT	0.1–0.3 ml/kg of 1:10 000 (10 μg/kg) repeated as needed every 3–5 minutes
	0.1 ml/kg of 1:1000 (100 μg/kg) if required after two doses as above
Glucose 10% IV	2 ml/kg
Blood/4.5% albumin	10–20 ml/kg
Sodium bicarbonate (4.2% soln) IV	1 mmol/kg
Naloxone IM, IV, ETT	10 μg/kg

ETT sizes and lengths

Weight	ETT size	ETT length (tip-to-lip)
1 kg	2.5	7 cm
2 kg	3.0	8 cm
3 kg	3.5	9 cm
4 kg	3.5/4.0	≥9 cm

APGAR SCORES

The Apgar score is used to describe the condition of the infant at varying times from birth but it is poorly predictive of later adverse outcome.

	Score		
Physical sign	0	1	2
Appearance	Pale	Blue extremities	Pink
Pulse	Absent	<100 bpm	>100 bpm
Grimace on suction	None	Grimace	Cry, cough
Activity	Flaccid	Some limb flexion	Active
Respiratory effort	Absent	Irregular	Regular

HIGH-RISK DELIVERIES

Fetal/delivery	Maternal conditions
Fetal distress	Diabetes
Meconium-stained liquor	Hyperthyroidism
Preterm delivery	Myaesthenia gravis
Breech delivery	SLE
Multiple pregnancy	AITP
Antenatal US detection of anatomical abnormality	Drug abuse
Emergency caesarean section	Severe preeclamptic toxaemia

Normal neonate

NEONATAL EXAMINATION

Examination of the newborn includes the following.

Measurements	Gestational age, birth weight, centiles (head circumference, weight, length)
General	Appearance, posture, movements
Skin	Colour (cyanosis, jaundice, anaemic, plethoric), birth marks
Head	Fontanelles (normal size and pressure? fused sutures?), shape
Face	Signs of dysmorphism
Ears	Size, formation, position
Mouth	Size, other abnormality (cleft?), neonatal teeth?
Eyes	Red reflex (cataracts?), discharge, colobomas, size
Palate	Inspected and palpated (cleft palate?), sucking reflex checked
Neck	Any swellings (cystic hygroma?, sternomastoid 'tumour')
Respiratory	Respiratory movements, rate, auscultation
Cardiovascular	Auscultation, femoral pulses
Abdominal	Palpation (masses?)
Genitalia	Inspection (malformations, ambiguous genitalia?), testes (descended?)
Anus	(Patent?). NB. Meconium normally passes within 48 hours of birth (within 24 hours in 95%)
Back	Check spine (midline defects?)
Muscle tone	Observation, holding baby prone
Reflexes	Moro reflex may be checked
Hips	Checked for CDH (see below)

NEONATAL HIP EXAMINATION

The baby should be relaxed while this is carried out. The pelvis is stabilised with one hand and the middle finger of the other hand is placed over the greater trochanter and the thumb around the femur. The hip is held flexed and adducted. Then:

1. **Barlow manoeuvre**. *To check if the hip is* dislocatable. *The femoral head is gently pushed downwards. The femoral head will be pushed out of the acetabulum if the hip is dislocatable.*
2. **Ortolani manoeuvre**. *To see if the hip is* dislocated and can be relocated *into the acetabulum. The hip is abducted and upward pressure is applied. If the hip is dislocated it will clunk back into position. NB. Clicks are insignificant and due to ligaments.*

VITAMIN K

Prophylactic vitamin K is recommended for all newborns to prevent haemorrhagic disease of the newborn. The vitamin K is given IM 1 mg at birth or a course of oral vitamin K (at birth, seven days and six weeks) may be given as an alternative (efficacy unknown).

Haemorrhagic disease of the newborn

- *Due to low vitamin K-dependent factors at birth (immature liver, gut bacteria low) and a further fall in breastfed babies (poor source of vitamin K)*
- *Bleeding on day 2–6, usually mild, may be catastrophic*
- *Late presentation may occur at around six weeks (rare)*
- *If bleeding occurs, give IV vitamin K, FFP, blood and plasma as needed*

GUTHRIE TEST

This is a biochemical screen performed on all infants at the end of the first week of life via a blood test (usually a heel prick sample). The test can detect:

Disease	Compound detected
Phenylketonuria	Phenylalanine
Hypothyroidism	TSH level
Galactosaemia	Galactose
Maple syrup urine disease	Leucine
Homocystinuria	Methionine
Histidinaemia	Histidine

Haemoglobinopathies and cystic fibrosis may also be screened for using the Guthrie card. Some of these diseases are routinely screened for in certain areas of the country only.

INFANT FEEDING

Purely milk feeding is used for the first four months and solids are then introduced (weaning).

Infant requirements

Energy (kcal/kg/day)	Term	100
	Premature	120
	SGA	140

Recommended daily dosage for vitamin supplementation:

Vitamin A (iu)	500–1500
Vitamin D (iu)	400
Vitamin E (iu)	5
Vitamin C (mg)	35
Folate (μg)	50

Breastfeeding

Breast milk is composed of *colostrum* for the first few days (protein, phospholipid, cholesterol and immunoglobulin content are high).

Advantages of breastfeeding:

- *Helps establish maternal–infant bonding*
- *Transfer of immunological protection (IgA especially)*
- *Convenient and cheap*
- *Nutritional components optimum for infant (eg. fatty acids, arachidonic acid and docosohexaenoic acid, needed for infant brain development)*
- *Contraceptive (lactation amenorrhoea)*
- *Uterine involution (oxytocin release)*

Reasons for not breast feeding

Maternal	Neonatal
Maternal acute illness	Acute illness
Maternal chronic illness (eg. TB, HIV)	Cleft lip/palate (may be able to breastfeed)
Inverted nipples (may be able to manage)	Metabolic disease (eg. galactosaemia)
Breast abscess (may use other breast)	
Maternal dislike	
Certain drugs eg. antithyroid drugs, lithium	

Comparison of human milk with cow's milk and formula feed (per 100 ml)

	Human milk	Formula milk	Cow's milk
Energy (kcal)	70	60–65	67 (↓)
Protein (g)	1.3	1.5–1.9	3.5 (↑↑)
Casein: whey	40:60	40:60–63:37	63:37 (↑↑)
Carbohydrate (g)	7	7–8.6	4.9 (↓)
Fat (g)	4.2	2.6–3.8	3.6 (↓)
Sodium (mmol)	0.65	0.65–1.1	2.3 (↑↑)
Phosphorus (mmol)	0.46	0.9–1.8	3.2 (↑↑)
Calcium (mmol)	0.88	0.88–2.1	3 (↑↑)
Iron (mmol)	1.36	8–12.5	0.9 (↓↓)

Formula feeds

These are usually made from modified cow's milk. **Special formulas include**:

1. *Soyabean*   *Cow's milk protein intolerance (30% overlap NB.)*
                                             Lactose intolerance
                                             Galactosaemia
2. *Lactose-free milk*   *Lactose intolerance*
3. *Low protein milk*   *Certain inborn errors of amino acid metabolism eg.*
                                             PKU, MSUD
4. *Premature infant and low birth*
   weight infant milks
5. *Casein and whey-hydrosylase*   *CMP sensitivity/soya*
   milks
6. *Elemental milks*   *Multiple antigen sensitivity*
7. *Modular milks*   *Specific diseases such as terminal liver failure*

Birth injuries

HEAD INJURIES

Caput succedaneum   Bruising and oedema of the presenting part of the head
Chignon   Bruising from a Ventouse delivery
Cephalhaematoma   A bleed beneath the periosteum due to torn veins (there-
                            fore limited to one skull bone)
                            Resolves over several weeks
                            Complications: Underlying skull fracture
                                           Jaundice
                                           Calcification
                                           Associated intracranial haemorrhage
Subaponeurotic haemorrhage An uncommon bleed beneath the occipitofrontalis
                            aponeurosis. This may spread over the scalp to become
                            large and result in shock

NERVE INJURIES

Facial nerve palsy   LMN: Forceps injury, prolonged pressure on maternal sacral
                       promontory
                       UMN: Uncommon, due to brain injury or nuclear agenesis
                       (Moebius syndrome)
                       The lesions are difficult to distinguish clinically and result in an
                       asymmetrical face when crying and inability to close the eye in the
                       affected side
Erb palsy   Common injury to the upper (C5 + 6, ± 7) nerve roots of the
                       brachial plexus. Arm is held in adduction, elbow extended, inter-
                       nally rotated, forearm pronated and wrist flexed: '*waiter's tip*' posi-
                       tion. 5% also have phrenic nerve involvement causing ipsilateral
                       diaphragmatic paralysis

| *Klumpke palsy* | Injury to the lower (C7 + 8 + T1) nerve roots of the brachial plexus. A wrist drop and paralysis of the small muscles of the hand result in 'claw hand'. Around 30% also have a Horner syndrome. |

Management

This is conservative, with physiotherapy to prevent contractures. For facial nerve injury, eye patching and artificial tears if eye closure incomplete. Most spontaneously recover over weeks to months.

BONE INJURIES

Clavicle fracture	This is the most common fracture occurring during delivery. Seen in large babies with impacted shoulders (eg. infant of diabetic mother) and in breech deliveries
Humerus fracture	Upper third usually fractured; deformity and radial nerve injuries occur. Treatment with immobilisation is necessary.
Femur fracture	Seen with breech delivery (particularly extended breech). Orthopaedic treatment with immobilisation is needed

Twins

Monozygotic (identical)	Single fertilised egg 1 : 80
	Separate chorion, separate amnion (division of egg <72 hours)
	Mixed (separate amnion, monochorionic, division 4–8 days)
	Single chorion, single amnion (division of egg >8 days)
Dizygotic (non-identical)	Variable rate, familial
	Two fertilised eggs
	Dichorionic placenta (may be fused and therefore clinically confusing)

RISKS ASSOCIATED

- *Mortality ↑ (× 9 monozygotic, × 3 dizygotic)*
- *Prematurity*
- *IUGR, discordant growth*
- *Asphyxia*
- *Sharing of the chorion + amnion – twin-twin transfusion, cord entanglement, discordant growth*
- *Monozygotic – congenital anomalies, low birth weight*
- *2nd twin at particularly increased risk of RDS and asphyxia*

Congenital infections

TRANSPLACENTAL

Congenital rubella, CMV and toxoplasmosis

These produce similar multiple abnormalities when the fetus is clinically affected. In toxoplasmosis and CMV approximately 10% of infected infants are clinically affected. Rubella infection has a high incidence of producing congenital rubella syndrome if the infection occurs <18 weeks gestation and particularly <8 weeks gestation.

Relative clinical features

Abnormality		Rubella (<18 weeks)	CMV	Toxoplasmosis
Eyes	Microphthalmia	+	−	+
	Chorioretinitis	+	++	+++
	Cataracts	+++	−	+
Brain	Epilepsy	−	++	−
	Microcephaly	+	++	+
	Hydrocephalus	−	−	++
	Calcification	−	++ (periventricular)	++ (widespread)
	Deafness	+++	++	+
Heptosplenomegaly		+++	+++	++
Petechiae		++	++	+
Cardiac malformations		++	−	−
Pneumonitis		+	++	+
Bony involvement		++	−	−
IUGR		+++	+++	+

Diagnosis

1. *Maternal history of immunisation and exposure to infections and clinical picture*
2. *Urine, throat, NPA – CMV culture, rubella*
3. *Serology – IgM levels for suspected infections and serial raised IgG in toxoplasmosis*
4. *Maternal serology – specific IgM levels*

Congenital varicella infection

Maternal infection in the first or second trimesters in pregnancy may rarely produce *congenital varicella syndrome*:

Skin	Cicatrix (zigzag scarring)
Limbs	Malformation and shortening
Eyes	Cataracts, chorioretinitis, microphthalmia
CNS	Microcephaly, hydrocephaly, brain aplasia

Maternal chicken pox developing between *five days before and two days after* birth may result in potentially fatal neonatal varicella (no protective maternal antibodies will have crossed the placenta). This is managed with:

- *Anti-varicella zoster IgG (VZIG) IM to infant*
- *If any vesicles develop, commence IV acyclovir*

Listeria monocytogenes

This may be acquired transplacentally or from ascending infection, the mother acquiring it from unpasteurised cheeses and uncooked meat products.

Clinical features	Premature delivery, abortion or stillbirth
	Meconium passed *in utero* (seen in premature delivery)
	Meningitis, septicaemia and pneumonia
	Hydrocephalus common sequelae
	Disseminated infection – fits, rash, hepatosplenomegaly
Treatment	Ampicillin IV and gentamicin IV

Other congenital infections:

- *Syphilis (see p. 70)*
- *Hepatitis B (see p. 204)*
- *HIV (see p. 41)*
- *Parvovirus B19 (see p. 59)*

Intrapartum infections

These are acquired from the maternal genital tract during birth and include group B β-haemolytic streptococcus, herpes simplex, *Chlamydia trachomatis*, gonococcus and HIV.

GROUP B β-HAEMOLYTIC STREPTOCOCCUS (GBS)

Colonisation of the vagina with GBS occurs in 20–30% of women; 10% of babies become colonised and only 0.3 in 1000 become unwell due to this.

GBS produces serious disease:

1. *early sepsis and shock, pneumonia, meningitis*
2. *late-onset meningitis (at 5–7 days)*

Investigations	FBC, CRP and septic screen (blood culture in particular)
	CXR (diffuse or lobar changes)
Treatment	Ampicillin and gentamicin IV on suspicion. Supportive therapy

HERPES SIMPLEX

Clinical features	Skin vesicles within the first week, with rapid CNS involvement
	Mortality 80% untreated
Treatment	Acyclovir IV

CHLAMYDIA TRACHOMATIS

Chlamydia is found in the vagina in 4% of pregnant women and 70% of babies infected are asymptomatic.

Clinical features	Conjuctivitis (purulent, like gonococcal)
	Pneumonia (may be present at 1–3 months of age), middle ear infection

Diagnosis	Organism identified on Giemsa staining and culture on special medium
Treatment	Oral erythromycin, tetracycline eye drops

Postnatal infections

It can be difficult to distinguish intrapartum or ascending infection from postnatally acquired infections and many can be acquired either way.

NEONATAL SEPTICAEMIA

Common causes	Group B streptococcus
	E.coli
	Staph.epidermidis
Clinical features	Lethargy, poor feeding, irritability, jaundice, features of shock (late)
Investigations	Septic screen (blood cultures, CSF, urine), FBC, CRP
	If E.coli infection, consider UTI, bowel disease and galactosaemia
Management	IV antibiotics (eg. penicillin and gentamicin) and supportive therapy

NEONATAL MENINGITIS (see p. 52)

NEONATAL CONJUNCTIVITIS

This may be due to:

- *Staph. aureus* (purulent)
- *Chlamydia trachomatis* (purulent)
- *Neisseria gonorrhoeae* (purulent)
- haemophilus, *Strep. pneumoniae* (purulent)
- aseptic causes (usually chemical)

Ophthalmia neonatorum is any purulent conjunctivitis occurring in the first three weeks of life.

Diagnosis

Eye swab   Gram stain, PCR (chlamydia and gonorrhoea require special media)

Management

- *Frequent eye toilet*
- *Choramphenicol or neomycin eye drops*
- *Chlamydia: oral erythromycin (two weeks) plus tetracycline eye drops*
- *Gonococcus: eye irrigation with crystalline penicillin hourly. IV penicillin 10-day course*

OMPHALITIS AND FUNISITIS

Omphalitis = umbilical stump infection
Funisitis   = umbilical cord infection

These are usually due to *E.coli* or *Staph.aureus* and may lead to portal vein infection with subsequent portal hypertension.

Investigations   Swab umbilicus for M, C + S

Management   IV antibiotics to cover staphylococcal infection if signs of spread (cellulitis around umbilicus)

Small for gestational age (SGA)

These are infants with a birth weight <10th centile for age. They may be:

Asymmetrical   Weight on a lower centile than head circumference due to relative sparing of brain growth

Results from placental failure late in pregnancy

Causes: maternal pre-eclampsia, cardiac or renal disease, uterine malformation, multiple gestation

Rapid weight gain after birth

Symmetrical   Head and body equally affected

Results from prolonged intrauterine growth failure. The fetus is usually small but normal, though may be abnormal

Causes: chromosomal abnormalities, congenital infection, maternal drug abuse, smoking, chronic illness, malnutrition

Poor postnatal growth also

ASSOCIATED PROBLEMS OF SGA INFANT

- *Hypoxic ischaemic encephalopathy (HIE)*
- *Hypoglycaemia (poor fat and glycogen stores)*
- *Hypocalcaemia*
- *Polycythaemia*
- *Hypothermia (large surface area: weight ratio)*
- *Pulmonary haemorrhage*
- *Infection*

Large for gestational age (LGA)

These are infants whose birth weight is >90th centile for age.

Causes   Diabetic mother

Familial

Beckwith–Weidemann syndrome

ASSOCIATED PROBLEMS

- *HIE (difficult delivery)*
- *Birth trauma (difficult delivery)*
- *Hypoglycaemia (hyperinsulinism)*
- *Polycythaemia*

Prematurity

Any infant born <37 weeks gestation is premature. Many premature infants are small but appropriate for gestational age (AGA) due to prematurity.

Survival rates have increased dramatically over recent years but a significant proportion of extremely premature infants will have chronic disability if they survive.

SPECIFIC PROBLEMS ASSOCIATED WITH PREMATURITY

Temperature	Thermal instability
Liver	Jaundice
Kidneys	Inability to concentrate urine, inability to excrete acid load
Lungs	Apnoea, TTN, RDS, pneumothorax, BPD
Cardiac	PDA, PPHN
CNS	HIE, intracranial haemorrhage, lack of primitive reflexes
Gastrointestinal	NEC, intolerance of enteral feeds, gastrooesophageal reflux
Immunity	Susceptibility to infections
Eyes	Retinopathy of prematurity
Metabolic	Hypoglycaemia, electrolyte imbalances (eg. hypocalcaemia), osteopenia of prematurity
Haematological	Iron deficiency anaemia, physiological anaemia
Surgical	Undescended testicles, inguinal and umbilical hernia

Neonatal intensive care

Sick or preterm infants on the neonatal unit are monitored and supported according to their own special needs.

THERMAL STABILITY

Incubators provide a stable thermal environment.

MONITORING

HR, RR and temperature are continuously monitored.

Oxygenation	Pulse oximetry (saturation), transcutaneous (O_2 tension)
CO_2 levels	Transcutaneous (CO_2 tension)
Blood gases	Umbilical arterial catheter (UAC) or peripheral arterial line
	Capillary analysis from heel prick samples
BP	UAC or peripheral arterial line (most accurate) or BP cuff

VENTILATION

Ambient oxygen may be sufficient or one of the methods of ventilation may be required.

Continuous positive airway pressure (CPAP)

Via face mask, nasal cannulae or endotracheal tube (ETT). This keeps the terminal bronchioles open in expiration, preventing their collapse.

Intermittent positive pressure ventilation (IPPV)

Paralysis and sedation may be required for ventilation if a baby is struggling and 'fighting' the ventilator.

Ventilators

Ventilators are pressure and time cycled. Adjustments may be made to:

FiO_2	As low as able to avoid retinopathy of prematurity	
Rate	A fast rate will reduce CO_2	
Pressure	**PIP**	Peak inspiratory pressure
	PEEP	Positive end expiratory pressure. Used while ventilating, acts as CPAP does
		High pressures needed for stiff lungs (low compliance) but risk of pneumothorax
Time		Inspiratory and expiratory times and their relative ratio may be altered

Inspiratory: expiratory (I: E) ratio

Normal	$1:2$
RDS	$1:1, 2:3$
Severe RDS	$2:1$ (ie. ratio reversed)

Examples of ventilator settings

	RDS	PHHN
Rate (/min)	60	80
PIP (cmH_2O)	25–30	20–25
PEEP (cmH_2O)	5	4
I: E ratio	2:3	1:1
Inspiratory time (s)	0.4	0.4
FiO_2	0.7	0.7

Ventilation types

Continuous mandatory ventilation (**CMV**)	Used for full ventilation
Intermittent mandatory ventilation (**IMV**)	Occasional breaths given by ventilator. Used to wean a baby who is making some effort
Patient-triggered ventilation (**PTV**)	Ventilator assists breath after triggered by baby. Used for weaning

High-frequency oscillatory ventilation (HFOV)

Very high frequency rates (720–1500/min) are used. This type of ventilation is useful in infants with severe homogeneous lung disease, but its use is becoming more widespread in milder lung problems also.

Extracorporeal membrane oxygenation (ECMO)

This is used when other ventilatory methods fail (eg. in meconium aspiration syndrome, PPHN, severe RDS, pneumonia). The extracorporeal circuit oxygenates the blood and returns it to the baby. Complications include intracranial haemorrhage (heparinisation necessary for ECMO). Contraindications to ECMO include uncontrolled bleeding and IVH grade II or greater.

Nitric oxide (NO)

This is a neurotransmitter, made by vascular endothelium and macrophages. It also acts as a vasodilator via increasing cGMP levels, particularly on the pulmonary artery smooth muscle. It also inhibits platelet function. It is used in PPHN to decrease pulmonary hypertension.

Side-effects   Methaemoglobinaemia
               Platelet function affected

Blood gas acid–base monitoring

Regular arterial gases or transcutaneous measurements need to be taken whilst ventilating. The following *disturbances* may exist.

Acidosis   Respiratory acidosis occurs with high CO_2
           Metabolic acidosis occurs with low bicarbonate
Alkalosis   Respiratory alkalosis occurs with low CO_2
           Metabolic alkalosis occurs with high bicarbonate

These will be **compensated** for (*but never enough to bring the pH to normal*) by:

- *metabolic means by altering the bicarbonate level*
- *respiratory means by altering the CO_2 level*

To calculate the disturbance present:

1. *look at the pH to decide if acidosis or alkalosis*
2. *look at the CO_2 and bicarbonate to see which one has caused this primary defect*
3. *Look at the other agent (CO_2 or bicarbonate) to confirm that it is trying to compensate (if not, a mixed picture exists).*

CIRCULATORY SUPPORT

Intravenous fluids are given as 10% dextrose with added electrolytes (sodium 2–3 mmol/kg/day, potassium 2 mmol/kg/day and calcium 1 mmol/kg/day). Inotropes (dopamine, dobutamine) are given as required if the MAP remains low. TPN can be given from day 1 if prolonged stay is anticipated.

Example of parenteral fluid regimes (ml/kg/day) (vary between units)

	Day 1	2	3	4	5	Up to
Term infant	60	90	120	150	150	150
Preterm infant	60	90	120	150	180	180

If nursed with phototherapy, an extra 30 ml/kg/day is given. Certain criteria increase or decrease fluid requirements (eg. hypoglycaemia, shock).

FEEDING

Enteral feeds   If tolerated, breast or formula feeds given by bottle (usually able if >34 weeks) or bolus nasogastric (NG) tube if unable to feed. Special formulas for premature infants

Parenteral feeds   Total parenteral nutrition (TPN) is used if enteral feeds contraindicated (eg. NEC, extreme prematurity). This is given via an umbilical venous catheter (UVC) or a peripheral long line.

Complications: *Sepsis*

TPN cholestasis

Microemboli

Supplements

Children's vitamin drops   Commenced when enteral feeds commenced until two years. Contain vitamins A, C and D

Iron   Commence oral supplements (if BW <2.5 kg or <36 weeks gestation) when four weeks old until on solid feeds

Folic acid   Give if haemolytic anaemia from incompatible blood group until eight weeks

Neonatal systems

APNOEA AND UPPER AIRWAY DISORDERS

Apnoea

This is cessation of breathing for >20 seconds and may be accompanied by bradycardia and cyanosis. The apnoea may have a central cause due to chemoreceptor failure or an obstructive cause. Reflex causes are due to protective mechanisms to close the airway, which lead to apnoea. Premature neonates have poorly developed central chemoreceptors and respiratory centres.

Causes of Apnoea

Central	Obstructive	Reflex
Prematurity	Choanal atresia	Vagal response (eg. suctioning, physiotherapy)
Hypoxia	Pierre–Robin sequence	
Metabolic eg. hypoglycaemia	Laryngeal nerve palsy	Gastrooesophageal reflux
Drugs eg. maternal narcotic		
Sepsis		
Intracranial haemorrhage		
Hyper/hypothermia		
Polycythaemia		
Convulsions		
Developmental brain abnormalities		

Investigations

These depend on the clinical condition. Gastrooesophageal reflux is important to exclude. They may include investigations for sepsis, CXR, arterial blood gases, barium swallow and neurological investigations.

Management

Treat underlying cause.

Acute episode	Stimulation, manual ventilation, apnoea monitoring
Recurrent episodes	CPAP, methylxanthines (eg. theophylline, caffeine)
	Intubation and ventilation if severe
	Home apnoea monitor only in special circumstances (eg. sibling of SIDS child, hypoventilation condition)
	Resuscitation skills for the parents

Choanal atresia

This is failure of the bucconasal membrane to cannulate. It may be uni- or bilateral. It presents with difficulty in breathing from birth (babies are obligate nasal breathers until they cry).

Diagnosis	Inability to pass a NG tube in the affected nostrils
Management	Provide an airway (pharyngeal or ETT) until surgery performed

Laryngomalacia

This common condition is caused by a floppy larynx, which narrows on inspiration and so causes stridor. (For other causes of stridor see p. 132.) The stridor is worse or only present on crying. Diagnosis is by direct laryngoscopy. The condition resolves over the first few months of life.

RESPIRATORY DISORDERS

Features of respiratory distress

- *Tachypnoea – RR >60/min*
- *Expiratory grunt*
- *Nasal flaring*
- *Recession – intercostal, subcostal, sternal*
- *Cyanosis*

Investigations of respiratory distress

- *Oxygen saturation*
- *Chest transillumination (?pneumothorax)*
- *Pass NG tube (if choanal or oesophageal atresia suspected)*
- *CXR*
- *Nitrogen washout test (to differentiate cause of cyanosis; see p. 103)*

Bloods	Blood gases
	FBC (anaemia, WCC $\uparrow$ or $\downarrow$), haematocrit ($\downarrow$)
Infection screen	Blood, urine, CSF, gastric aspirates (bacterial and viral cultures), swabs (ear, throat, umbilicus), maternal high vaginal swab result
	Serology

Transient tachypnoea of the newborn (TTN)

This is due to retained fetal lung fluid and is a self-limiting condition. Incidence 1–2% of newborns.

Predisposing factors	Caesarean section, HIE, heavy maternal analgesia, breech, asphyxia
	Infant of diabetic mother
Clinical features	Respiratory distress resolving over the first 48–72 hours
CXR	Generalised streakiness, fluid in the fissures, pleural effusions
Treatment	Oxygen, CPAP if necessary. Ventilation rarely necessary
	Antibiotics until pneumonia/sepsis excluded

Respiratory distress syndrome (RDS)

A specific disease due to *insufficient surfactant* in the alveoli. Surfactant is produced by type II pneumocytes and acts to lower the surface tension of the alveoli and so increase the compliance. It is a phospholipid composed of lecithin and sphingomyelin. The lecithin: sphingomyelin (LS) ratio is altered in RDS:

LS ratio	Risk of RDS
<1.5	70%
1.5–2	40%
>2	Very small

It is secreted by the lungs from 30–32 weeks. A low compliance leads to hypoxia and acidosis and if severe causes PPHN.

Predisposing factors	Prematurity, diabetic mother, APH, second twin, male, hypoxia, acidosis, shock, asphyxia.
Protective factors	IUGR, maternal drug addiction, stressful pregnancy.
Clinical features	Respiratory distress from 6 hours of age.
	Worsening course with a peak at 2–3 days, lasting 5–10 days.
CXR	Fine reticular 'ground glass' appearance, air bronchograms present.

Management

Surfactant replacement therapy	Administered via the ETT; more than one dose may be needed
Ventilatory support	Oxygen, CPAP, IPPV as needed, physiotherapy
Antibiotics	If infection suspected
Prevention	Maternal oral dexamethasone commenced 48 hours prior to delivery
Complications	Pneumothorax, IVH, BPD

Pneumonia
Causes
Common *Group B b-haemolytic strep.* Gram-negative bacteria (*E.coli*, klebsiella, pseudo-
   monas, serratia), *Staph. saprophyticus*
Rarer Listeria, chlamydia, mycoplasma, CMV, coxsackie, RSV, rubella, fungal

Clinical features
Non-specific, respiratory distress features.

CXR Patchy opacification

Treatment
Antibiotics, physiotherapy and respiratory support.

Meconium aspiration syndrome
Meconium is present at 10% of deliveries. If resuscitation is required, the airway must
be aspirated prior to ventilation (as described in Resuscitation above). Inhaled meconium can produce airway plugging with distal atelectasis, air leaks, secondary pneumonia, chemical pneumonitis, hypoxia, PPHN and acidosis (respiratory and
metabolic).

Clinical features

- *Respiratory distress worsening, severe acidosis*
- *Hyperinflated chest*
- *Signs of cerebral irritation*

CXR Hyperinflation, diffuse patchy opacification

Management

- *Respiratory support (high pressures or high-frequency oscillatory ventilation may be needed)*
- *Management of PPHN*
- *Antibiotics, physiotherapy*

Pneumothorax
Causes   Idiopathic (1% term infants)
        IPPV, PEEP (particularly for meconium aspiration and hypoplastic
        lungs)
        RDS
Clinical features Mostly asymptomatic
        Those of respiratory distress
        Rapid deterioration suggests a tension pneumothorax
Diagnosis   Chest transillumination with fibreoptic cold light
        CXR
        Diagnostic chest tap

Management	Chest drain insertion (anterior axillary line, 4th intercostal space)
Other airleaks	Pneumopericardium, pneumomediastinum, pulmonary interstitial emphysema (PIE), pneumoperitoneum

Pulmonary haemorrhage

Haemorrhagic pulmonary oedema due to elevated pulmonary capillary pressure from acute left ventricular failure or increased fluid (eg. from lung injury or hypoproteinaemia).

Associations	Prematurity
	RDS
	Pneumonia
	Asphyxia
	Acute cardiac failure
	Coagulopathies
Clinical features	Frothy pink sputum
	Low haematocrit
	Acutely unwell neonate
Management	Ventilation
	Correct coagulation defects
	Antibiotics

Bronchopulmonary dysplasia (BPD)

This is the prolonged requirement for oxygen (traditionally >28 days) with persistent X-ray changes and occurs after severe RDS or other neonatal lung disease. There are areas of emphysema and collapse, fibrosis and thickening of pulmonary arterioles.

Clinical features	Chest hyperinflation, recession, crepitations
	Oxygen requirement
CXR	Cystic pulmonary infiltrates, reticular pattern, 'honeycomb lung'
Management	Steroids and diuretics
	Bronchodilators if wheezy
	Long-term home oxygen (may be needed for 2–3 years)
	Pertussis vaccination from two months

Wilson–Mikity syndrome

Clinical features	Respiratory distress, hypoxia and apnoea developing slowly during the first month in premature infants who have no history of severe respiratory disease
CXR	Streaky infiltrates and cysts
Management	Respiratory support, long-term oxygen may be required
	Resolves over weeks-months usually, with susceptibility to chest infections for the first few years of life

Congenital diaphragmatic hernia

Incidence 1: 4000. These may be:

1. *posterolateral (Bochdalek) type: common type, 80% on the left side*
2. *anteromedial (Morgagni) type.*

Clinical features

- *Severe respiratory distress at birth*
- *Cyanosis*
- *Scaphoid abdomen*
- *Apex displaced to the right*

Diagnosis

CXR and AXR Loops of bowel in the thorax

Management

Resuscitation NG tube and aspirate

Intubation and ventilation, circulatory support

PPHN management

Surgical correction When fully resuscitated

Complications

Pulmonary hypertension with PPHN, pulmonary hypoplasia

Congenital lobar emphysema

Uncommon condition due to a cartilaginous defect of a lobar bronchus. *Upper lobe* most commonly affected.

Clinical features Insidious onset respiratory distress in first few weeks

Mediastinum displaced away from lesion

Hyperesonant with decreased breath sounds over affected lobe

Management Lobectomy

Oesophageal atresia and tracheo oesophageal fistula (TOF)

Incidence 1: 3000. A condition of oesophageal atresia usually associated with tracheo-oesophageal fistula.

Associations VACTERL = **V**ertebral, **A**nal, **C**ardiac, Tracheoo**E**sophageal, **R**enal and **L**imb abnormalities

VATER = **V**ertebral, **A**nal, Tracheoo**E**sophageal, **R**enal or **R**adial anomalies

Clinical features

- *Maternal polyhydramnios (60%)*
- *Recurrent aspiration pneumonia*
- *Coughing episodes with cyanosis*
- *Abdominal distension (air passing into GIT)*
- *Choking with feeds intermittently (H-type fistula)*

Investigations

1. *Inability to pass a radiopaque catheter into the stomach*
2. *AXR – no gas in stomach (A and B)*
3. *CXR – areas of collapse*
4. *Non-irritant radiopaque contrast study (to define lesion)*
5. *Cine contrast swallow with prone oesophagogram (for H-type fistula)*

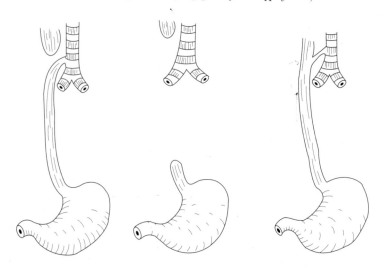

Proximal oesophageal atresia, distal tracheo-oesophageal fistula

Pure oesophageal atresia

H-type tracheo-oesophageal fistula

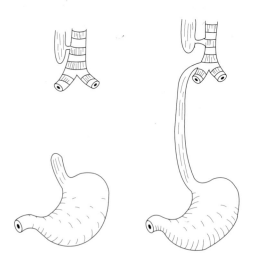

Oesophageal atresia, proximal tracheo-oesophageal fistula

Oesophageal atresia, double tracheo-oesophageal fistula

Figure 16.1 Types of oesophageal artresia and tracheo–oesophageal atresia

Management

1. *Nurse head up and prone*
2. *Surgical correction: division of fistula and anastomosis of oesophageal segments. If large defect, temporary oesophagostomy and gastrostomy may be made, with definitive surgery later*

CARDIAC DISORDERS

For detail on congenital heart disease, see Chapter 13.
General cardiac conditions include the following.

Causes of cyanosis

Severe lung disease
Cyanotic congenital heart disease
PPHN
Methaemoglobinaemia
Others: Sepsis, airway problem
Neurological (eg. asphyxia, seizures, neuromuscular)

See p. 103

Persistent pulmonary hypertension of the newborn (PPHN)

This is also known as persistent fetal circulation. It is the most difficult condition to distinguish clinically from cyanotic congenital heart disease. There is failure of the pulmonary vascular resistance to fall after birth and blood is shunted via the ductus arteriosus (right to left) and the foramen ovale. This results in central cyanosis.

Predisposing factors Hypoxia, acidosis, metabolic disturbance
Severe lung disease
Small for dates, asphyxiated babies, polycythaemia

Clinical features and diagnosis

1. *Central cyanosis*
2. *Loud P2 heart sound*
3. *Arterial blood gases: pO_2 low, pCO_2 relatively normal*
4. *Little improvement in saturations with 100% O_2*
5. *Preductal blood pO_2 is >5 mmHg higher than postductal pO_2 (demonstrate by transcutaneous pO_2 measurements on right chest and lower abdomen)*
6. *CXR: normal heart and well-expanded oligaemic lung fields*

Management

1. *Correct acidosis:*
Respiratory – ensure CO_2 is low
Metabolic – sodium bicarbonate or THAM (if Na ↑)
2. *If cyanosis remains, options include:*
Tolazoline IV (side-effects include hypotension and gastrointestinal bleeding)
Prostacyclin IV
Inhaled nitric oxide
ECMO

Persistent ductus arteriosus (PDA)

Commonly seen in premature infants. For features and treatment, see p. 98.

Cardiac failure

Common complication of PDA. Seen in certain congenital heart diseases. For features and treatment, see p. 91.

Duct-dependent circulations

Emergency treatment includes prostaglandin E_2 (see p. 104).

NEUROLOGICAL DISORDERS

Hypoxia-ischaemia

Hypoxia (insufficient arterial oxygen concentration) and ischaemia (insufficient blood flow to cells) can damage the fetus, affecting many organs and resulting in a collection of features. On delivery these infants are depressed and they fail to breathe adequately. They are resuscitated as necessary at birth and then, if needed, managed on the neonatal unit.

Fetal hypoxia may occur as an intrauterine or intrapartum event. *Intrauterine hypoxia* may be acute, presenting with signs of fetal distress, chronic (often not obvious, resulting in IUGR) or acute on chronic. *Intrapartum hypoxia* may be acute (often prolonged) or acute on chronic.

Signs of fetal distress include bradycardia, lack of beat-to-beat variability, late decelerations (type II dips), reduced fetal movements and meconium.

Causes of hypoxia-ischaemia

Maternal	Acute hypotensive episode, maternal cyanotic heart disease or respiratory disease
	Preeclampsia, eclampsia, inadequate uterine relaxation during delivery
Placental	Chronic insufficiency (many causes eg. pre-eclampsia), abruption, cord prolapse
Fetal	Obstructed labour, prematurity, postmaturity, hydrops fetalis

After birth, hypoxia may result from several causes including severe anaemia, severe shock, failure to breathe adequately or cyanotic cardiac disease.

Effects of hypoxia-ischaemia

System	Effects
CNS	Hypoxic-ischaemic encephalopathy
Renal	Acute tubular necrosis
Cardiac	Ischaemic changes, cardiac failure
Respiratory	Respiratory distress syndrome, PPHN, pulmonary haemorrhage
Gastrointestinal	NEC
Metabolic	Metabolic acidosis, hypoglycaemia, hypocalcaemia, hyponatraemia
Other	Adrenal haemorrhage, DIC

Hypoxic ischaemic encephalopathy (HIE)

This is a disturbance of neurological behaviour due to ischaemic damage to the brain. The condition involves *watershed zone* infarcts (the zones between the major arteries, susceptible to hypoperfusion) in the cortex and periventricular white matter. These can result in cortical and subcortical necrosis and cysts, and periventricular leucomalacia (PVL). Particularly in premature infants, *germinal matrix haemorrhages* occur, with intraventricular haemorrhage.

PVL is cystic changes in the white matter, with later reduction in myelin around the ventricles secondary to ischaemic insults. Diagnosis is on USS, CT and MRI scan. A high risk of cerebral palsy follows.

Clinical severity of HIE

Mild	Moderate	Severe
Irritability, hyperalert	Lethargy	Coma
No seizures	Seizures	Prolonged seizures
Normal tone	Differential hypotonia	Severe hypotonia
Jittery	(legs > arms, neck extensors > flexors)	Need for ventilation
Weak sucking	Poor suck, NG feeds required	No sucking reflex
Sympathetic dominance	Parasympathetic dominance	Respiratory support needed

The condition develops over a period of a few days. In the first 12 hours infants are usually hypotonic with irregular breathing and seizures in 50%. They may remain hypotonic or become hypertonic in the next few hours and cerebral oedema may develop.

Management

- *Initial resuscitation*
- *General support as necessary (eg. NG feeding, metabolic balance, renal support)*
- *Brain oedema management (fluid restriction, mannitol, ventilatory control)*
- *Seizure management*
- *Management of complications*

Prognosis

This is related to the severity of HIE. Mild encephalopathy generally resolves within two days, moderate encephalopathy usually begins to resolve in the first week and full recovery (if it occurs) over a few weeks. Severe encephalopathic infants may die in the acute phase or may show a complete recovery but if abnormal neurology is present after six weeks, cerebral palsy is likely.

Periventricular haemorrhage (PVH)

This is a generic term encompassing several types of intracranial haemorrhage in neonates. Bleeds occur when there is an unstable cerebral circulation, most commonly into the germinal matrix at the head of the caudate nucleus.

Predisposing factors

- *Prematurity*
- *Low birth weight*
- *Hypercapnoea*
- *RDS*
- *IPPV*
- *Metabolic acidosis*
- *Coagulation disorder*

Clinical features

- *Asymptomatic*
- *Subtle neurological signs (eg. roving eye movements)*
- *Slow deterioration – apnoeas, bradycardias, metabolic acidosis, seizures, anaemia*
- *Massive collapse – bulging fontanelle, hypotension*

Diagnosis
Cranial USS.

Grades of PVH
Grade I   – subependymal bleed
Grade II – intraventricular haemorrhage (IVH)
Grade III – IVH with distension of the ventricle
Grade IV – bleeding into the brain parenchyma

A new classification has been formulated with GMH-IVH denoting bleeding into the germinal matrix and ventricle and all other bleeds being carefully described.

Complications

1. *Hydrocephalus*
2. *Porencephaly*

Management
Supportive.

Neonatal convulsions and jitteriness
Causes

Seizures	Jitteriness
Asphyxia	Hypoglycaemia
Infections	Hypocalcaemia
Drug withdrawal	Sepsis
Pyridoxine deficiency/ other inborn errors	Drug withdrawal
Metabolic eg. glucose ↓, Ca ↓, Mg ↓	
CVA, subarachnoid haemorrhage	

Clinical features

NB. Neonatal seizures are not always obvious and may manifest, for example, as apnoea.

	Seizures	Jitteriness
Predominant movement	Multifocal, tone alteration, apnoea	Rhythmic, tonic-clonic, no facial involvement
Conscious state	Altered	Alert or asleep
Eye movements	Eye deviation occurs	Normal
Movements stop when limb held	No	Yes

Investigations

Infection screen	Blood, CSF and urine, M, C + S, serology (NB. CSF is persistently bloodstained throughout the CSF in IVH or CVA)
Electrolyte disturbance	Urea and electrolytes including Ca and Mg
Metabolic screen	Glucose, metabolic work-up (see p. 286)
USS brain	
EEG	Often unaffected

Management

1. *Treat cause, eg. glucose IV, calcium IV, magnesium IV, IV antibiotics, IV pyridoxine*
2. *Anticonvulsants used in neonatal seizures:*

Phenobarbitone	*IV, IM, oral*
Phenytoin	*IV*
Diazepam	*IV*
Paraldehyde	*PR*
Clonazepam	*IV*

Drug withdrawal (Maternal drug abuse)

Clinical features

Wakefulness
Irritability
Temperature instability, tachypnoea
Hyperactivity, high-pitched cry, hypertonia, hyperreflexia
Diarrhoea, disorganised suck
Respiratory distress, rhinorrhoea
Apnoea, autonomic dysfunction
Weight loss, failure to thrive
Alkalosis
Lacrimation

Management

This includes close observation for the above signs. Naloxone contraindicated at delivery.

Conservative measures   Decreased sensory stimuli, frequent feeds, swaddling

Drug treatment	These include opiates (eg. morphine) and sedatives (eg. diazepam, chlorpromazine). These are weaned over a few weeks

NB. Increased incidence of SIDS.

Retinopathy of prematurity

This is due to a proliferation of blood vessels at the junction of the vascular and non-vascular retina secondary to reoxygenation after hypoxia.

Associations	Prematurity and oxygen therapy	
Complications	Retinal detachment	
	Decreased acuity, blindness	
Stages	Stage I	Demarcation line separating vascular and avascular retina
	Stage II	Ridging of demarcation line
	Stage III	Fibrovascular proliferation
	Stage IV	Partial retinal detachment
	Stage V	Total retinal detachment

Management

- *Screening of all premature infants at risk from 32 weeks of age by ophthalmologist*
- *Spontaneous resolution of most lesions*
- *Laser or cryotherapy may be required*

GASTROINTESTINAL DISORDERS

Intestinal obstruction

Causes

- *Atresia: Oesophageal*
  Duodenal
  Jejunal
  Colonic
  Imperforate anus
- *Congenital hypertrophic pyloric stenosis*
- *Hirschsprung disease*
- *Volvulus neonatorum (malrotation)*
- *Meconium plug (eg. cystic fibrosis)*
- *Hernial obstruction (internal or external)*
- *Duplication cyst*
- *NEC (stricture, ileus)*
- *Annular pancreas*

Clinical features

- *Polyhydramnios*
- *Bile-stained vomiting*

- *Abdominal distension*
- *Visible peristalsis*
- *Delayed or absent passage of meconium*
- *Features of dehydration*

Investigations
These include electrolyte status, CXR and AXR and contrast studies.

Management
Dependent on the condition (often surgical).

Necrotising enterocolitis (NEC)
A disease of bowel wall inflammation, ulceration and perforation due to many causes. An ischaemic or hypoxic insult causes mucosal sloughing leading to bacterial invasion and gastrointestinal gangrene and perforation.

Risk factors

- *Hypoxia*
- *Prematurity*
- *Hyperosmolar feeds*
- *Sepsis*
- *Hypovolaemia*
- *Venous and umbilical catheters*
- *Exchange transfusion*
- *Polycythaemia*

Clinical features
General   Apnoeas, lethargy, vomiting, temperature instability, acidosis, shock
Abdominal   Distended, shiny abdomen, bile aspirates, rectal fresh blood

Complications
Short term   Perforation, obstruction, gangrenous bowel, intrahepatic cholestasis Sepsis, DIC
Long term   Short bowel syndrome, stricture, lactose intolerance

Diagnosis
AXR   Distended loops of bowel, fluid levels, *pneumostasis intestinalis* (intramural gas), portal vein gas, pneumoperitoneum
FBC   Neutrophils ($\uparrow$ or $\downarrow$), platelets ($\downarrow$), DIC
Blood, stool   M, C + S

Management

1. *Manage shock, acidosis, electrolyte and clotting disorder and anaemia and ventilate if necessary*
2. *Parenteral feeds only*

3. *Gastrointestinal decompression (NG tube with aspiration)*
4. *Systemic antibiotics*
5. *Surgical intervention if surgical complication occurs*

Prognosis

10% mortality, higher if perforation occurs.

Meconium ileus

Intestinal obstruction of terminal ileum due to thick, inspissated meconium. There is failure to pass meconium within 48 hours of birth and clinical features of obstruction; 90% have cystic fibrosis.

Diagnosis

AXR	Foamy pattern seen around plug
Gastrograffin enema	Microcolon
Immune-reactive trypsin	NB. This falls after surgery
Sweat test	At 2–3 months to confirm diagnosis
Genetics	Genotype for cystic fibrosis

Management

1. *Conservative*
2. *Gastrograffin enema or surgical decompression*

NB. *Meconium plug syndrome* is a lower bowel obstruction or delayed passage of meconium due to a plug of meconium around 10 cm long. Seen in premature infants, Hirschsprung disease and cystic fibrosis.

Congenital atresias

These may occur anywhere along the gastrointestinal tract (see p. 484). Features are those of obstruction, which vary according to the level of obstruction. Diagnosis is on imaging studies, in particular:

Duodenal atresia 'Double bubble' of air seen on plain AXR
Imperforate anus Air bubble seen on plain AXR with baby held inverted

Management is with initial resuscitation and then surgical repair.

Imperforate anus

Incidence 1 : 2500. Low and high forms exist ± fistula to urethra or vagina. Air bubble seen on AXR after first 12 hours of life, baby with bottom up

Management is often with an initial colostomy, with further repair later. Rectal inertia is a long-term problem.

Gastroschisis and exomphalos

Exomphalos

Incidence 1: 5000. An evisceration of gastrointestinal contents *through the umbilicus*. This is covered by peritoneum. Other abnormalities are often associated:

- *trisomy 13, trisomy 18*
- *Beckwith–Weidemann syndrome*
- *renal malformations including bladder exstrophy, Wilms tumour (40% incidence)*
- *congenital heart disease*

Gastroschisis

Incidence 1: 30 000. This is evisceration of gastrointestinal contents through a right *paraumbilical* defect. There is no peritoneal covering and hypoalbuminaemia occurs. Bowel atresias are associated. Bowel may be scarred and have adhesions resulting in stenosis, strictures and atresias.

Complications: Short bowel syndrome, failure to thrive.

gut & cardiac abn.

Management

Preoperative Gastric decompression, resuscitation with IV albumin, antibiotics, TPN Wrap abdominal contents in moist antibiotic-soaked gauze

Operative Small lesions (<5 cm) are surgically treated with primary closure. Larger defects treated with a staged repair, using a non-reactive silicon sheeting to cover bowel contents in gastroschisis

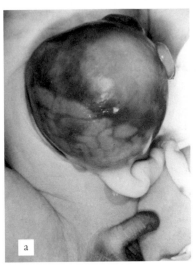
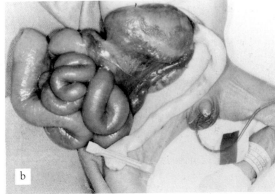

Figure 16.2 (a) Exomphalos (an umbilical defect) and (b) gastroschisis (a para-umbilical defect)

HAEMATOLOGICAL DISORDERS

Hydrops fetalis

This is severe oedema, ascites and pleural effusions present at birth.

Causes

Idiopathic (50%)

Severe anaemia	Severe haemolytic disease of the newborn (rhesus, ABO)
	Chronic twin-twin transfusion
	Fetomaternal haemorrhage
	α-thalassaemia
Congenital infections	eg. Parvovirus B19
Cardiac failure	SVT
	Severe CHD
	Premature closure of ductus arteriosus and foramen ovale
Hypoproteinaemia	Congenital nephrotic syndrome, maternal preeclampsia
Congenital malformations	Chromosomal anomalies (eg. Turner syndrome), obstructive uropathy, pulmonary adenoma, fetal or placental angioma

Investigations of cause

FBC, serum albumin and other proteins, Coombs' test, congenital infection screen. Kleihauer test on maternal blood is checked for fetomaternal haemorrhage.

Management

1. *Resuscitation – transfusions, abdominal and chest drainage as necessary, ventilatory support*
2. *Treat the cause*

Twin-twin transfusion

This occurs in monozygous twins who have a shared placenta.

Acute fetofetal transfusion	Similar size twins, one anaemic, one plethoric
Chronic fetofetal transfusion	Anaemic twin has IUGR

The plethoric twin is often the most at risk as diminished blood flow through small vessels may cause multiorgan damage.

Twin	Complications
Anaemic	Severe anaemia
	Hydrops fetalis
	IUGR
Plethoric	Neurological – jitters, apnoea, seizures
	Cardiac-failure, pulmonary hypertension
	Gastrointestinal-NEC
	Renal-renal vein thrombosis
	Others-hypoglycaemia, Ca ↓, platelets ↓, jaundice
	Dilutional exchange transfusion

Management

- *Anaemic twin may require transfusion*
- *Plethoric twin may require dilutional transfusion (if venous haematocrit >70 or symptomatic)*

ENDOCRINE/METABOLIC DISORDERS

Hypoglycaemia
There is no universally accepted definition, but blood glucose levels <2.6 mmol/l at any age are hypoglycaemic. See p. 272 for persistent hypoglycaemia.

Causes of transient neonatal hypoglycaemia

Substrate deficiency (ketotic)	IUGR, prematurity, asphyxia, hypothermia, sepsis, malformation
Hyperinsulinism (non-ketotic)	Diabetic mother, gestational diabetes, rhesus iso-immunisation

Clinical features

- *Asymptomatic*
- *Apnoeas, jitteriness, seizures, lethargy, hypotonia*

Investigations

- *Blood glucose*
- *If persistent and recurrent, screen for ketones, hormone levels and metabolic disorders (see p. 272)*

Management

If asymptomatic	Oral feed 3 ml/kg (milk), then hourly feeds with monitoring of blood glucose
If symptomatic	IV 10% glucose 2 ml/kg bolus, then 10% glucose infusion 60–90 ml/kg/day
	If remains low, may need 15–20% glucose infusion
	Frequent monitoring of blood glucose throughout

Persistent hypoglycaemia is managed according to cause.

Osteopaenia of prematurity
Most of the calcium and phosphorus of the skeleton is formed in the third trimester. Premature infants therefore have high requirements for phosphate and calcium. Changes of both rickets and osteoporosis are seen.

Investigations

Serum	Alk phos ↑ (up to × 6 adult levels)
	PO_4 ↓, Ca N or ↑
X-ray changes	From six weeks old (reduced density, fraying and cupping, fractures)

Management

- *Phosphate supplements to feeds*
- *Prevention with preterm formulas (contain high phosphate and calcium) and vitamin D for first three months*

Maternal diabetes

Problems associated with maternal diabetes.

Foetal	Neonatal
Congenital malformations:	Hypoglycaemia (from fetal hyperinsulinism)
risk increased × 3	RDS
Macrosomia (difficult labour)	Hypertrophic obstructive cardiomyopathy
Hypoplastic left colon	Polycythaemia
Caudal regression syndrome (sacral agenesis)	
Renal venous thrombosis	
CHD, eg. VSD, coarctation, TGA,	
hypertrophic subaortic stenosis	

CRANIOFACIAL DISORDERS

Cleft lip and palate

Incidence 1 : 1000 babies, polygenic inheritance. Subsequent pregnancy risk 5%.

Associations   Older mothers

Syndromes eg. Patau syndrome

Drugs eg. maternal anticonvulsant therapy, alcohol

They may be unilateral or bilateral and isolated or combined.

Problems

- *Inability to feed*
- *Choking episodes*
- *Otitis media*
- *Speech problems*

Management

A multidisciplinary approach involving plastic surgeons, ENT surgeons, geneticists, paediatricians, speech therapists, audiologists, orthodontists. Special feeding teats, speech therapy.

Surgical repair   Lip may be repaired early (first week of life), though some surgeons prefer to wait until three months old

Palate usually repaired at several months of age

Pierre–Robin sequence

A sequence of:

1. *midline cleft of soft palate*

2. *micrognathia*
3. *glossoptosis (posterior displacement of the tongue).*

These result in difficulty feeding and upper airway obstruction.
Management includes:

- *nasopharyngeal airway*
- *special feeding teat*
- *surgical repair of palate (mandible grows)*

ORTHOPAEDIC DISORDERS

Congenital dislocation of the hip (CDH)

Incidence 2 : 1000, female > male, left side > right side. Polygenic inheritance, recurrence risk 1 in 30.

Associations   Breech position
Positive family history
Oligohydramnios
Chinese (as a result of neonatal carrying position)
Muscular or neurological problems eg. spina bifida
Syndromes eg. trisomy 13 and 18
Multiple congenital abnormalities

Clinical features

- *Diagnosed on screening (Ortolani and Barlow tests)*
- *Asymmetrical buttock creases*
- *Only becomes obvious when walking develops*

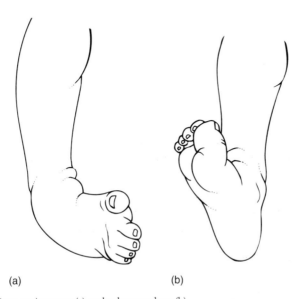

(a)   (b)

Figure 16.3 Talipes equinovarus (a) and calcaneovalgus (b)

Investigations
USS hip. NB. This may be used as a screen in high-risk babies.

Management
Immobilisation of the hip in abducted position allows improved acetabular and ligament development. Gallows traction, splintages (eg. Aberdeen, Van Rosen), plaster casts and Pavlik harnesses are used, depending on the age at diagnosis. Late diagnosis may require major orthopaedic involvement.

Talipes
This may be of two types:

1. *talipes equinovarus (club foot)* – *more common than calcaneovalgus*
2. *talipes calcaneovalgus.*

Management is with orthopaedic correction, by conservative means (serial plasters) or operative if conservative measures fail.

NB. *Positional talipes* is common and involves no bony deformity. It is easily correctable by movement and treated with physiotherapy.

FURTHER READING

Avery GN, Fletcher MA, MacDonald MG *Neonatology. Pathophysiology and management of the newborn*, 5th Ed. Lippincott, Williams & Wilkins, Baltimore, 1999

Levene M, Tudehope D, Thuearle D *Essentials of neonatal medicine*, Blackwell Sciences, London, 2000

Robertson NRC *Textbook of neonatology*, 3rd Ed, Churchill Livingstone, Edinburgh, 1999

17

Surgical conditions and emergencies

- *Gastrointestinal conditions*
- *Genitourinary conditions*
- *Emergencies*

- *The Children Act*
- *Statementing*
- *Consent*

Gastrointestinal conditions

THE ACUTE ABDOMEN

This is a clinical diagnosis indicating potentially serious intraabdominal pathology which demands urgent management through resuscitation and usually surgical intervention.

Peritonitis is an inflammation or irritation of the peritoneum resulting in clinical signs either localised to a specific area or generalised throughout the abdomen.

Surgical acute abdomen causes

Upper GIT	Oesophageal, gastric or duodenal perforation
Hepatobiliary	Cholecystitis
	Ruptured liver, spleen or gall bladder
Lower GIT	Appendicitis
	Inflamed Meckel's diverticulum
	Inflammatory bowel disease causing obstruction, perforation, severe exacerbation, megacolon
	Ischaemic bowel eg. intussusception, volvulus
	Incarcerated hernia causing ischaemia or obstruction
	Neoplasia causing obstruction or perforation
Retroperitoneum	Pancreatitis
	Ureteric obstruction (renal colic)
Pelvic	Rupture or torsion of ovarian cyst
	Testicular torsion

Clinical features

General   Malaise, fever, rigors
Abdominal   Pain – enquire about location, duration, severity, constant or intermittent
Other features Anorexia, nausea, vomiting, dysuria, bowel habit

Examination

- *Temperature, pulse, BP, HR*
- *Specific systems (abdominal – examine for tenderness location, guarding)*
- *General (eg. nutrition, jaundice, anaemia)*

Investigations

These will depend on the probable cause. Some important considerations are:

Urine   Urinalysis and microscopy if indicated, pregnancy test
Bloods   FBC, U&E, amylase, glucose
          ABG, LFTs, Ca, PO_4
CXR   (Erect)
AXR   (Supine)

Medical causes of acute abdominal pain

Renal   Urinary tract infection
                  Henoch–Schönlein purpura
Respiratory   Lower lobe pneumonia
Metabolic   Diabetic ketoacidosis
                  Acute porphyrias
Liver   Acute viral hepatitis
Haematological Sickle cell disease crises
                  Congenital spherocytosis (haemolytic episodes)
Other   Lead poisoning

ACUTE APPENDICITIS

Common acute surgical condition, rare <5 years, peak age 10–20 years.

Typical clinical features

Abdominal pain   Commencing paraumbilically and moving to the right iliac fossa
                   Worse on movement, gradually worsening
                   Guarding indicates peritonitis
Vomiting and anorexia
Low-grade fever

Examination

- *Pain localised to McBurney's point in the right iliac fossa*
- *In young children pain is poorly localised and peritonitis features may be absent*
- *Retrocaecal and pelvic appendix may not present with classic signs*
- *Flushed, foetor, tachycardic*

Investigations

The diagnosis is clinical.

FBC   Mild neutrophilia may be present
Urine   Check to exclude UTI

Management

Appendicectomy.

MESENTERIC ADENITIS

This is thought to be due to a viral infection (eg. adenovirus) or bacterial infection (*Yersinia enterocolitica*) with inflammation of the mesenteric lymph nodes. It can be difficult to distinguish clinically from appendicitis. Management is conservative.

INTUSSUSCEPTION

This is invagination of one segment of bowel into an adjacent lower segment. It most commonly occurs proximally to the ileocoaecal valve. The blood supply to the intussuscepted bowel is then compromised and it will become necrotic if not reduced promptly. Most commonly occurs at 6–9 months of age. Male > female.

Associations (<10%)   Intestinal polyp, lymphoma, Meckel's diverticulum, cystic fibrosis, Henoch–Schönlein purpura, inflamed Peyer's patch.

Clinical features

Abdominal pain   Episodes of screaming and pallor, infant draws up its knees during these episodes

Abdominal   Distension, sausage-shaped abdominal mass, rectal examination may reveal blood-stained mucus

Other   Vomiting, diarrhoea (the classic '*red currant jelly*' stools are rare) Dehydration progressing to shock. Infant may be very unwell

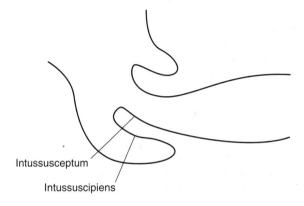

Intussusceptum

Intussuscipiens

Figure 17.1 Intussusception

Investigations

Abdominal USS	This may reveal the mass (target-shaped) if radiologist is skilled
Plain AXR	Signs of small bowel obstruction, reduced gas in right iliac fossa
Air enema	This may be therapeutic as well as diagnostic

Management

- *Fluid resuscitation as required*
- *Air enema reduction (contrast may be used instead) successful in 75%*
- *Contraindications to enema: Rectal bleeding*
                              Peritonism
- *Surgical reduction ± resection if enema unsuccessful or contraindications to enema*

MALROTATION

This is a result of abnormal movement of the intestine occurring during the third month of gestation. The most common type is incomplete rotation with the caecum in the midline. In this case the duodenum does not pass posteriorly to the superior mesenteric artery. The base of the small bowel is not fixed from the ligament of Treitz to the caecum but is anchored on the superior mesenteric artery and the caecum is fixed in the right upper quadrant by fibrous tissue (Ladd's bands) crossing the second part of the duodenum. Obstruction may occur due to Ladd's bands crossing the second part of the duodenum or a volvulus occurring around the superior mesenteric artery.

Associations	Diaphragmatic hernia
	Gastroschisis and exompholos

Clinical presentation

1. *Acute neonatal obstruction*
2. *Episodic intestinal obstruction – distension, bilious vomiting, pallor, abdominal mass, bloody stools*
3. *Midgut volvulus*
4. *Protein-losing enteropathy (secondary to bacterial overgrowth)*
5. *Asymptomatic to adolescence (25–50%)*

Investigations

Radiological	AXR (abnormal gas pattern, signs of obstruction)
	Contrast studies (upper gastric series and enema)
	A failure of the third part of the duodenum to cross the midline may be seen

Management

This is surgical, with release of Ladd's bands and fixation of the bowel. NB. If an asymptomatic malrotation is discovered it should be treated to avoid volvulus in the future.

MECKEL'S DIVERTICULUM

This is an ileal remnant of the vitellointestinal duct, which may contain ectopic gastric mucosa or pancreatic tissue.

Approximately:

- *2% of people affected*
- *2 inches long*
- *2 feet from the ileocaecal valve*

Clinical features

- *Mostly asymptomatic*
- *May present as rectal bleeding, intussusception, volvulus or acute appendicitis*

Investigations

Technetium scan. Increased uptake by gastric mucosa seen (70%). False negatives common post-haemorrhage, as gastric mucosa then often ulcerated. Therefore, perform scan 3–4 weeks post bleed.

Management

Surgical resection.

CONGENITAL HYPERTROPHIC PYLORIC STENOSIS

This is due to a hypertrophy of the muscle layer of the pylorus of unknown cause.

Associations   Males > females
Most common presentation age 4–6 weeks
Caucasian
Family history (especially maternal)
Syndromes: Trisomy 18, Turner Syndrome, Cornelia de Lange Syndrome.

Clinical features

Vomiting	Persistent, not bile stained, may be projectile
Feeding	Hungry, thin infant
Abdominal examination	Visible peristalsis
	Olive-shaped tumour in upper abdomen

Investigations

Diagnosis is made on a test feed or USS, both of which are operator dependent.

Test feed	Palpate abdomen for olive-shaped tumour, observe for peristalsis
Abdominal USS	May outline tumour as a 'doughnut' ring (muscle thickness >4 mm, pyloric length >14 mm)

Serum electrolytes and pH: Signs of dehydration may be present, jaundice is seen in 5–10%. A *hypochloraemic hypokalaemic metabolic alkalosis* is seen. NB. Serum potassium is usually maintained but total body potassium is depleted.

rehydration: 0.45% D saline + 40 mmol KCl/l over the first
12 hours until bicarbonate corrected, then standard fluid replacement

,lar U&E and ABG measurement (6–12 hourly)

decompression

Surgery .en rehydrated and alkalosis corrected, a pyloromyotomy (*Ramstedt's procedure*) is performed.

ACHALASIA

This is a motility disorder of the oesophagus with lack of normal peristalsis in the oesophagus and a relative gastrooesophageal junction obstruction. It generally presents in adolescence or adulthood. The underlying pathology is of a decrease in the number of ganglion cells in the oesophagus, with an increase in inflammatory cells.

Associations Chagas' disease and adrenal insufficiency

Investigations
Upright CXR Air–fluid level in dilated oesophagus and/or absence of gastric air bubble
Barium swallow Abnormal motility and dilatation of oesophagus
Oesophageal manometry Abnormal

Management
Medical Calcium channel blockers, eg. nifedipine ⎫
⎬ Temporary measures only
Intrasphincteral botulinum toxin injection ⎭
Surgical Heller myotomy (division of the muscle fibres at gastrooesophageal junction)
Balloon dilatation (less effective than myotomy in childhood)

NB. Surgical management often results in gastrooesophageal reflux.

Genitourinary conditions

UNDESCENDED TESTES (CRYPTORCHIDISM)

This is seen at birth in approximately 3.5% of boys. At three months the total incidence is 1.5%. The testes descend through the inguinal canal in the third trimester of pregnancy.

The testes may be: Palpable or impalpable along the normal line of descent
Ectopic

Most commonly they are in the superficial inguinal pouch.

Investigations

Imaging techniques	USS (this may detect testes in the inguinal canal difficult to palpate in fat boys)
	CT/MRI scan
Laparoscopy	The most accurate method to identify the site of intraabdominal testes
Serum hormones	Testosterone response to IM HCG (if bilaterally impalpable)
Karyotype	If bilaterally impalpable

Management options

Surgical correction	Reasons for correction:
(orchidopexy)	increases fertility
	allows early detection of malignant change (increased risk in undescended testes)
	cosmetic result
	Correction is generally done by two years
Staged orchidopexy	If unable to bring down in one stage
Orchidectomy	If unilateral intraabdominal and unable to correct

HYDROCOELE

Commonly present at birth secondary to a patent processus vaginalis.

Clinical features

Scrotal swelling: usually fluctuant (may be tense), variation in size, transilluminates.
NB. A hydrocoele of the cord is a harder lump associated with the spermatic cord.

Management

Infant hydrocoeles may be observed for one year, during which time most spontaneously resolve. Persistent hydrocoeles are treated with surgical ligation of the processus vaginalis.

TESTICULAR TORSION

This is a twist of the testis and causes vascular compromise of the testis. It is an emergency as testicular necrosis occurs within six hours of onset of symptoms.

Clinical features

- *Acute scrotal pain, nausea, vomiting*
- *Firm, dusky scrotal swelling, relatively painless*

Investigations

A clinical diagnosis. Doppler ultrasound of testes can show reduced testicular blood flow but is relatively inaccurate.

Management

Surgical   Untwist the torted testis and fix *both* testes. If testis is non-viable an orchidectomy is performed

EPIDIDYMOORCHITIS

This is the main differential diagnosis of testicular torsion. It may be seen in young children associated with UTI or secondary to viral infections (mumps) or in adolescents related to sexually transmitted disease. The pain is of rapid onset and increasing in severity; there is not usually any nausea and vomiting and pyrexia is often present.

Management is with antibiotics. In doubtful cases, surgical exploration is performed.

INGUINAL HERNIA

In children these are usually indirect due to a patent processus vaginalis.
Males > females; right side > left side.

Associations   Preterm infants
Cryptorchidism
Connective tissue disorders, eg. Marfan syndrome

Clinical features
- *Intermittent scrotal swelling, more prominent on crying or straining*
- *Irreducible hernia   Painful swelling*
  Risk of bowel obstruction or strangulation

Management
- *Elective surgical repair*
- *Irreducible hernias must be reduced urgently (usually possible by gentle pressure and analgesia, otherwise urgent surgery is necessary)*

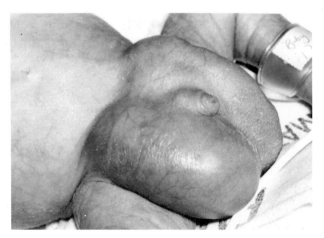

Figure 17.2 Inguinal hernia

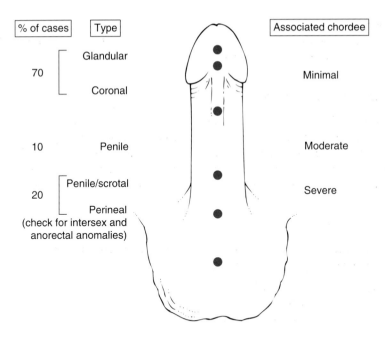

Figure 17.3 Hypospadias

HYPOSPADIAS

Incidence 2–3: 1000. Hypospadias comprises:

1. *ventral urethral meatus*
2. *hooded prepuce*
3. *chordee (a fibrous ventral curvature)*

Management
Surgical correction by two years to enable normal micturition and a straight erection.

NB. The foreskin must be preserved as it may be required for the correction process and so the parents must be informed not to have the child circumcised.

CIRCUMCISION

Medical indications for circumcision:

Phimosis   This results from scarring, usually due to lichen sclerosis et atrophicans also known as balanitis xerotica obliterans (BXO), a chronic inflammatory process.

Recurrent balanitis

Recurrent UTIs   Particularly if associated renal abnormality or damage

NB. Non-retractile foreskin is normal in young children, 90% are retractile by four years.

Emergencies

Whatever the underlying cause, in an acutely unwell child, any compromise of the airway, breathing or circulation must be attended to using basic resuscitation measures.

The procedures outlined for basic and advanced life support are regularly updated by the European and UK Resuscitation Committees and thus current guidelines should be checked.

BASIC LIFE SUPPORT

	Infant	Child
Check area is safe		
Responsiveness	Shake gently and call for help	Shake gently and call for help
A Airway	Head tilt to *neutral position*	Head tilt to sniffing position
	Chin lift/jaw thrust (trauma)	Chin lift/jaw thrust (trauma)
B Breathing	Look, listen, feel for breathing	Look, feel, listen for breathing
	Mouth-to-*mouth-and-nose*	Mouth-to-mouth
	5 breaths	5 breaths
C Circulation	*Brachial or femoral pulse*	Carotid pulse
	If *<60/min* commence CPR	If no pulse commence CPR
	Chest compressions: *2 fingers*	Chest compressions: heel of one
	1 cm below nipple line, 1/3	hand to lower sternum, depth of
	depth of chest	1/3 depth of chest

Continue CPR using ratio 5:1 chest compressions:breaths, 20 cycles per minute (pulse rate 100/min). Go for help if none has arrived by one minute (take a small child with you).

Choking

If foreign body aspiration is suspected back blows or chest thrusts are used to dislodge the object in an infant; abdominal thrusts are also used in a child >1 year old. See Figure 17.4.

ADVANCED LIFE SUPPORT

Airway	Oral airway (Guedel)
	Nasal airway (not if risk of basal skull fracture)
	Endotracheal intubation if necessary { ETT internal diameter = [age of child/4] + 4; ETT length = [age/2] + 12
Breathing	Bag and mask ventilation with 100% oxygen
	Connect to ET tube if intubated
	Monitor with pulse oximeter and ECG leads
Circulation	Assessment of output and cardiac rhythm. Drugs given as per protocols

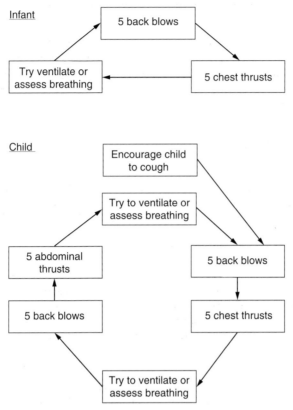

Figure 17.4 Protocol for management of choking
Adapted from: UK Resuscitation Council, 1998 Resuscitation guidelines for use in the United Kingdom.

Cardiac arrest protocols

Most cardiac arrests in children are respiratory in origin, with a secondary cardiac arrest. There are three basic cardiac rhythms seen: ventricular fibrillation, asystole, and electromechanical dissociation (the latter two classed as non-VF).

It is important to check the blood sugar during cardiac arrest as children have low glycogen stores and thus rapidly become hypoglycaemic. The European resuscitation council regularly revises the protocols for cardiac arrest, and the latest guidelines should be viewed.

Defibrillation is given on initial shock as 2J/kg, then 2J/kg then 4J/kg and further shocks at this level.

Adrenaline is given as 10 μg/kg (0.1 ml/kg of 1 : 10 000) first dose, via direct venous or intraosseous access or 100 μg/kg by ETT, then subsequent doses 100 μg/kg (0.1 ml/kg of 1 : 1000).

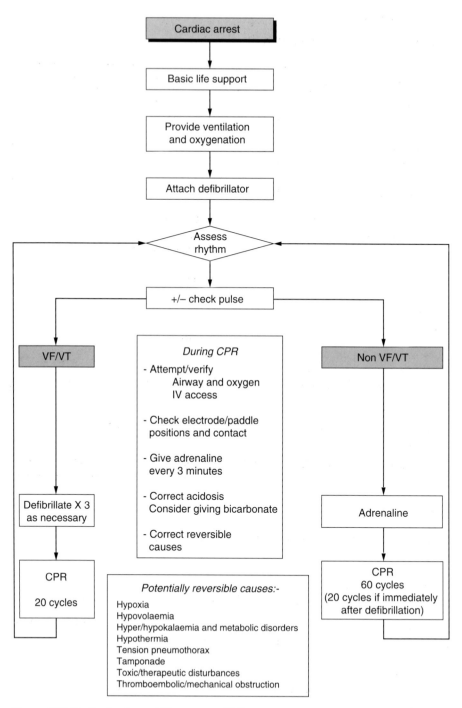

Figure 17.5 Paediatric advanced life support guidelines
ref: From 1998 resuscitation guidelines for use in the United Kingdom, Resuscitation Council
(UK).

COMA SCALES

Maximum score 15, minimum score 3.

Children's Coma Scale	<4 years	Glasgow Coma Scale	4–15 years
Eye opening			
Spontaneous	4	Spontaneous	4
To speech	3	To speech	3
To pain	2	To pain	2
None	1	None	1
Best motor response			
Spontaneous or obeys command	6	Obeys command	6
Localises pain	5	Localises pain	5
Withdraws from pain	4	Flexion with pain	4
Abnormal flexion (*decorticate* posture)	3	Abnormal flexion with pain	3
Abnormal extension to pain (*decerebrate* posture)	2	Extension	2
None	1	None	1
Best verbal response			
Smiles, orientated to sound, interaction	5	Orientated, converses	5
Crying *Interaction*			
Consolable Innapropriate	4	Disorientated, converses	4
Inconsistently Moaning consolable	3	Inappropriate words	3
Inconsolable Irritable	2	Incomprehensible sounds	2
None None	1	None	1

NB. The Children's Coma Scale, unlike the Glasgow Coma Scale, has *not* been validated.

BRAIN DEATH

This is the irreversible *loss of consciousness* and the *capacity to breathe*.

The coma state must:

1. *be apnoeic*
2. *be of diagnosed cause*
3. *exclude: poisons, drugs, temperature <35° C, metabolic or endocrine disturbance*

Diagnosis involves absence of brainstem reflexes, being performed by two senior doctors, >6 hours into the coma. It is repeated, at least >1/2 hour apart.

Brainstem reflexes

Pupils	Fixed, dilated, no direct or consensual reflexes
Corneal reflex	Absent
Occulocephalic reflex	'Doll's eye reflexes'. Absent
Caloric tests	Vestibulo-ocular reflexes. Absent

Painful stimulus	No response to central and peripheral stimuli (primitive reflexes may be present)
Gag reflex	Absent
Apnoea	10 minutes disconnected from ventilator, with 100% high-flow O_2 and ABG pCO_2 > 6.7 kPa (50 mmHg)

HEAD INJURY

This is the single most common cause of death in children. The causes include automobile accidents and NAI.

Concussion	A brief, reversible impairment of consciousness
Extradural haematoma	From a bleed into the middle meningeal space due to rupture of middle meningeal artery or dural veins
Subdural haematoma	A bleed between the dura and the cerebral mantle, due to rupture of cortical veins. Seen in shaken infants
	Chronic subdurals may gradually enlarge with a long history of irritability, poor feeding and lethargy
	Acute subdurals often associated with other brain injuries
Intracerebral contusion	Insult to the brain substance

A skull fracture is not always present with severe intracerebral injury. Subdural haematoma is more common in head injuries without skull fracture.

Skull fractures

Non-depressed, linear	Most common fracture seen
Depressed	Need surgical treatment if >3–5 mm depressed
Basal skull fracture	CSF rhinorrhoea and bilateral eyelid ecchymoses: 'panda eyes'
	Difficult to demonstrate on SXR, CT views helpful

Management

- *Basic resuscitation as needed and check for and treat any other injuries*
- *Monitor closely with neurological observations using the Glasgow Coma Scale*
- *Raised intracranial pressure and seizure management as necessary (see p. 356 and 378)*
- *Surgical intervention by neurosurgeons as necessary*

SHOCK

Shock is the failure of adequate perfusion of the tissues.

Causes

Hypovolaemic	Blood loss, gastrointestinal loss, skin loss (burns)
Distributive	Septicaemia, anaphylaxis, spinal cord injury
Cardiogenic	Arrhythmias, cardiac failure, myocardial infarction
Obstructive	Tension pneumothorax, flail chest, cardiac tamponade, pulmonary embolism
Dissociative	Profound anaemia, carbon monoxide poisoning

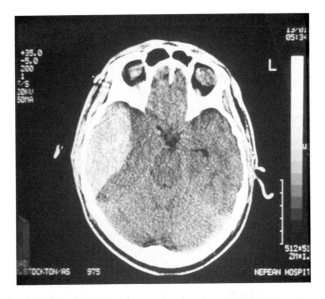

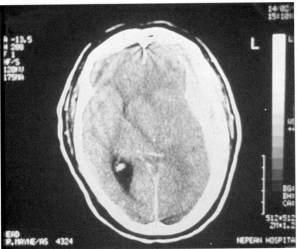

Figure 17.6 Extradural (top) and subdural (bottom) haematoma

Three stages of shock

1. *Compensated shock — perfusion to vital organs is maintained at the expense of non-essential tissues*
2. *Uncompensated shock — the mechanisms start to fail, tissue hypoxia and acidosis occur*
3. *Preterminal — the situation is becoming irreversible*

Early treatment of shock and thus recognition of compensated shock is vital. The following are features of shock in the various stages.

	Compensated	Uncompensated	Preterminal
HR	↑	↑↑	↑ then ↓
Systolic BP	N	N or ↓	Falling
RR	N or ↑	↑↑	Sighing
Pulse volume	N or ↓	↓	↓↓
Capillary refill time	N or ↑	↑	↑↑
Skin	Pale, cool	Mottled, cold	Pale, cold
Mental status	Agitation	Lethargic	Deeper coma
Urine output	↓	Absent	Absent
Peripheral temperature	Low	Low	Low
Estimated fluid loss	<25%	25–40%	>40%

Management

The immediate treatment is the same for all types of shock.

- *100% oxygen via face mask*
- *IV fluid replacement in 20 ml/kg boluses (crystalloid or colloid, then blood) as required*

If there is no improvement mechanical ventilation, inotropic support, intensive monitoring and correction of any biochemical and haematological abnormalities are carried out as necessary.

SEPTICAEMIA

The commonest causes of septicaemia in children are Gram-negative infections and causes of meningitis.

Clinical features

- *Fever, lethargy, irritable, focal infection*
- *Shock, purpuric rash (meningococcal infection), multiorgan failure*

Initial investigations

Serum	FBC, glucose, electrolytes and creatinine, coagulation screen (may be deranged), ESR and CRP (↑)
Infections screen	Urine, blood, CSF (if not contraindicated), skin swabs, any suspected infective sites for microscopy and culture
Arterial blood gas (acidosis)	

Management

- *IV broad-spectrum antibiotics, choice depending on likely source of infection*
- *Treatment of shock as above*

ANAPHYLAXIS

Clinical features

These include:

- *uticaria, pruritis, flushing, facial swelling*
- *bronchospasm*
- *hypotension*

Management

- *Removal of the cause and basic assessment of airway, breathing and circulation and 100% oxygen*
- *Adrenaline 1:1000 IM (dose age-dependant)*
- *Adrenaline dose repeated after 5 mins if no clinical improvement*
- *Chlorpheniramine IM (dose age-dependant)*
- *In addition for severe/recurrent reactions and patients with asthma, hydrocortisone IM or IV (dose age-dependant). Inhaled B$_2$-agonist may be used as an adjunctive measure.*
- *If clinical manifestations of shock do not respond to drug treatment 20 ml/kg IV fluid (crystalline may be safer than colloid) is given, which may be repeated and infusion given if necessary*
- *In profound shock CPR/ALS is given as necesssary and slow IV adrenaline may be given by experienced practitioners*

Ref: Adapted from: The emergency medical treatment of anaphylactic reactions, Resuscitation council (UK) 1999 (see latest resuscitation guidelines)

BURNS

Assessment

Burns are assessed by depth, extent and location.

Depth	Partial thickness – blistering, skin pink or mottled, painful
	Full thickness – white or charred skin, painless
Extent	See Figure 9.7
Location	Facial burns and hand burns are of particular cosmetic and functional significance. Airway involvement with smoke inhalation must be checked for.

Management

1. *Analgesia – strong IV analgesics usually necessary for anything other than minor burns*
2. *Shock – management with fluids and close monitoring of status. Burns >10% will need IV fluid replacement*
3. *Wound care – specialist burns unit management for significant burns (eg. inhalational injury, >10% area, full thickness, cosmetic significance). Removal of dead tissue, sterile dressings. Antibiotics if concern of infection (have high index of suspicion)*
4. *Definitive care is then carried out in a paediatric burns unit.*

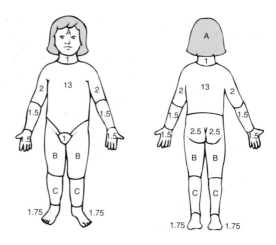

Percentage surface area at different ages					
Area	0 years	1 year	5 years	10 years	15 years
A	9.5	8.5	6.5	5.5	4.5
B	2.75	3.25	4.0	4.25	4.5
C	2.5	2.5	2.75	3.0	3.25

Figure 17.7 Assessment of burns

POISONING

Poisoning in children is generally accidental though may be deliberate.

General management
Specific advice should be obtained from a local poisons information centre. Methods of elimination:

Activated charcoal	Considered with recent ingestion, given orally (nasogastric if necessary) it reduces intestinal absorption of drugs
	Not appropriate after caustics (eg. acid or alkalis)
Gastric lavage	Rarely indicated in children. The airway must be protected. Contraindicated after ingestion of corrosives or hydrocarbons

Specific remedies

Substance	Effects	Specific management
Alcohol	Hypoglycaemia	Blood glucose monitoring
		IV glucose if necessary

Paracetamol	Gastric irritation	Check plasma levels 4 hours since ingestion
	Liver failure (>2–3 days)	If plasma concentration high or >150 mg/kg thought to have been taken, give IV acetylcysteine as per protocol
		Monitor liver function (LFTs, prothrombin time)
Salicylates	Nausea, vomiting	Check plasma salicylate concentration
	Dehydration	Empty stomach <12 hours of ingestion
	Tinnitus, deafness	(salicylate delays gastric emptying)
	Disorientation	Correct dehydration, fluid and electrolyte imbalance
	Hyperventilation	
	Respiratory alkalosis	Forced alkaline diuresis
	Metabolic acidosis	Dialysis
	Hypoglycaemia	
Button batteries	Gastrointestinal upset	CXR and AXR to monitor gut progress
	Gut wall corrosion	Remove if signs of disintegration, not moving,
	Oesophageal stricture	or not passed few days (not always
	Mercury release if broken	recommended)
Bleach	Local erosions	Avoid emesis. Oral milk and antacids
		Endoscopy and ventilatory support if necessary
Iron	Vomiting, diarrhoea	AXR to view number of tablets
	Haematemesis, melaena	Serum iron levels, management of shock
	Acute gastric ulcerations	Gastric emptying
	Drowsiness, liver failure, convulsions, coma within hours	Iron chelation (IV desferrioxamine)
	Gastric strictures	

Chronic lead poisoning

This is usually chronic poisoning, from the ingestion of lead-containing paint or water in lead pipes. Rare in the UK. It may result in permanent mental retardation.

1. *Chronic illness:* Bone features, developmental delay, gum involvement, constipation, neuropathy
2. *Acute:* Vomiting, ataxia, seizures, coma, anaemia, renal involvement

Clinical features

Gastrointestinal	Anorexia, nausea, vomiting, constipation, abdominal pain
Haematological	Hypochromic microcytic anaemia with basophilic stippling on red cells
Neurological	Peripheral neuropathy, eg. wrist drop, foot drop
	Lead encephalopathy (seizures and reduced consciousness)
Skeletal	Dense metaphyseal bands at the growing end of long bones – 'lead lines'
Renal	Fanconi syndrome
Other	Blue line on gums

Diagnosis

Serum	lead levels
	FBC (basophilic stippling, hypochromic microcytic anaemia)
Urine	Proteinuria, glycosuria, aminoaciduria

Management

Chelation therapy with dimercaptosuccinic acid (DMSA). Calcium EDTA and dimercaprol may be used instead. Removal of source

NON-ACCIDENTAL INJURY (NAI)

There are many forms of NAI.

Physical abuse

- *Unexplained or multiple injuries*
- *Inconsistent history*
- *Late presentation*
- *Unusual parental behaviour (hostile, unconcerned)*
- *Anxious withdrawn child ('frozen watchfulness')*
- *Injuries:* Lacerated oral frenulum
  Cigarette burns
  Bite marks
  Bruises: Finger tip bruises
                 Belt mark bruises
                 Unexplained multiple bruises or fractures
  Head injuries: Retinal haemorrhages (shaking injury)
                 Subdural (shaking injury)
                 Wide skull fractures
  Fractures: Spiral fractures, skull fracture with >3mm displacement, old
                 fractures

Emotional abuse and neglect

This may be more difficult to identify. Features include general neglect, dirty child, scruffy clothing, failure to thrive.

Sexual abuse

In most cases the perpetrators are male and the abused child a girl, though all variations exist. Features include:

- *sexually transmitted infection*
- *UTI, eneuresis*
- *anal fissure, pruritis ani, constipation, encopresis*
- *inappropriate sexual behaviour*
- *behavioural disturbance*
- *direct allegation*

Management

- *Detailed injury history, include direct quotes*
- *Detailed family and social history*
- *Involvement of senior paediatrician*
- *Full examination (genital examination by senior paediatricians)*
- *Detailed documentation of injuries seen*
- *Follow local procedures for social services, police and further management*

Differential diagnosis

Medical conditions to be considered:

Bruising   Coagulation disorders, leukaemia, ITP, HSP, mongolian blue spot

Fractures Osteogenesis imperfecta, copper deficiency, Coffey disease, rickets, local tumour

Munchausen by proxy

An uncommon form of abuse, where illness in the child is fabricated by the carer/parent(s). Features of the disorder include:

- *the condition may be difficult to diagnose*
- *features are only present when the parent visits*
- *multiple hospital admissions*
- *the mother often has healthcare connections (eg. a nurse)*

Examples include:

- *feeding salt to the child*
- *putting blood in urine, stool or vomit*
- *putting sugar in the urine*

The child may come to serious harm from these activities.

SUDDEN INFANT DEATH SYNDROME (SIDS)

This is the sudden unexplained death of a previously well infant, most commonly occurring at 2–4 months, with 90% occurring <7 months. Some of these deaths are now explained, for example, as metabolic disorders, eg. fatty acid oxidation defects, or deliberate suffocation by the carer. The risk of SIDS for subsequent children is slightly increased.

A significant decrease in SIDS occurred in the UK with the advice:

- *to put infants to sleep on their back or side*
- *to avoid overheating*
- *to avoid smoking near the infant*

Home apnoea monitoring for infants at risk may be considered, though it can be anxiety provoking for the parent and has not been proven to be of benefit. Basic resuscitation skills should be taught to parents of children at risk.

The Children Act

This is a document for the protection of children. It was fully implemented in October 1991 (given royal assent in 1989) and replaced the Children and Young Persons Act 1969. The act includes the following features.

- *The child's welfare is the court's paramount consideration, so any court order made should contribute positively to the child's welfare*
- *The prime responsibility for bringing up children lies with the parents*

- *Local authorities should provide supportive services to help parents in bringing up children.*
- *Local authorities should take reasonable steps to identify children and families in need.*
- *Every local authority should have a register of children in need.*
- *Sensitivity to ethnic considerations in assessing a child's needs and providing services.*
- *The local authority should work in partnership with the parents.*

The Children Act 1989 provides protection orders for 'at-risk' children:

1. **Emergency protection order (EPO)** – *any person may apply to a magistrates court for an EPO and then has parental responsibility for the child. Lasts eight days, extension of seven days possible. Appeal can be made after three days.*
2. **Police protection provision** – *a police constable may take a child into police protection without assuming parental responsibility. Lasts up to three days.*
3. **Child assessment order** – *allows proper assessment of a child over up to seven days. (Removal of the child from the family home does not necessarily occur.)*
4. **Care and supervision orders** – *these allow a child to be placed in the care of or under the supervision of the local authority. Maximum duration eight weeks.*

Statementing

The local education authority must provide a statement for children with special educational needs. This is part of the Education Act 1981 (updated 1993).

An initial assessment is made by interested professionals and then a statement of the child's educational and non-educational needs is made. The statement includes information given by the parents and professionals (including, as necessary, the teacher, paediatrician, educational psychologist, occupational therapist, physiotherapist and speech therapist). The services to be offered to the child are included within the statement (eg. one-to-one tuition, special transport to school).

The statement should be regularly reviewed and revised if necessary.

Consent

Consent to a procedure is normally given by the patient. However, where this is not possible (due to *age* or mental *capacity*) the consent can be authorised from other sources. Capacity is the mental process to deal with a matter.

THE COMPETENT CHILD

Children over 16 years are regarded as though they were adults for the purposes of consent. A child under 16 years may give consent if they are deemed to be competent. However, a refusal to consent by a competent child can be countermanded by those with 'parental responsibility'.

A competent child may thus give consent but *may not withhold it* in the same way.

THE INCOMPETENT CHILD

If a child does not have the capacity to provide consent a proxy may do so. The proxy is expected to act in the best interests of the child and they can include the following.

1. *A parent who has 'parental responsibility' in respect to the child.*
2. *A local authority that has acquired 'parental responsibility' and the power of consent. A local authority can only usurp this power by restricting their power as the parents.*
3. *The court can act as proxy in wardship, under inherent jurisdiction or via court orders. In this way it can review a parent's decision (eg. the refusal of a life-giving blood transfusion for a child of a Jehovah's witness).*

WARDSHIP

If the child is a ward of court 'the court is entitled and bound in appropriate cases to make decisions in the interests of the child which override the rights of its parents'. Wardship may not be invoked by the local authority or while a child is in care, but may be made by other interested parties (eg. a health authority) and ends when a child ceases to be a minor. This is a major step to take as, when evoked, 'no important step in the life of that child can be taken without the consent of the court'.

INHERENT JURISDICTION

This is more commonly used in medical law cases. The court does not take all the decisions relating to the child's life, but only in certain issues (eg. medical care). It can be invoked in an emergency and also by a local authority even while the child is in care.

COURT ORDERS

The court also has the power to make specific orders and prohibited step orders. A prohibited step order means that no step (specified in the order) can be taken by any person (including the parent) without the consent of the court. A specific issue order gives directions to determine a specific question in connection with any aspect of parental responsibility for a child. These orders cannot be made if a child is in care, or in an emergency, and are rarely made if the child is 16 years old. They do not represent a true order as they only allow a local authority to authorise and supervise a policy. As with all treatment, the final decision and duty of care still rests with the doctor in charge of the case.

FURTHER READING

Meadows R Ed. *ABC of child abuse.* 3rd Ed. BMJ Publishing Group, London, 1997
Spitz L, Coran AG Eds *Paediatric Surgery.* 5th Ed. Chapman & Hall Medical, London, 1995
Resuscitation Council (UK) Guidelines July/Sept 1999

Appendix 1

NB. Values vary from one laboratory to another

Normal ranges: haematology

Age	Hb (g/dl)	MCV (fl)	WBC ($\times 10^9$/l)	Platelets ($\times 10^9$/l)
Birth	14.5–21.5	100–135	10–26	150–450 at all ages
2 weeks	13.4–19.8	88–120	6–21	
2 months	9.4–13.0	84–105	6–18	
1 year	11.3–14.1	71–85	6–17.5	
2–6 years	11.5–13.5	75–87	5–17	
6–12 years	11.5–15.5	77–95	4.5–14.5	
12–18 years				
Male	13.0–16.0	78–95	4.5–13	
Female	12.0–16.0	78–95	4.5–13	

Appendix 2

Normal ranges: clinical chemistry

Test		Normal range (plasma or serum)	
Alanine aminotransferase (ALT)		<40 U/l	
Albumin	Neonate★	25–35 g/l	
	Child	35–55 g/l	
Alkaline Phosphatase (ALP)	Neonate★	150–700 U/l	
	1 m–1 yr	250–1000 U/l	
	2–9 yr	250–850 U/l	
	Yr	Females	Males
	10–11	250–950 U/l	250–730 U/l
	14–15	170–460 U/l	170–970 U/l
	>18	60–250 U/l	50–200 U/l
Ammonia	Neonate	<100 μmol/l	
	Infant/child	<40 μmol/l	
Amylase	Neonate	<50 lU/l	
	1–3 m	<100 lU/l	
	>1 yr	100–400 IU/l	
Aspartate amino transferase (AST)		<50 U/l	
Blood gas (arterial, not preterm)	pH	7.35–7.45 (Hydrogen ion 35–44 nmol/l)	
	pO$_2$	11–14 kPa (82–105 mmHg)	
	pCO$_2$	4.5–6 kPa (32–45 mmHg)	
	Bicarbonate	18–25 mmol/l	
	Base excess	−3 to +3 mmol/l	
Calcium (total)	24–48 h	1.8–3.0 mmol/l	
	>1 week	2.15–2.60 mmol/l	
Calcium (ionised)	24–48 h	1.00–1.17 mmol/l	
	>1 week	1.18–1.32 mmol/l	
Chloride		96–110 mmol/l	
Creatinine kinase	Infant/child	60–300 U/l	
Creatinine	Infant★	20–65 μmol/l	
	1–10 yr	20–80 μmol/l	
Creatinine clearance	1–3 months	27–69 ml/min/1.73 m^2	
	3–6 months	61–84 ml/min/1.73 m^2	
	6–12 months	77–126 ml/min/1.73 m^2	
	>2 yrs	110–200 ml/min/1.73 m^2	
C-reactive protein		<10 mg/l	
Ferritin	Child	<150 μg/l	
Gammaglutaryl transferase (GGT)	1–12 m	<80 U/l	
Glucose	1d★	2.2–3.3 mmol/l	
	>1d	2.6–5.5 mmol/l	
	Child	3.0–6.0 mmol/l	

Glycosylated haemoglobin (HbA$_{1c}$)	5–16y	3–6%
17-Hydroxyprogesterone (17-OHP)	>2d	0.7–12 nmol/l
	Child	0.4–4 nmol/l
Iron	Infant	5–25 μmol/l
	Child	10–30 μmol/l
Lactate (fasting)		0.5–2.0 mmol/l
Magnesium		0.6–1.0 mmol/l
Osmolality		275–295 mosm/kg
Phosphate	Neonate★	1.4–2.6 mmol/l
	Infant	1.3–2.1 mmol/l
	Child	1.0–1.8 mmol/l
Potassium	Infant	3.5–6.0 mmol/l
	Child	3.3–5.0 mmol/l
Protein (total)	Neonate★	54–70 g/l
	Infant	59–70 g/l
	Child	60–80 g/l
Pyruvate		40–70 μmol/l
Sodium		133–145 mmol/l
Thyroid stimulating hormone (TSH)	>1 week	0.3–4.5 mU/l
Thyroxine (T4, total)	Child	85–180 nmol/l
Urea	Neonate★	1.0–5.0 mmol/l
	Infant	2.5–8.0 mmol/l
	Child	2.5–6.5 mmol/l
Urate		120–350 μmol/l

★ *Depends on gestational age*

As the normal range for tests varies between laboratories, this must be checked with the local laboratory. (Values adapted with permission from Addy, D.P. Investigations in Paediatrics. WB Saunders, London, 1994 and other sources.)

Appendix 3

COMMONLY USED ABBREVIATIONS

For simplicity of reading, abbreviations and symbols are used in this book

M	male
F	female
↑	increased
↓	decreased
>	greater than
<	less than

Index

NOTES

NOTES

NOTES

NOTES

NOTES

NOTES